M. Postel M. Kerboul J. Evrard
J. P. Courpied (Eds.)

Total Hip Replacement

With the Collaboration of
S. André T. Arama B. Augereau R. Charon
A. Chevrot M. Cornic B. Coulondres P. Denier
P. Deplus C. Fayeton M. Forest C. Gaudillat
A. Gestraud C. Hedde A. Kindermans J. P. Lamas
D. Lance B. Loty M. Mathieu V. Pacault
G. Pallardy Ph. Sauzières L. Trévoux C. Viguie

Translated by R. Brueton

With 163 Figures in 317 Separate Illustrations,
Some in Color and 30 Tables

Springer-Verlag
Berlin Heidelberg New York
London Paris Tokyo

Prof. Michel Postel
Prof. Marcel Kerboul
Dr. Jacques Evrard
Prof. Jean Pierre Courpied

Clinique chirurgicale orthopédique et reparatrice, Hôpital Cochin
Pavillon Ollier; 27, rue du Faubourg Saint-Jacques,
F-75674 Paris Cedex 14

Translator: Richard Brueton, M. D.
St. Thomas Hospital, Lambeth Palace Road, S. E. 1 London

Title of the original French edition: *Arthroplastie totale de hanche*

ISBN 3-540-15030-7/0-387-15030-7

ISBN 3-540-13198-1 Springer-Verlag Berlin Heidelberg New York
ISBN 0-387-13198-1 Springer-Verlag New York Berlin Heidelberg

Library of Congress Cataloging-in-Publication Data. Arthroplastie totale de hanche. English. Total hip replacement. Translation of: Arthroplastie totale de hanche. Includes index. 1. Hip Joint-Surgery. 2. Artificial hip joints. I. Postel, M. (Michel) II. André, S. III. Title. (DNLM: 1. Hip Prosthesis. WE 860 A7865)
RD549.A7413 1987 617'.581 86-20421

Typesetting, Printing and Binding: Appl, Wemding. 2124/3140-543210

Foreword

Postel, Kerboul, Evrard, Courpied, and their coauthors take a completely objective attitude in describing the progress achieved in total hip replacement with reference to their own experience over the last 20 years. They avoid any triumphant fanfares, but not because of Pascal's dictum: "Do you want people to speak well of you? Don't do it yourself." Rather, they know that other surgeons, like themselves, are more concerned with efficiency than with laurels, and want that is, new ideas based on sufficiently wide experience and analyzed in a strict and uncompromising manner. In addition, surgeons are particularly anxious for in-depth study of the problems, complications, and failures encountered as well as for indications as to how these can be avoided and corrected. This book is sure to satisfy surgeons on both these counts. It is the exciting and almost incredible product of the work and the immense progress that have taken place in the 15 years since I retired.

The spirit behind this work has inspired it from the start. It is characterized by a determination to take constant study of the results as the only guide in matters of indications and technique, and the authors insisted on a system of documentation whose purpose (and perhaps merit) was to facilitate comparison both of the preoperative functional state and of the final result; they have also kept an open mind for interesting new insights from whatever quarter they might arise.

It was in this spirit that Postel and Kerboul came to put their confidence in the person who pioneered hip replacement surgery, John Charnley, and in particular in two features he had adopted following a long, detailed and objective study. The first of these was the small head of the prosthesis, which means a smaller friction area to compensate for the inevitable drawbacks of having an inert material instead of viable articular cartilage at the point of friction; and the second was the use of cement for fixation. The difficulties and setbacks encountered at first were resolved at the outset: Painstaking investigations to determine why they had arisen were not conducted in a completely different sample of patients, who would not have benefited from them, or of lengthy laboratory studies, or yet of years of experience in clinical practice; but they were directed at perfecting the Charnley prosthesis and especially at producing a range of sizes and models of it, so that each patient would be able to have the model and size best suited to his or her particular needs.

A study of the results and of the way they have developed, as presented in this volume, shows that the authors were right. Since they conducted their investigation with a laudable degree of rigor, they have been able to follow it through with a high level of continuity, even though almost half their patients, who were already advanced in years when they underwent surgery, were lost to follow-up owing to death or from other causes after 12–15 years. The group's experience encompasses 20 years and 8000 total

hip replacements, so that they have been in a position to appreciate the impact the improvements made have had on the results.
In the treatment of coxarthrosis they have obtained results that were very good in 98% of the cases (perfect in 85%). These were maintained at the end of 5 years and seemingly also at the end of 10 years and more. Despite the almost equally good results obtained in inflammatory coxitis, necrosis, and even ankylosis and persistent dislocations, the authors do not claim victory in this sector, but address the complications, devoting over half this volume to a painstaking study of them.
The frequency of postoperative periarticular ossification, which is a relatively common cause of failure, has been reduced by an improved technique, in particular by the application of trochanterotomy instead of section of the glutei. This has led to other problems, especially pseudarthrosis, but these have not been so frequent and can be more easily corrected when they affect function.
A very searching and original radiological study is presented to illustrate how another rare complication, dislocation, can be avoided. There is no doubt but that a high proportion of dislocations occur in connection with anomalous anteversion of the elements of the prosthesis.
Two complications that genuinely compromise the results that are theoretically possible with total hip replacement are loosening and infection. These have been the subject of such an interesting and detailed study that to give a summary of it here would amount to an act of betrayal. Nonetheless, I will take it upon myself to say that one of these dangers, loosening, has been overcome and the other, infection, which is more serious and watched for with greater apprehension, has been considerably reduced.
Up to 1970, loosening of the cup caused a 30% failure rate with metal-on-metal prostheses, which led to the discontinuation of their use in favor of prostheses with the cup made of polyethylene, whose fixation remained firm in almost all cases. However, there was play on the femoral element of Charnley's prostheses in over 5% of cases. These problems led some surgeons to invent and promote prostheses that were inserted without cement. Postel and Kerboul's work shows that this was not a good path to take. In fact, since they have been using they femoral elements commissioned by Kerboul and adapted to any form and size of femur, among 485 prostheses, 250 of which have been followed up for over 5 years, none has shown signs of loosening. Loosening of the cup has been observed in only 6 among over 800 cases.
The chapter on operations performed following loosening continues in the same vein. The impressive radiographs illustrating the text show several cases of nonfixation of the prostheses with cement. The plates also show amazing reconstructions of hips affected by virtually complete degeneration, and these results cannot fail to excite admiration. This is particularly true of those obtained with the use of a shaped metal element supporting homologous bone grafts that have taken and been incorporated into the iliac bone to a degree that surgeons had hardly dared to hope.
The study of the functional results has excluded the cases affected by infections; but this formidable complication has also been studied and is accorded an appropriately serious treatment. While all authors recognize the gravity of such infections, they estimate their frequency in very different ways. When the doubtful cases were included the frequency amounted to around 4% early in the Cochin experience. But technological advances, and especially the use of routine prophylactic antibiotic therapy, caused it

to fall to 1.8% in a series of 720 cases and to 0.4% in the 200 cases in the randomized series. The treatment of these infections is another source of amazement to me, since keeping the prosthesis in place after "cleaning" has resulted in recovery in 13 of 28 cases of acute early infection and a second operation with insertion of a complete new prosthesis has been successful in three-quarters of the 99 cases of chronic late infection in whom this was attempted.
The quality and duration of the results obtained with total hip replacement carried out with strict observation of the recommended indications, and the low incidence of complications and the possibility of their correction therefore combine to give an overall picture exceeding any hopes we might have entertained 15 years ago. But how much patient and strenuous work has gone into achieving this result, and what measure of vigilance and discipline will be needed to maintain it and improve it still further? These questions are now answered in a manner that cannot but satisfy even the most exacting workers.

R. Merle d'Aubigné

Contents

1 Introduction

M. Postel

Eighteen years have passed since the first total hip replacement was performed at Cochin, and I believe it was also the first in France. This coming of age is worthy of a summary of the experience accumulated during this time, in particular because after 13-14 years, the Charnley prosthesis and its derivatives seem to have lived up to their first promise (although signs of wear have appeared in some cases), and because the modifications made with regard to the shape and size of the femoral component 10 years ago seem to have achieved their aim.

It was in July, 1965, that R. Merle d'Aubigné and I were kindly invited to Norwich by Karl Nissen; there we discovered total hip replacement. The very British clinical presentation, organized by George McKee and John Watson Farrar, gave us the opportunity to examine a dozen of their patients. Their enthusiasm was exceeded only by our amazement at the quality of their results, the likes of which we had never seen in spite of our long experience with surgery for osteoarthritis.

Two months later, John Watson Farrar came to Cochin to help us carry out the first three total hip replacements. However, importation of the equipment was not easy; several months passed before further operations followed. Meanwhile, Georges Girard agreed to tackle the problems of manufacturing, and at the beginning of 1966 he produced the first French total hip replacement. The design of the femoral component was close to that of the Moore prosthesis, which we thought was mechanically more satisfactory than the Thompson prosthesis used by McKee; it was still a metal-on-metal prosthesis. This was a technically difficult achievement, but we were on our way.

At this time, after some years of trial and error, John Charnley had perfected his metal-on-plastic prosthesis, which seemed very attractive. But he gave authorization for the use of his prosthesis only to those who had spent 6 months in his department. Today, one can only be amazed at such strictness! After we had made two trips to Wrightington, in 1968 and 1969, he finally granted us this authorization and the implantation of imported Charnley prostheses could begin. They were soon replaced by a product from Benoist and Girard, who had overcome many technological problems. And so, after 1969, the use of this prosthesis of steel and high-density polyethylene with a 22.2 mm head became widespread in our department.

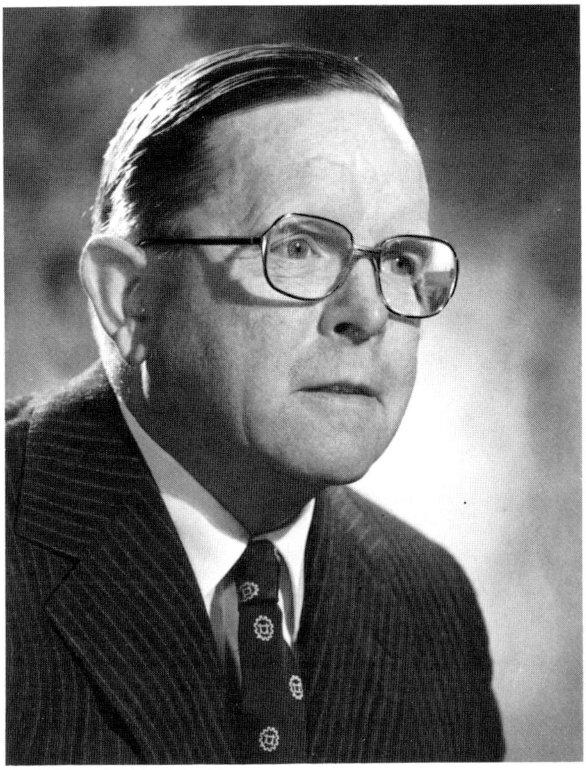

Sir John Charnley
(photo kindly provided by Lady Jill Charnley)

In 1970, the McKee and Charnley prostheses were used with equal frequency. For a while we used a modification of the McKee with greatly reduced friction, but this did not compare well with the Charnley prosthesis and was abandoned for good in 1974.

However, although problems with the cup seemed to have been overcome by the use of polyethylene, abnormalities appeared quite rapidly at the femoral site after 3 or 4 years of use. In 1972-1973, Kerboul proposed modifications in the shape and size of the femoral stem. It rapidly became apparent that these modifications were advantageous, and since 1974 the modified Charnley prosthesis has been the only prosthesis used at Cochin.

This book, a collection of the papers presented at Cochin on the 16th and 17th of February, 1984, summarizes the reasoning behind our development of the total hip prosthesis during the period between 1965 and 1982, when 8000 were implanted in our department. It also takes stock of the results that we have achieved and assesses the potential of the modified Charnley prosthesis that we have been using since 1974.

We think that, at a time when a multitude of other designs and other materials are being put forward and when the principle of cement fixation is being challenged, it is of interest to make an appraisal of the considerable experience of hip replacement acquired by one team of surgeons.

We have remained faithful to a cemented, metal-on-plastic prosthesis with a small head. We will not compare it with others, and will restrict ourselves to the results drawn from a study of our own prosthesis.

Finally, we should add that a new generation of modified Charnley prostheses has just been introduced, under the name of the Cochin prosthesis. The principle has not changed. The modifications are limited to a widening of the available choice of cross-sections and stem and neck lengths to enable a better fit to be obtained in each individual case. The cross-sections of the new stems make them slightly more solid and reduce the stresses imparted to the surrounding cement.

2 Methodology

J. P. Courpied and M. Postel

The results presented in this book are drawn from two sources, first from studies carried out within the department, some of which have been published or presented at teaching sessions at Cochin, and second from a recent retrospective computer study of 1500 total hip replacements, which allows the precise analysis of a large number of parameters.

The computer study covered 1300 items, assessed both radiologically and clinically. We have thus reviewed in great detail 100 McKee-Merle d'Aubigné prostheses representing a continuous series carried out in 1967, the first 500 Charnley prostheses implanted in our department during the period 1970–1971, and 700 modified Charnley prostheses representing samples from a variety of hip conditions operated upon between 1973 and 1980.

A separate study has been carried out on the problems of infection in total hip replacement.

The functional outcome has been assessed according to the Merle d'Aubigné and Postel classification, which assigns a score from 0 to 6 for pain, movement, and stability of the hip (Table 2.1). This last criterion is slightly different from the quality of walking and allows a better assessment of the hip itself, for in the case of polyarthritis, the ability to walk may be poor while the function of the hip remains good.

The outcome is assessed according to an annual radiological and clinical review. The long-term follow-up of our patients consists in principle of a clinical and radiological examination at the end of convalescence (that is to say at the 6th or 8th week), at 6 months, at 1 year, and then each year subsequently. At the 6th or 8th year, if all is well, and in view of the ever-increasing load of follow-up appointments, it is tempting to increase the time interval before the next assessment. However, this is perhaps not without its dangers. An annual follow-up becomes a routine. To disturb this routine risks the breaking of a pattern and thus seeing patients disappear. Perhaps it is from this moment that the risk of missing complications begins. These are often initially asymptomatic. We have therefore been strict in our routine of calling for all our patients every year.

Table 2.1. Scoring system for the assessment of hip function (Merle d'Aubigné-Postel classification)

	Pain	Movement[a]	Stability
6	None	Range of flexion $\geq 90°$	Perfect stability; walking unrestricted and normal
5	Minimal and infrequent, not preventing normal activity	Range of flexion 75°–85°	Imperfect stability; slight limp when tired; uses cane for long distances
4	Physical activity reduced, allowing ½ h or more of walking	Range of flexion 55°–70°	Slight instability; definite limp; often uses a cane out of doors
3	Prevents walking after 20 min	Range of flexion 35°–50°	Unstable; gross limp; always uses a cane
2	Prevents walking after 10 min	Range of flexion $\leq 30°$	Marked instability; two canes, occasionally one crutch
1	Very acute on movement and on weight bearing; can take only a few steps	Reduced flexion + significant deformity	Weight bearing impossible on one leg; two crutches
0	Very acute and continuous, preventing walking; patient confined to bed; insomnia	Reduced flexion + significant deformity	Impossible to stand; weight bearing impossible; bedridden

[a] No deformity, considering only the range of flexion; deformity, subtract 1 point for 20° or + of fixed flexion or ER 2 points for 10° or + of abd., add., IR

Unfortunately, as the years pass, some patients die or are lost to follow-up. In other words, the last examination in our series was carried out more than 2 years ago, in spite of several appointments.
And so, among our patients (1300 prostheses) 11% died and 20% were lost to follow-up. Of course, age is very important. We noticed a correlation between the ages of the patients who died and those who were lost to follow-up. Of those patients operated upon when under 60 years of age, 13% were lost to follow-up and 5% had died by the end of the study. Of those who had their operations at 80 years of age or older, the corresponding figures were 39% and 30%. This correlation continues as the time that has elapsed since operation increases (Fig. 2.1). We wondered whether the patients who were not followed up as long as we would have wished (whether they died or were lost from view) would have had an influence on the statistical value of the results of our study of known patients. To elucidate this point we carried out two studies:

1. A comparison, at similar postoperative times, of the function of those patients regularly followed and those who were eventually to be lost to follow-up.
2. Meticulous in-depth research into three groups of patients who were lost to follow-up.

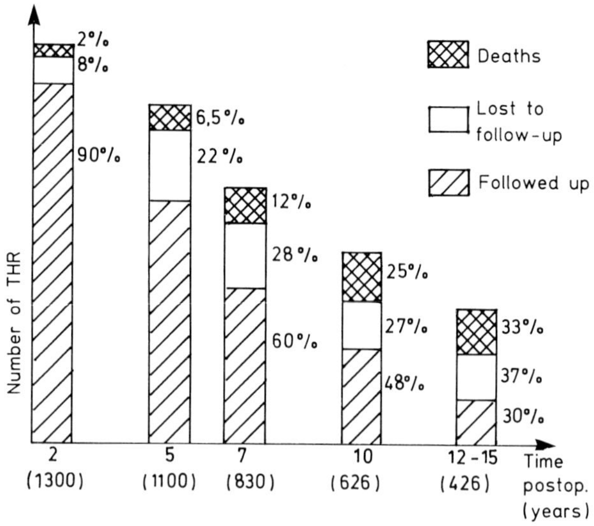

Fig. 2.1. Outcome of patients in relation to time elapsed after surgery. *THR*, Total hip replacements

2.1 Statistical Survey Comparing Patients Followed Up with Patients Later Lost to Follow-up

This was carried out on different samples of patients included in our computer study. The function of each hip had been assessed by the sum of the scores for pain, movement, and stability.
The results were as follows:

1. Patients between 60 and 79 years of age operated upon for primary osteoarthritis of the hip were assessed at 1 year. Of these 388 arthroplasties, the average scores at 1 year were 16.8 for those who would be followed for more than 5 years, 16.7 for those who were to be lost to follow-up between 1 and 5 years (68), and 17.1 for those who died between 1 and 5 years postoperatively (20). There is no significant difference between these three average scores.
2. The group of patients between 60 and 79 years of age operated upon for primary and secondary osteoarthritis of the hip and followed up for at least 3 years consisted of 356 arthroplasties with an average function of 17.5 at 3 years. For those patients among whom the latest assessment was made at least 8 years postoperatively (250) the score at this time was 17.4, while the score was 17.3 at the last assessment of those patients who were to default from appointments between 3 and 8 years, whether they died (34) or just did not appear (72). Once more, there is no significant difference between these three scores.
3. Among patients operated upon in 1970 for primary of secondary osteoarthritis, i.e., 270 total hips, the score at 10 years of those regularly followed up (137) was 17. The scores of function taken at the last examination of patients lost to follow-up between 1 and 10 years (71) was 16.9, and for those who died over the same time interval it was 16.8. Once again, there is no significant difference.

This comparative study, which was also carried out for other age ranges and for other etiologies, shows that the population of patients who were later lost to follow-up was in no way different from the overall population at the outset. Also, the function of patients who were eventually lost to follow-up was identical to the function of those who were followed up regularly, whether assessed early on or at their last examination.

2.2 In-depth Research on Patients Lost to Follow-up

Three series of 100 sets of consecutive files corresponding to the three types of prostheses were chosen. We did our utmost to find all those patients who had been lost to follow-up by sending letters to the patients and their doctors and by inquiring at the city hall in the town of their last address or of their place of birth.

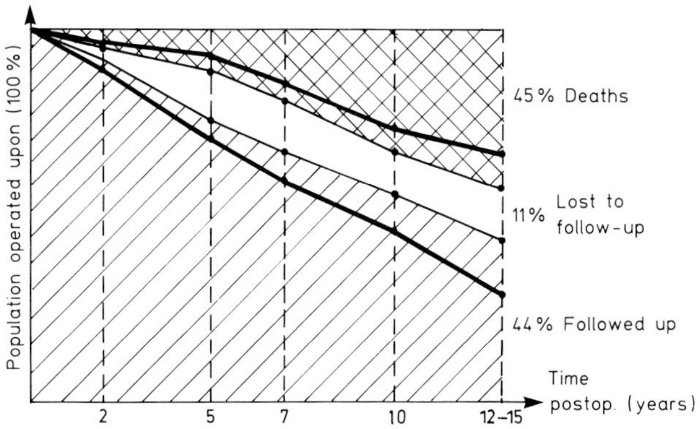

Fig. 2.2. Theoretical diagram shows that the percentage of deaths and of patients lost to follow-up rises progressively. Roughly one-third of the population falls into each category. After research the one-third lost to follow-up can be divided once more into three. At 12–15 years, this finally gives 45% died, 11% lost to follow-up, and 44% under review

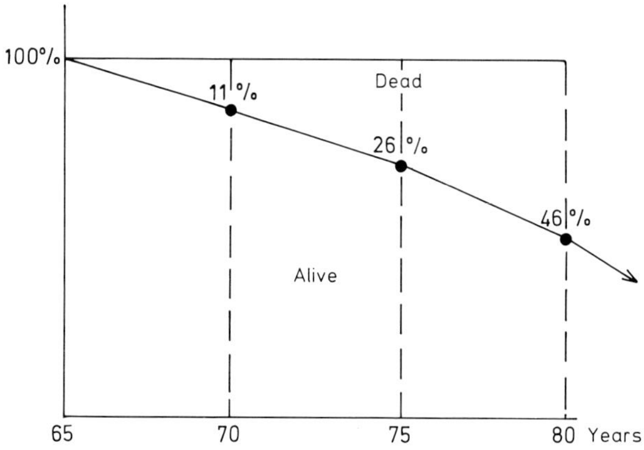

Fig. 2.3. Public survey published by L'Insee, showing the percentage of deaths after 5, 10, and 15 years for those aged 65 years (average age of our patients) during the period 1973–1980

The first series researched in this way involved 100 patients with McKee-Merle d'Aubigné prostheses operated upon in 1967. An initial review in 1983 showed that 37 had been regularly assessed, 13 had died, and 50 had not been followed up for as long as would have been wished. Concerning these 50 patients, the inquiry ended by finding 16 with usable new information and by discovering that 18 patients had died. So this survey finally gave us 53 usable sets of notes and 31 deaths. Only 16 patients remained lost from view.

Comparison of the files on those patients who had been followed up regularly and on those who had been retrieved by the survey showed that the two populations were similar. The Merle d'Aubigné-Postel average score was 13.6 for the former and 13.8 for the latter. Taking the two groups together, approximately one-third of the replacements were failures, one-third had developed complications, and one-third were still functioning well.

We had slightly less success in our search for the 100 patients operated upon in 1970 with the Charnley prosthesis. However, the results are remarkably similar. A review of the files showed that 33 patients had been followed up regularly, 17 had died, and 50 had been lost to follow-up. Our inquiries concerning these last 50 patients enabled us to rediscover 13 patients for further assessment; 13 others had died. This gave us final figures of 46 patients followed up, 30 deaths, and 24 patients lost from view.

The distribution of patients with good results and those with problems was the same among the patients regularly followed up and those rediscovered in our survey, i. e., 26 of the 33 patients followed up regularly and 10 of the 13 rediscovered patients had good results. This is 77% in both groups.

The results obtained from our research into the series of modified Charnley prostheses were approximately the same. They will be described in detail later.

The outcome of this research into the patients who were lost to follow-up shows that, overall, after 15 years one-third of our patients had been followed up, one-third had died, and one-third had been lost to follow-up. Our further research into those lost to follow-up showed that one-third had died, one-third had been found again, and one-third remained lost (Fig. 2.2). Those whom we found again gave us information that put them in the same category of results as those who had been followed up regularly. The files on those who had died showed that before their death the patients had a function that fell within the average distribution curve.

We therefore think that although it is unsatisfactory to be left with 11% untraceable patients, they would not greatly modify the figures of the results even if they were found. In summary, we consider the figures that we have arrived at valid, these being taken from those files within the department which have been kept up to date. The figures quoted throughout this study will be expressed as a function of the known population, and not as a function of all the patients on whom we have operated.

It should be noted that the distribution curve of those patients who died is similar to the 5-, 10-, and 15-year survival rates shown by the *Institut National de Statistique et d'Etude Economique* for 65-year-olds, and this is the average age of our patients operated upon between 1973 and 1980 (Fig. 2.3).

3 The Development of Total Hip Replacement

3.1 The Different Total Hip Prostheses Used at Cochin

M. Postel

It is instructive to look back at our motives for using certain types of prostheses, at their results, and at how the lessons we drew from them directed the development of our future choice. The changes made were few and were motivated only by the hope of providing a solution to a specific problem (Fig. 3.1).

The first prostheses that we used were of the metal-on-metal type, derived from the McKee prosthesis and called the McKee-Merle d'Aubigné prosthesis. From the beginning of 1966 the number implanted per year rose very quickly, reaching 363 by 1969.

However, from 1969 on, the Charnley prosthesis began to hold an important place. The metal-on-metal low-friction band prosthesis was introduced in 1971, and for several years it was used along with the modified version of the Charnley prosthesis. In 1975, the modified Charnley prosthesis became the only prosthesis in use in our department. The only exceptions were trials with aluminum prostheses and with linked cemented cups.

A long time is necessary in order to judge the defects of one type of prosthesis, and advances must be made very carefully if all that has been gained is not to be lost. The better the results, the slower the change.

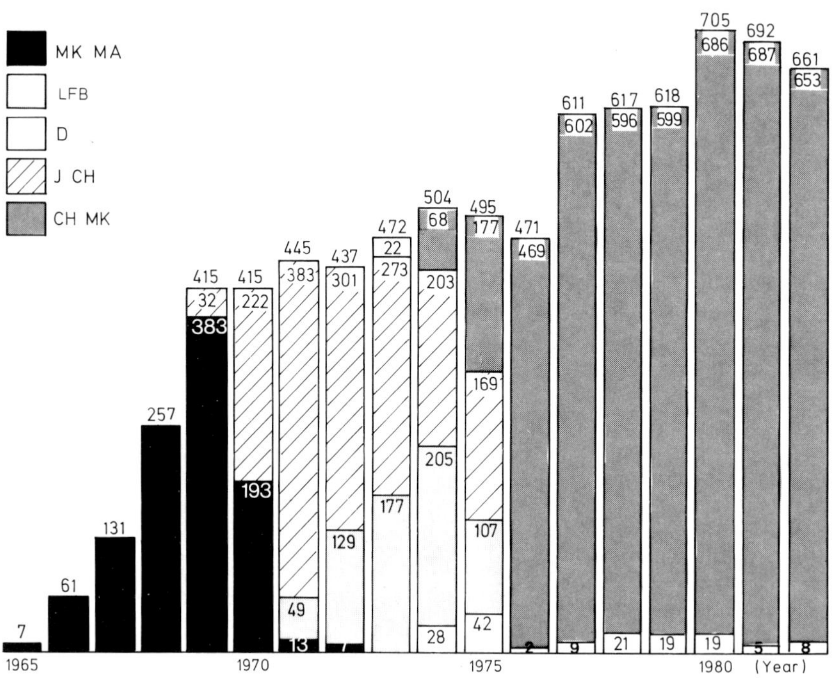

Fig. 3.1. Types of prostheses used each year from 1965 to 1982 in 8000 THRs at Cochin. *MK MA*, McKee-Merle d'Aubigné prosthesis; *LFB*, low-friction band prosthesis; *J CH*, Charnley prosthesis; *CH MK*, Charnley prosthesis modified by Kerboul; *D*, a variety of prostheses used in several partial revisions, aluminum prostheses, linked cemented cup

3.2 The McKee-Merle d'Aubigné Prosthesis

M. Postel and C. Fayeton

The first total hip replacement used in large numbers in our department was a metal-on-metal, slightly modified McKee prosthesis known as the McKee-Merle d'Aubigné prosthesis (MK MA; Fig. 3.2).
The initial results were excellent and as good as those that we had seen in G. McKee's own department. This led us to widen our indications for surgery, which had been very restricted. The number rose rapidly, with 245 prostheses implanted in 1968 and 380 in 1969.
Here we will study the outcome of 113 of these replacements, which represent nearly the total sum of our work in 1967. The average age of the patients was 64 years. Half of the patients (53%) suffered from primary osteoarthrosis and a quarter (26%) from secondary osteoarthrosis. One-third were followed up for the maximum possible period of 15 years, and the average follow-up was 9 years.
Overall, this series produced 44% poor or bad results and 56% good or very good results. Twenty-two hips had to be revised. Eighteen of these showed aseptic loosening and four were both loose and infected.

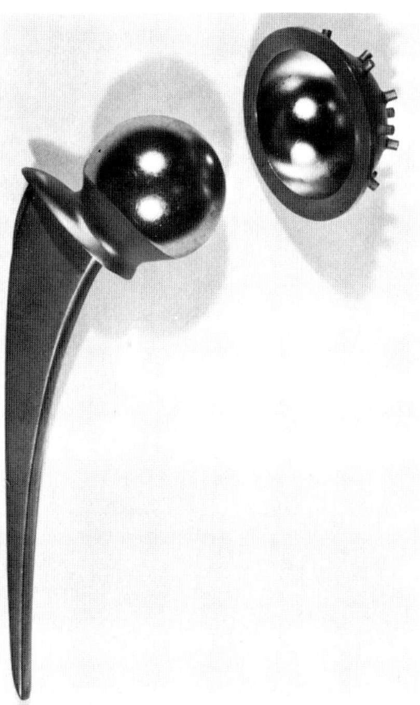

Fig. 3.2. The McKee-Merle d'Aubigné prosthesis. The features of this prosthesis in chromium cobalt are: a head of 41 mm diameter; a short neck; a femoral stem similar to that of the Moore prosthesis but with no window; a smooth cup, machined to take the head; only one component size

Table 3.1. Aseptic loosening of the McKee-Merle d'Aubigné prosthesis

	Cups	Femoral components
Revised	18	1
Not revised	17	4
	35 (31%)	5

For the 91 hips that were not revised, and with an average follow-up of 9 years, the sum of the pain-movement-stability score was an average of 14.8 out of a possible 18. One-third of the patients had poor or bad results while two-thirds had good results. We should point out that in this series there were 17 loosenings that we were not able to revise. This was because of the age and general condition of the patients or because they died or became lost to follow-up before the revision could be carried out.
However, the particular features of these loose prostheses were most interesting. On reviewing all of the case histories, we found that 33 patients (29%) presented with serious mechanical problems related to the cup. This is an impressively large proportion (Table 3.1).
The majority of the problems became apparent during the 2nd or 3rd year. Not all of them were diagnosed at that time, and it often took several more years for us to be sure. However, the clinical and radiological signs of loosening – which we now understand better – and a retrospective stucy of these patients' files show us that the problems appeared very early (Table 3.2). They continued to appear as the years passed and occasionally presented in quite an acute way. A hip that seemed to be progressing very well would suddenly deteriorate over a few months. In fact, a careful examination of the old roentgenograms showed us that all had not been completely satisfactory in the roof of the acetabulum (Fig. 3.3).
What was the reason for this large number of loosenings? There is no doubt that our operative technique in 1967 contained many faults of which we are now

Table 3.2. Time of onset of acetabular loosening

Onset (years post-op)	1	2	3	4	5	6	7	?[a]
No. of loosenings (among 113 THRs)	4	10	7	2	2	1	2	3

[a] Date not available from case files

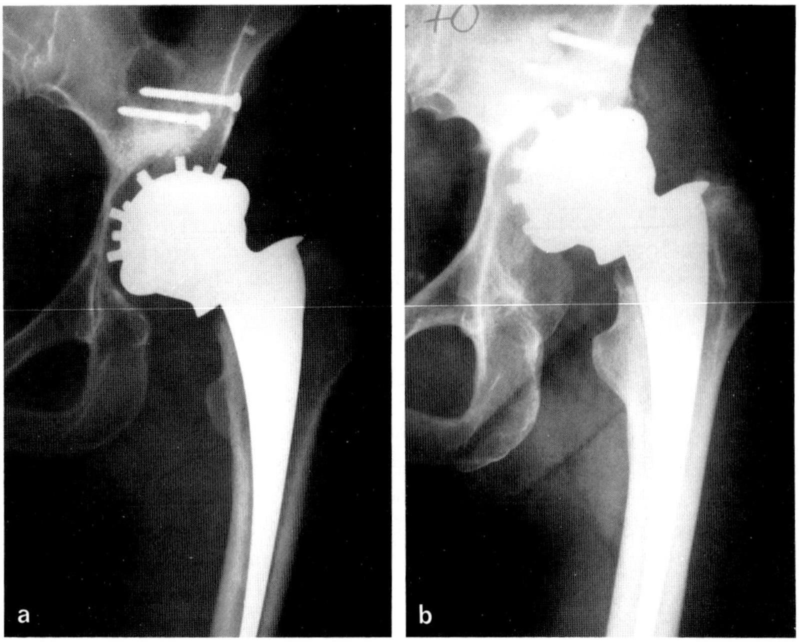

Fig. 3.3 a, b. Two years after implantation this McKee prosthesis shows several abnormalities around the cup (**a**). At 4 years there is definite loosening (**b**)

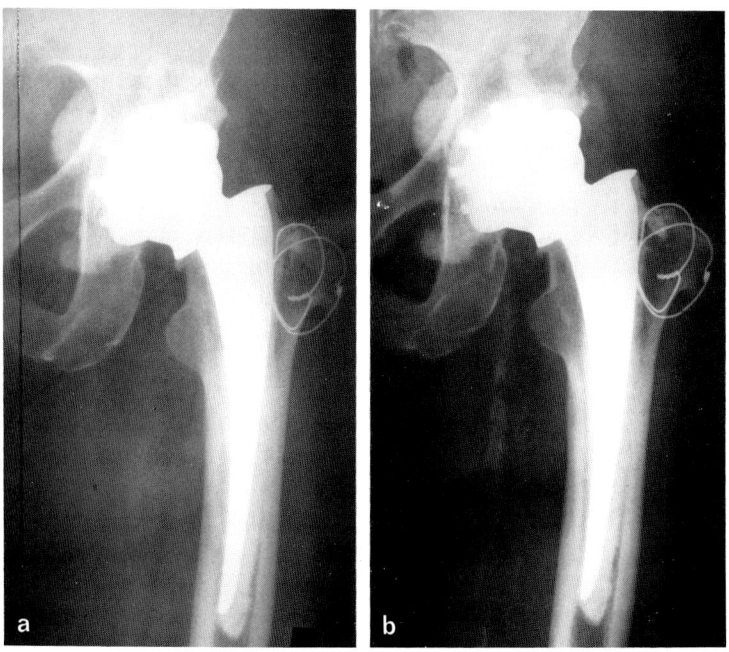

Fig. 3.4 a, b. A good clinical and radiological result at 4 (**a**) and 14 years (**b**) after surgery

aware in the light of experience, especially in relation to the preparation of the acetabulum. It is also clear that being limited to only one size of prosthesis prevented us from achieving the precision of technique required.

But it was definitely the very poor quality of friction of this prosthesis that was the most frequent cause of loosening. This was mainly the result of the high friction associated with a metal-on-metal prosthesis, however good the precision of the machining. There was also a strong couple acting to loosen the prosthesis, owing to the large diameter of its head.

On the other hand, this series includes only five femoral loosenings (with or without a loose cup), only one of which needed to be revised. At 15 years, the great majority of femoral components are seen to be intact and unchanged from the day of implantation (Fig. 3.4). This can frequently be confirmed today during revisions for acetabular loosening when the femoral cement is seen to be holding perfectly throughout its length.

This provides us with proof of the ability of cement to last for a long period without aging, or at least without its mechanical properties in relation to bone being called into question. Of course, the stem of these prostheses is large and occasionally produces an autoblocking effect. However, this is far from always the case, and it is the cement that is responsible for the good quality of fixation.

Thus, the metal-on-metal prosthesis that we used out of necessity at the beginning enabled us to observe to what extent methylmethacrylate cement was capable of providing a firm and lasting fixation.

3.3 The Low-friction Band Prosthesis

M. Postel and T. Arama

During 1969–1970, therefore, we were disturbed by the problem of loosening of the cup associated with the McKee prosthesis. However, the combination of metal with polyethylene in the Charnley prosthesis was still in its infancy and the possibility of wear caused us a little worry.

It was this that made us look for a way to modify the metal-on-metal prosthesis in the hope of avoiding the problems associated with friction. The idea came from the belief that, geometrically, the head could not possibly have exactly the same diameter as the cup. The head was either smaller and the contact area reduced to one point, thus giving rise to significant wear, or it was larger and made contact with the whole circumference at the opening of the cup thus causing maximum loosening. We therefore made a cup with raised concentric bands within its inner surface that could be easily adapted to the spherical surface of the head and would redistribute the load. Machine testing showed that this design produced less friction than completely smooth cups, very close to the friction of the Charnley prosthesis. Measurements of wear in vitro appeared favorable, in that the cup hardly seemed to become worn, and the quantity of loose particles produced was small (Fig. 3.5).

In order to quantify the development of this prosthesis, of which we implanted 600, we selected 100 consecutive case files of patients operated upon in 1973 and 1974 under the same technical conditions. The septic prostheses were excluded, as we were interested only in studying the functional outcome.

The patients in this study had an average age of 67 years and suffered from hip pathology justifying arthroplasty for a variety of indications but in the usual proportions.

The average length of follow-up was 6 years and this proved to be more than adequate time for complications to appear.

3.3.1 Clinical Progress

The outcome of this series was disastrous. Of 100 hips, 26 had to be revised at an average of 5.5 years postoperatively; 13 others required revision, but this could not be carried out because of the patients' poor condition, age, or the presence of other contraindications.

The average functional results of those prostheses which are still in place are the same as those of the other prostheses regarding pain and movement. Strangely, the stability score seems to be slightly worse (an average of 5.2).

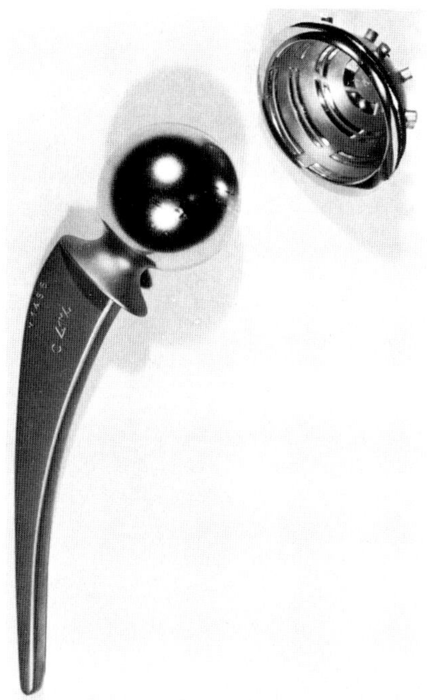

Fig. 3.5. The low-friction band prosthesis. Inside the hemispherical cup are raised circular bands to allow sliding, and the corresponding head is carefully machined to reduce friction. The femoral stem comes in only one size, and its outline is very similar to that of the McKee-Merle d'Aubigné prosthesis. In cross-section it is slightly narrower, and so it poses fewer problems with small femora but frequently requires more cement. There are three head sizes: 37, 39, and 41 mm, corresponding to three external cup sizes, and two choices of neck length. This improves the mechanical function of the reconstructed joint

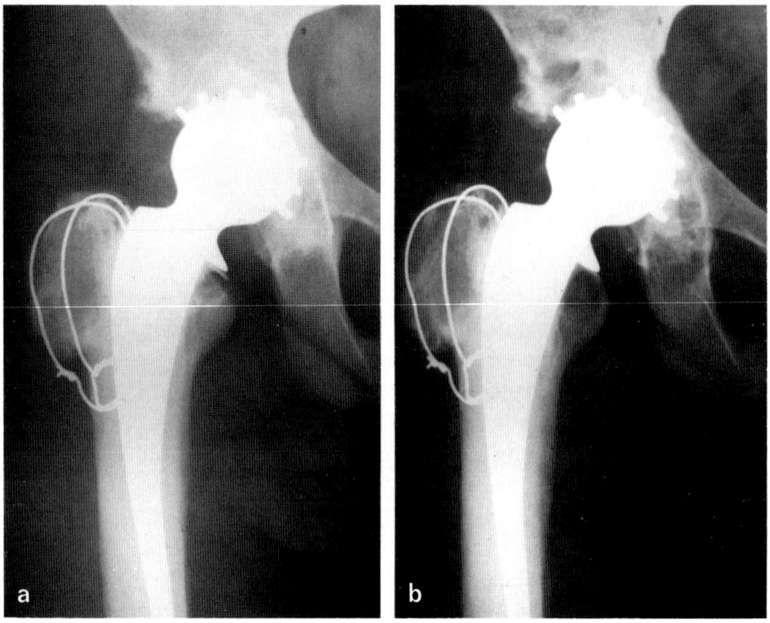

Fig. 3.6 a, b. One year after this prosthesis was implanted a localized ischiatic lucent area appeared together with a cyst of the calcar (**a**). At 4 years, these complications had progressed and eroded the roof of the acetabulum, causing loosening (**b**)

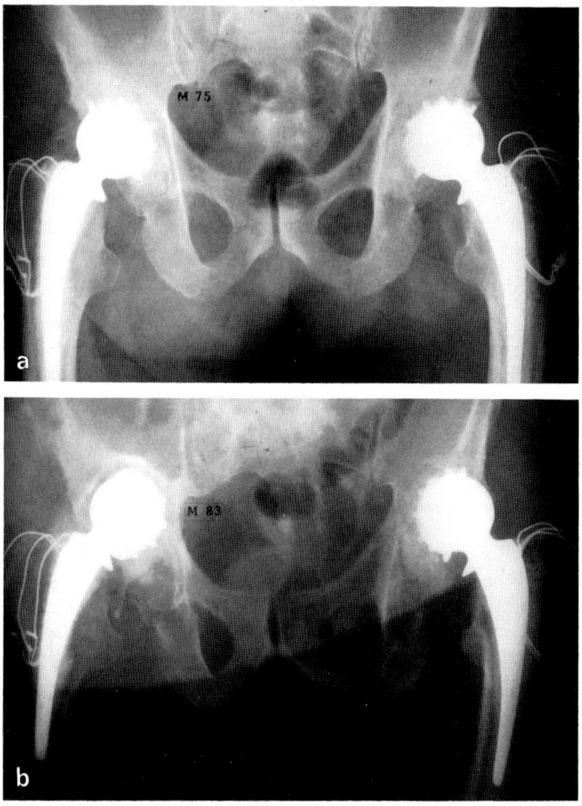

Fig. 3.7 a, b. These two prostheses were implanted in 1974. In 1975 the radiological appearance was satisfactory (**a**). In 1983 (**b**) they were completely loose and had a correspondingly poor clinical result. However, they caused almost no pain, and as a result of the very poor general condition of the patient, revision was postponed for the time being

3.3.2 Radiological Development

Worrying radiological signs appeared toward the 3rd year, and these were usually followed rapidly by obvious loosening of the cup. Clinical symptoms usually developed 1 year after the appearance of radiological signs.

The development of these radiological features was characteristic. First to appear was a lucent area in the ischiatic region that rapidly increased in size (Fig. 3.6). Then other changes and often cysts appeared in the roof. This could result in tilting of the cup together with its surrounding block of cement. But occasionally, before this change in position occurred there was further destruction of the acetabulum, leading to medial protrusion of the cup that could result in complete loss of bony continuity (Fig. 3.7).

The femoral component rarely loosened; when it did, it was only at a late stage. Lesions began at the calcar, which was destroyed in 23 of 100 cases. These then extended distally, as if a metallic granuloma had inserted itself between femur and cement to produce loosening.

Experience showed us that once these lesions appeared, their progression was inevitable, leading to bony destruction of increasing severity. This produced defects that became increasingly difficult to repair. We were therefore forced to advise several patients to have revisions while they still had little in the way of symptoms, in spite of the psychological problems that this engendered.

3.3.3 Reasons for Failure

At the latest follow-up of these 100 patients, 39 were failures, while 61 had satisfactory results. What was the cause for this unsatisfactory progression? Our first hypothesis was that it resulted from an allergy, as suggested by Freeman at that time in the first articles published on this subject [2, 3]. The amount of metallic debris that accumulated in the tissue around the prosthesis was found to be considerable. This was 17 mg per 50 g of tissue, compared with 0.13 mg around metal-on-plastic prostheses. Skin tests for cobalt allergy are positive in 1% of the general population. They were found to be positive in one in five patients with a metal-on-metal prosthesis, almost one in two when the prosthesis was loose. But we could produce no biological evidence of an intra- or extracellular allergy to the metallic constituents of the prosthesis. It therefore seemed unlikely that an allergic phenomenon was the basic cause of our loosenings.
A more likely cause seemed to be either a toxic reaction directed at the debris produced by wear, or a reaction to the granuloma provoked by the resorption of this debris [1]. This "metallosis" necessitated revision of one-quarter of all these prostheses. Such a high failure rate made us abandon the prosthesis completely.

References

1. Langlais F, Postel M, Berry JP, Le Charpentier Y, Weill BJ (1980) L'intolérance aux débris d'usure des prothèses. Int Orthop 4: 145-153
2. Mervin Evans E, Freeman M, Miller A, Vernon Roberts B (1974) Metal sensitivity as a cause of bone necrosis and loosening of the total prosthesis in total joint replacement. J Bone Joint Surg [Br] 56: 626-642
3. Swanson S, Freeman M, Heath J (1973) Laboratory tests on total joint arthroplasties. J Bone Joint Surg [Br] 55: 759-773

3.4 The Charnley Prosthesis

J. P. Courpied and M. Postel

We began to use the Charnley prosthesis in our department at the beginning of 1969, once it became available to us. However, this was not without a degree of apprehension. What would be the outcome of combining metal with plastic, and how would it stand up to wear? It seemed much more unstable than prostheses with large heads, and would this not lead to frequent dislocation?
The low coefficient of friction resulting from this new combination was very attractive, and, together with a small head, the loosening force acting on the cup was reduced. So it was in the hope of reducing loosening of the cup that we began to implant the Charnley prosthesis, although the metal-on-metal prosthesis was still in use at the same time. At that stage, of course, only 4 years after its introduction, the McKee prosthesis had not yet produced the impressive number of acetabular problems that we have just discussed, but they were already present in sufficient numbers to arouse anxiety. Thus, from 1969 onward, the Charnley prosthesis was more and more frequently used in our department. We shall look here at the results of a series of 439 Charnley arthroplasties carried out in 1970 and 1971, solely for osteoarthritis. Two important points emerge from this study. The first is the quality and long-lasting fixation of the cup. This Charnley series has the longest follow-up in our study and so is the only one that could give us this information. The second point is the quite rapid appearance, within a few years, of radiological signs at the junction of the cement and the femoral component. Their incidence was considerably larger than the femoral problems associated with the McKee-Merle d'Aubigné prosthesis.
In such a long study of 439 prostheses the number lost to follow-up must obviously be considerable, and 129 patients have been lost. The remaining series of 300 prostheses for which long-term progress is known includes 150 patients (some with bilateral arthroplasties) who have died.
There remain 162 prostheses which have been followed up for 12 or 13 years. We must also, unfortunately, report that this series includes 12 infected hips (4%), all of which have been revised, and nine revisions for aseptic loosening four femoral and three acetabular).
Excluding these revisions, the average scores for pain, movement, and stability are very good, being 5.9, 5.7, and 5.8 respectively, with an average of 17.5 out of a possible 18. This represents a very good standard of functional results in the long term. This could be expressed in another way: If only perfect hips are considered, which score 6, 6, and 6, these represent 74% of the total operated upon, when assessed 10 years postoperatively. Considering only those patients operated on for primary osteoarthritis who had had no surgery prior to their total hip arthroplasty, this figure is 85%.
Up to now we have considered only the functional results as a whole. Further study shows that radiological signs were present in 25% of cases. These are occasionally minimal but usually extensive, and we must question what are their effects on long-term function.

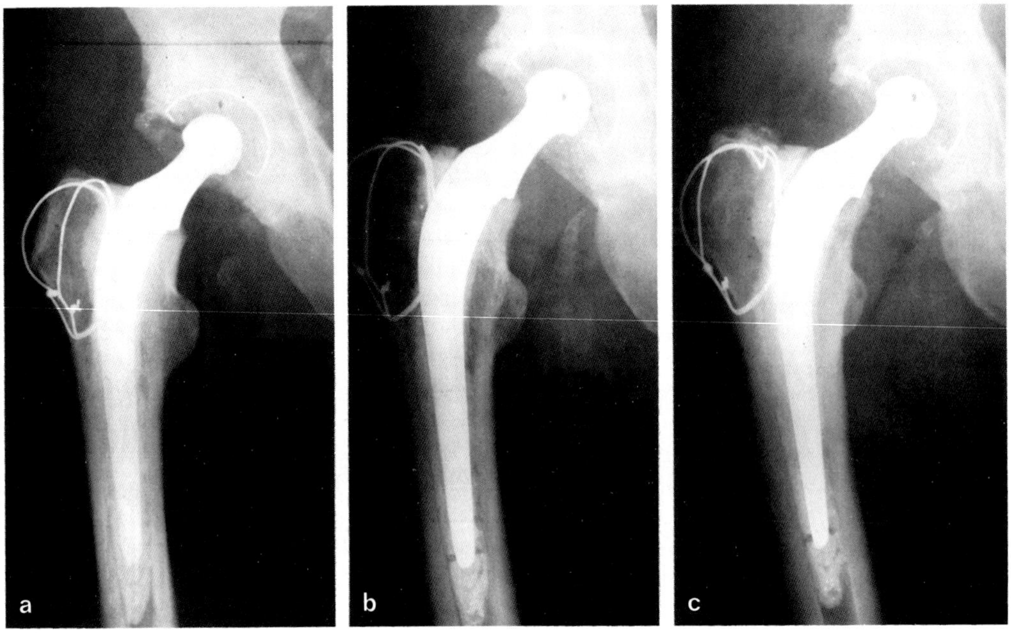

Fig. 3.8. **a** Charnley prosthesis implanted in 1971. **b** Several months later a localized dorsal lucent area appeared between the cement and the prosthesis, along with a fracture of the distal part of the cement. **c** In 1982 the situation had hardly progressed and function was excellent

Table 3.3 Incidence of lucent zones in the femoral component of the Charnley prosthesis and its relationship to alignment of the stem (400 THRs)

Alignment of femoral component *n*	No. with lucent areas
Varus (158)	66
Valgus (22)	3
Neutral (220)	23
Fit of femoral component into diaphysis	
Stem too narrow (383)	92
Stem well aligned and a good fit (17)	0

Serious radiological signs (excluding sepsis) are in effect the signs of loosening. In this series there were four acetabular and 16 femoral loosenings, i.e., 1.3% and 5.5% respectively.

We also noted that the number of problems related to the cup was very small. Obviously, this can be confirmed only in the long-term. However, it became evident after the first few years that the transition to the combination of metal with polyethylene had transformed our problems with the cup. Problems that did appear were the exception, whereas the metal-on-metal prosthesis would already have given rise to many complications.

We had fears that this prosthesis would have produced many more dislocations, more because of the small head than because of its material. There were a few, but at a level that we found acceptable.

We shall return to the problem of wear later on; for the moment, suffice it to say that we found this to be quite tolerable.

Signs related to the femoral component were much more worrying. The 16 true femoral loosenings did not all present in the early years. On the other hand, a long-term review of this series shows that radiological signs whithout true loosening were present in 60 cases and that they appeared early on. For the large majority, this required only careful subsequent monitoring by radiology. The signs nevertheless caused considerable concern for the future.

The radiological signs involved the appearance of a clear space on the dorsum of the prosthesis, at the level of its convexity and separating it from the cement. This dorsal lucent zone sometimes appeared within the first few months, and most commonly before the end of the 1st year. These initial observations were obviously most worrying, but fortunately, the situation usually remained stable. Two movements of the prostheses could explain them. One is the descent and impaction of the femoral component into the femur. This is demonstrated by the coexistence of a fracture frequently visible at the tip of the surrounding sheath of cement. The other is a varus tilt which implies a fracture of the cement in its concavity, along the length of

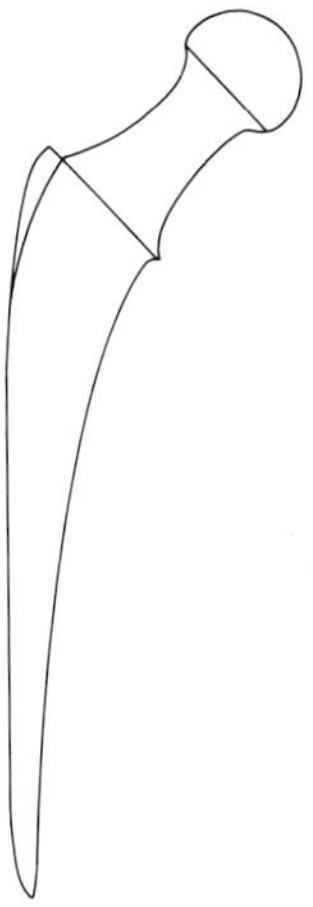

◁ **Fig. 3.9.** Scale drawing of the hybrid prosthesis; the head and neck of the Charnley with the stem of the McKee

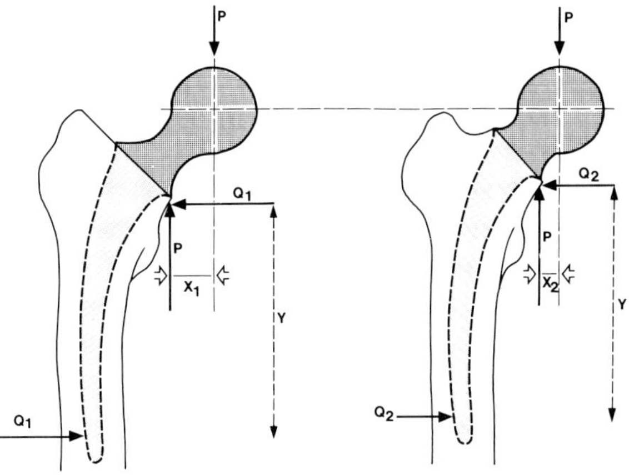

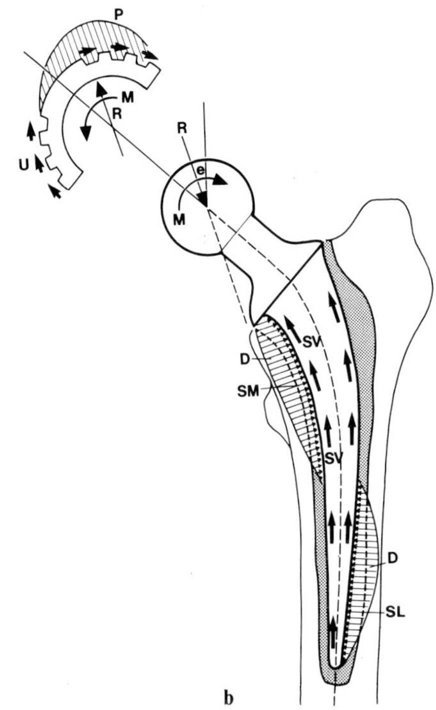

Fig. 3.10. **a** The flexion forces (Q) acting on the prosthesis increase as the length of the lever arm (X) is increased. **b** Compression and shearing forces at the level of the cement-bone interface. *D* and *P*, Compression; *M*, friction couple; *R*, resultant of forces acting on the hip; *SM* and *SL*, compression forces; *SV* and *U*, shearing forces

the calcar, and this has been found at several revisions. These two movements can occur simultaneously (Fig. 3.8).

A study made of the conditions under which these lucent zones between the cement and the prosthesis occur demonstrated the importance of the position of the femoral component within the femur. Stems that were perfecty aligned produced fewer problems than did those that were not. A varus position was, by far, the most unsatisfactory, but a prosthesis in valgus was not without disadvantages. On the other hand, it was most unusual for a lucent zone to appear if the size of the prosthesis was such that it apparently filled the whole medullary canal. It should be remembered that only two stem diameters were available, and that their fit within the femur was therefore completely unpredictable (Table 3.3).

Thus, the Charnley prosthesis proved early on to be a most important advance over the metal-on-metal prosthesis, as far as the cup was concerned. However, problems related to the femoral component rapidly became evident. Often this was demonstrated solely as a radiological feature, and we did not know what the outcome would be in the long term, but several were seen to be significant or progressive from their onset.

3.5 The Charnley-Kerboul Prosthesis

M. Kerboul

3.5.1 Historical Review

Our modifications to the original Charnley prosthesis find their justification in retrospect, in the study of the long-term results of the McKee-Merle d'Aubigné and Charnley prostheses. However, the situation was far from being as clear as this in 1971.

Of course, we already knew that the fixation of the femoral component of the McKee-d'Aubigné prosthesis was solid and long lasting, as it had been in use since 1965. On the other hand, the fixation of the cup was relatively precarious, as evidenced by the already large percentage of acetabular loosenings at that time (10% at 2 years).

We progressively reduced our use of this prosthesis from 1969 onward, because we believed that the loosening of the cup was the unfortunate result of two factors - high metal-on-metal friction and a large head. In its place we used the Charnley prosthesis, whose small head and low-friction steel-polyethylene combination appeared to be convincing mechanical features that would protect the cup from these severe stresses. Two years later, the situation was completely reversed but did not seem to be better. There was no longer any aseptic loosening of the cup, but in 8% of cases the roentgenogram of the femoral fixation was abnormal. At 6-12 months, a clear zone appeared between the cement and the convexity of the prosthesis that was usually associated with a distal transverse fracture of the tube of cement. This was evidence of movement of the prosthesis in its cement sheath. This partial loosening had no immediate clinical manifestation, but we thought it was a precursory sign that would lead to a true failure of femoral fixation. This worried us to the extent that in 1971 we began to search for a solution to this mechanical problem.

The first idea was to make a hybrid prosthesis, using the Charnley cup and a femoral component consisting of a small head with a McKee stem. A scale drawing of this prosthesis was even produced (Fig. 3.9). But as this did not seem to allow us to achieve our object of producing an exact reconstruction of the joint, we did not pursue this line. We therefore tried to understand the reasons for the precarious fixation of the femoral component of the Charnley prosthesis.

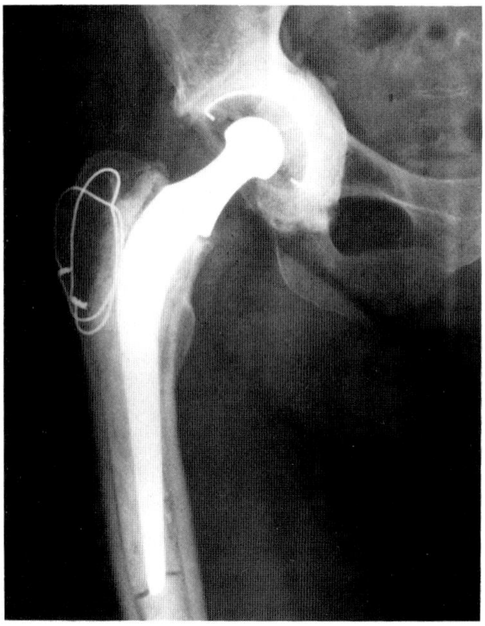

Fig. 3.11. Tilting into varus and impaction of a Charnley prosthesis inside its cement sheath after it has been weakened by a vertical fracture medially (not visible) and a transverse fracture distally

3.5.2 The Femoral Component of the Charnley Prosthesis

Charnley had produced a femoral component with a relatively closed neck-stem angle (125°) and a strong lever arm to reduce the overall forces on the cup. The femoral stem had a narrow cross-section so that it would fit all femora, and in all cases the constraining forces were transmitted to the bone via the intermediary of cement. He hoped to thus distribute the stresses transmitted to the bone in a satisfactory way. This was far from being illogical, but in many cases it resulted in submitting the cement to forces that exceeded its capabilities.

The forces acting on the femoral stem can be schematically resolved into two components. One is horizontal and tends to flex the stem. The longer the lever arm of the prosthesis, the greater the force, and it is transmitted to the bone via the cement at two zones (superomedial and inferolateral) which are subjected to compressive forces. The other component is vertical and transmits shearing forces to the cement along the whole length of the prosthesis. It also subjects the end of the tube of cement at the distal tip of the femoral stem to traction forces (Fig. 3.10). This brief mechanical analysis accounts for the deterioration of the fixation.

The superomedial layer of cement cannot resist these compressive forces for long, especially if it is separated from the cortex by a layer of deformable cancellous bone. A vertical fracture of the superomedial layer of cement will result. The proximal enlargement in the tube of cement will considerably increase the force acting distally on the cement sheath. The shearing forces exerted on a Charnley prosthesis, whose stem has the same thickness for its whole length, are badly absorbed laterally; the cement cannot long resist this excessive traction force and so breaks transversely (Fig. 3.11).

In order to diminish the flexion forces, Charnley suggested that the femoral stem be implanted in valgus. This would allow a thicker layer of cement to be interposed which would be more resistant to the superomedial and inferolateral compressive forces, especially if the medullary canal had already been emptied of any remaining cancellous bone at these points.

However, this valgus position, apart from other disadvantages, increased the resultant force on the acetabu-

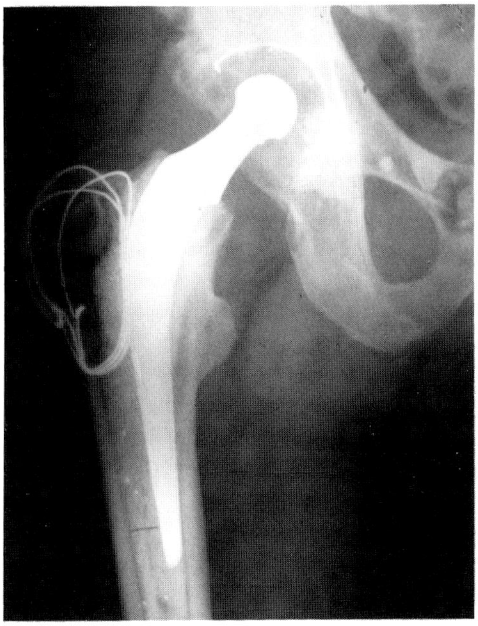

Fig. 3.12. Distal transverse fracture of the tube of cement despite implantation of the prosthesis in valgus

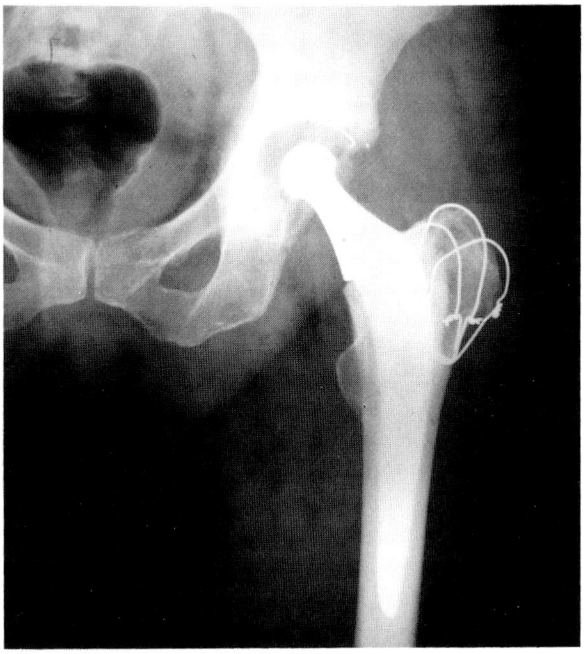

Fig. 3.13. The prosthetic stem is well adapted to the femur and exactly fills the medullary cavity

lum and also the vertical constraints exerted on the terminal part of the tube of cement. A transverse fracture was therefore the first sign of deterioration. Although it appears later and less frequently, its presence demonstrates the inadequacy of this clever technique (Fig. 3.12).

3.5.3 A New Series of Prostheses

Because of the relatively poor physical qualities of methylmethacrylate, we preferred to try and resolve the problem in a different way, one that did not exceed the capabilities of the cement, the function of which is to fill the irregularities between the prosthesis and bone. That led us in 1972 to design a new series of prostheses that retained the original Charnley small head (indispensable for its low-friction effect and allowing the cup to be thick) but would reduce the flexion and impaction forces acting on the femoral component. This was achieved by adjusting the neck-stem angle to 130° and changing the section of the femoral stem so that its thickness was greatest proximally and decreased distally.

To ensure that the prosthesis was still aligned, that no cancellous bone remained at the compression zones, and that the cement was not subjected to forces that it could not withstand, the simplest solution seemed to be to completely empty the medullary canal of cancellous bone and to force in a well-fitting prosthetic stem that would almost completely fill the medullary cavity prior to the addition of cement. This would also allow forces to be transmitted directly from the prosthesis to the bone, thus relieving the cement from harmful stresses (Fig. 3.13).

We decided to create a whole range of femoral components so that the prosthesis would exactly fit the shape of the bone, in spite of the diversity of sizes of femora or of the damage caused by disease or previous surgery. We could thus reconstruct an artificial hip as near to the normal as possible in every case, or one that was at least capable of good mechanical function and that took the balance of the periarticular muscles into account. At present, this series consists of 30 femoral components. A similar concern to fit the prosthesis exactly to the bone led us to increase the number of acetabular components to five cups of increasing sizes (Fig. 3.14).

We believe that over the past 12 years total hip replacement has become an extremely reliable operation, when performed using the above principles and a rigorous operative technique. At last, we seem to have overcome the technical problems that we previously encountered. Although other problems will no doubt appear in time, we think that here we have made an important advance.

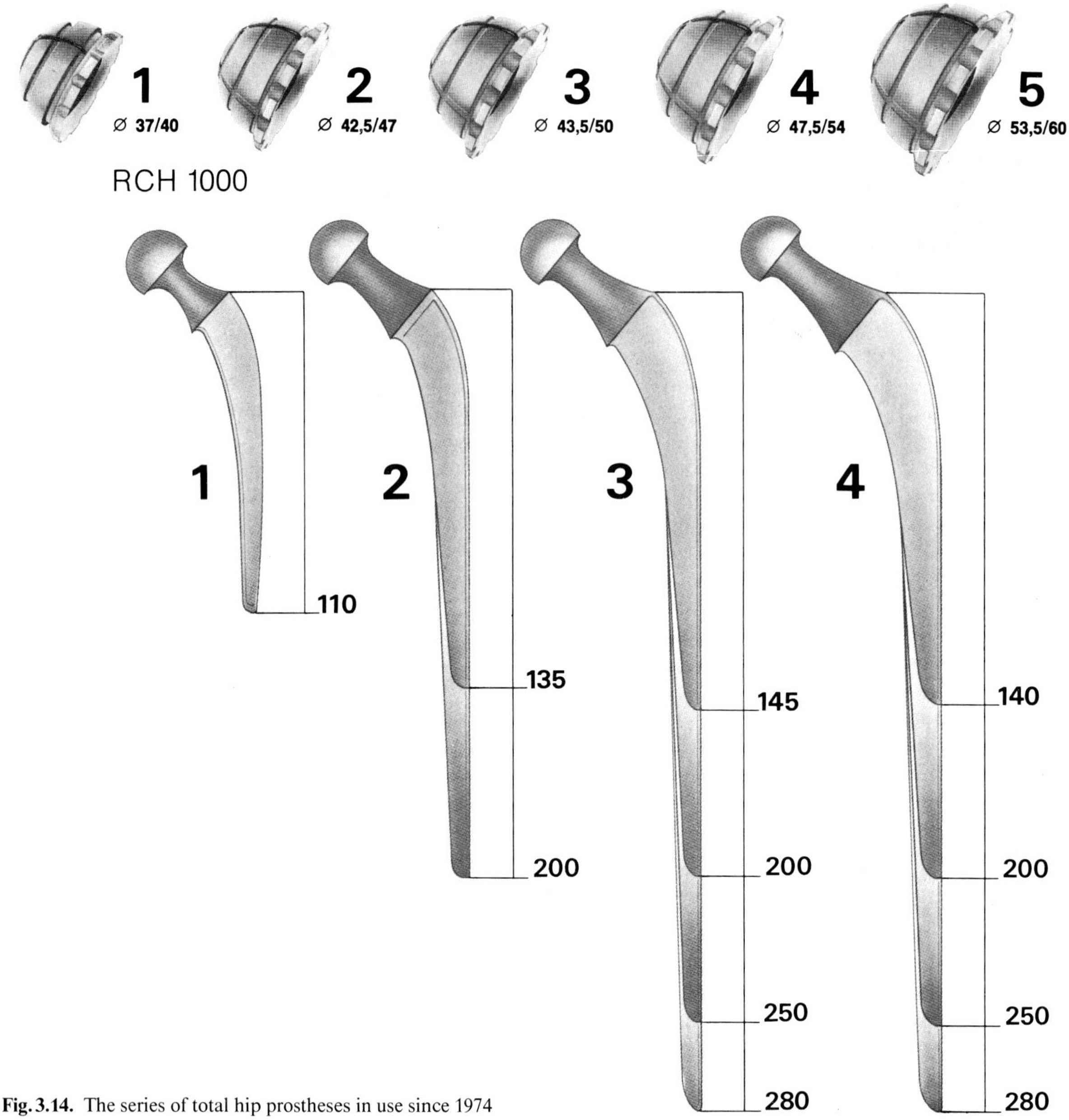

Fig. 3.14. The series of total hip prostheses in use since 1974

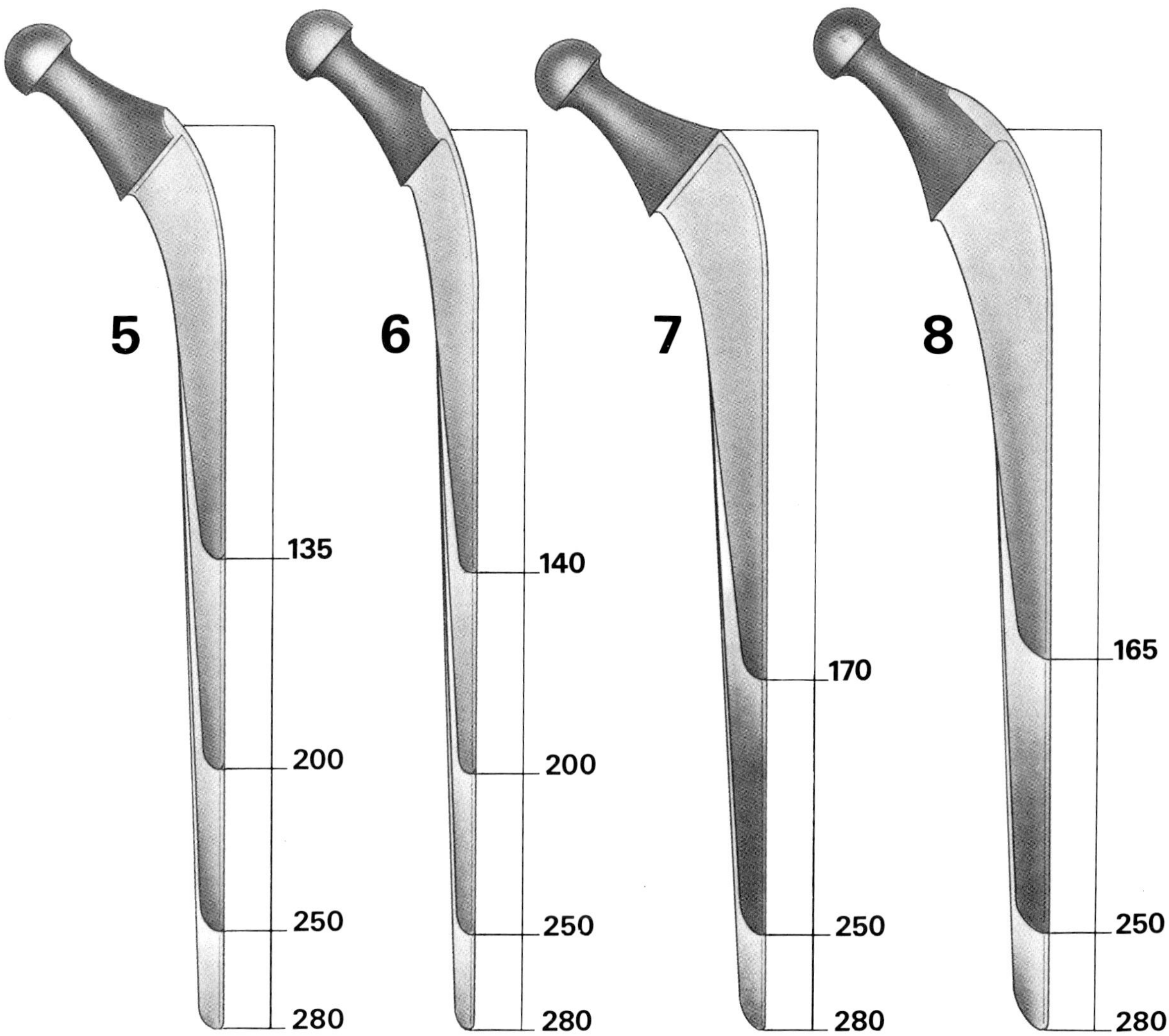

Fig. 3.14 *(continued)*

4 The Routine Operation

4.1 Indications for Total Hip Replacement and Preparation of the Patient for Surgery

M. Kerboul

Total hip replacement is never an emergency procedure. Even when the indication for surgery is clear and the patient is pressing for an operation, it is always preferable to prepare the patient so that he or she may approach surgery in the best possible circumstances.

4.1.1 Indications

Total hip arthroplasty is indicated above all where there is massive joint destruction. This may be the result of rapidly progressive osteoarthritis, advanced primary or secondary osteoarthritis, inflammatory arthritis, or damage following previous surgery, such as an acrylic arthroplasty, a Moore hemiarthroplasty, or a single or double cup, whether this is cemented or not. But it also has a place following failures of previous nonseptic surgery (i.e., femoral or pelvic osteotomy, the Voss procedure, or a shelf operation), in ankylosing spondylitis, following unsatisfactory arthrodesis or resections of the femoral head and neck, in tuberculosis, and even in high dislocations of the hip that are poorly tolerated.

In other cases, such as primary or secondary osteoarthritis, early inflammatory arthritis, or aseptic necrosis, or following fractures of the acetabulum or the neck of the femur, other effective forms of treatment are available. So total hip arthroplasty may for a while run in parallel with either medical treatment or another surgical procedure such as a shelf, femoral or pelvic osteotomy, cup arthroplasty, or, more rarely, an arthrodesis.

When the indication for surgery is not well defined, open-minded discussion and the exchange of different opinions may occasionally give rise to a useful line of thought that may help us to arrive at the best solution for the patient involved. It is in these cases that such diverse factors as the personality of the patient, the clinical and radiological features of the arthropathy, and the expected benefits of the proposed procedure will all enter into the discussion.

The personality of the patient can be defined by his or her physiological state, physical fitness, social, professional, and family obligations, intellectual capacity, and psychological makeup. The clinical presentation of the arthropathy is very wide ranging. The functional impairment is very variable, with no direct relationship to anatomical damage. Its repercussions upon the patient's life and family circle are felt in various ways, and we must be wary of two false candidates for surgery. First, the neurotic who cannot stand the slightest reduction in function and who demands operation as an emergency. Second, the apathetic patient who comes to the clinic only because he has been pushed by his family or his doctor. The first sets us a trap, and the second does not want to fall into ours. Both are in danger of not being satisfied by our attentions and it is better to put them off, at least temporarily.

The radiological features of the diseased hip must also be taken into account. In particular we must consider the disease in its overall context, its progression, the possibility of reversing the lesions, its morphology, and the extent of serious damage to the joint. Finally, an understanding of the potential benefits of this procedure must include two other factors: knowledge of the limits of the operation and the competence of the individual surgeon. It is not without relevance to the patient that his chances of a good result may be 99 out of 100, or only 70.

Each case is individual, but when it is reasonable to expect that a conservative procedure will produce a significant improvement in function that will enable the patient to take up an active life again, then there is no doubt about the treatment of choice.

The high quality of the results of hip arthroplasty is not an adequate reason, even today, to extend its indications to cover incipient coxarthrosis in patients in their fifth decade, when other less risky procedures can be genuinely effective in the long term.

4.1.2 Contraindications

Contraindications may be local or general. The presence of infection in the hip or of previous sepsis, especially if caused by *Staphylococcus aureus,* is a contraindication to surgery. One cannot be dogmatic, but the risk of reawakening latent infection, even if it has been dormant for several years, remains sufficiently significant, and the consequences are severe enough to warrant mature reflection before making any decision on hip arthroplasty. Exceptions to this rule are the sequelae of septic arthritis in infancy, an infection that genuinely seems to have been cured before the patient's becoming adult, and the sequelae of tuberculosis of the hip where medical treatment seems sufficiently effective to prevent recrudescence of the infection.

The presence of an infective focus far from the hip (in the skin, larynx, teeth, ears, lungs, bronchi, or in the gastrointestinal or genitourinary tract) presents a real risk of contamination of the artificial hip during or after the operation. It must therefore be eradicated before surgery is considered.

A poor state of general health can also be a contraindication to surgery. In the general preoperative assessment one must try to estimate the risk of this procedure, which is far from insignificant in patients who are old, atherosclerotic, hypertensive, obese, diabetic, or have limited cerebral perfusion or latent renal or respiratory insufficiency.

There is no doubt that better preparation of the patient, together with more meticulous anesthesia and postoperative care, has allowed us to considerably extend the indications for total hip arthroplasty without too much danger to the safety of the patient. But we must take care not to forget that this operation, carried out with the aim of gaining an improvement in function, can be fatal, for instance following the rare but very real possibility of massive fat embolism. Whatever one may have heard or read, it is nearly always surgery and not anesthesia that kills.

4.1.3 Preparation of the Patient

Preparation is essential, and although it should logically be carried out by the general practitioner or by the rheumatologist, it is no doubt preferable that the surgeon take the greatest part of the responsibility. It should begin with the first outpatient consultation. It requires a full and thorough medical assessment, which, if methodical and organized, can be brief and productive. This will include careful clinical examination, laboratory investigations, and possibly the opinion of several specialists. All factors must be assessed and it is vital to reduce excess weight by an adequate, balanced diet, to correct hypertension and arrhythmias, and to treat chronic bronchitis and improve respiratory function by reduction or preferably cessation of smoking. Glaucoma, diabetes, gout, and latent renal insufficiency must be treated, and hepatic function and clotting factors must be checked.

One must look for, and possibly treat surgically, symptomatic calculi which could give rise postoperatively to an acute and even occasionally gangrenous cholecystitis. Kidney stones may coexist with a chronic urinary infection, and a prostatic adenoma may result in acute postoperative urinary retention.

One must also especially look for, treat, and eradicate all foci of infection before contemplating total hip arthroplasty. This includes cutaneous infection from varicose ulcers, folliculitis, discharging eczema, and dermatitis, possibly treated with the aid of a dermatologist. Urinary gynecological, orolaryngeal, and dental infections must be treated. It may be necessary to extract teeth, and X-rays should be used to detect devitalized roots that must be removed in the presence of apical cysts. In spite of such an extensive assessment, one will sometimes be surprised to discover, or see revealed postoperatively, an infection that had hitherto remained dormant.

Psychological preparation is also important, if only to avoid any misunderstanding at a later date. Many candidates for hip replacement have a false idea of this procedure, often created by previous patients who are doing very well and who have completely forgotten the immediate postoperative period. They expect much more from this operation than it can provide.

It is not always an easy, benign procedure with an uncomplicated, short postoperative course that automatically guarantees excellent hip function. The future patient must understand this. He must also understand that this operation will not rejuvenate him. All other pain, especially that from lumbar spondylosis or from osteoarthritis of a distal joint, will persist. He must finally understand that in order to walk better he is going to put his life in jeopardy. Even if the risk is statistically minimal, it is not zero.

All this physical and psychological preparation should preferably be carried out on an outpatient basis, before admission, in order that the patient be fully aware of the situation and not run the risk of being turned down for surgery at the last moment.

4.2 The Psychiatrist's View Point

V. Pacault

These few lines are intended to point out the importance of the consultation with the patient prior to hip replacement. This will enable one to discover:

1. The possible presence of a depressive illness.
2. Those queries and anxieties that the patient has not yet outwardly expressed.

Depression can be a response to the physical handicap, but it can also be more serious and related to an existential malaise of the patient. We often notice that the moment chosen by the patient to ask for surgery is of significance. It may, for example, be at the time of a family conflict or at the beginning of retirement that the request becomes more urgent. Suffering and physical discomfort are then more poorly tolerated, even apart from objective deterioration.

If these depressive elements are not recognized and not treated prior to surgery, they may subsequently become worse and compromise the rehabilitation of the patient. It is therefore important to recognize serious depression that is over and above a reactive depression in response to physical pain, and so enable the patient to approach surgery in a satisfactory condition.

During the consultation, it is also important to determine the difference between what the patient openly asks for, through his organic symptoms, and what he implicitly expects. These secret expectations are rarely expressed immediately, and may be the desire to please or the wish to erase the signs of aging, rather like cosmetic surgery. If we can identify these motives prior to surgery, we may avoid seeing the patient returning to complain, as did one lady: "I thought that with a new hip, everything would be marvellous."

Finally, let us recall these words of Aristophanes: "No man can be truly healthy if he is unhappy."

4.3 The Cardiologist and the Candidate for Total Hip Replacement

C. Viguie

Total hip replacement is major surgery aimed at the relief of symptoms, and in the old patient this may have serious implications.

The high incidence of cardiovascular pathology in the retired age-group puts a special responsibility on the cardiologist in his preoperative assessment of the serious risks involved. The expected benefits of the operation, in terms of the increased physical activity of the patient, require the cardiologist to assess in perspective the circulatory repercussions that may result from an improvement in the range of walking, and whether these are beneficial or not.

The preoperative assessment by the cardiologist must be carried out some time before the proposed date of operation in this type of planned, elective surgery. This will enable additional investigations to be carried out and specific medical treatment to be begun if indicated. Recent advances in the field of noninvasive cardiovascular investigation, together with the availability of new treatments, have enabled us to extend the reliability of assessment of the cardiovascular risks during surgery and to present patients to the surgeon who would previously have been turned down.

We shall consider here the preoperative problems of selection and preparation of candidates for surgery.

4.3.1 Cardiovascular Risks and Fitness for Surgery

Although cardiac complications form a large part of the cardiovascular risks encountered during surgery, other problems, such as peripheral artery disease and venous thromboembolism, must also be taken into account. A multifactorial system of scoring cardiac risk in noncardiac surgical procedures has been devised by Goldman et al. [2]. The various risk factors and their relative scores are set out in Table 4.1 [5]. There is a good correlation between the total score and the occurrence of perioperative complications (pulmonary edema, myocardial infarction, ventricular tachycardia), which are significantly higher in groups III and IV.

Table 4.1 confirms the poor prognosis associated with aging but also underlines the adverse effect of certain conditions, such as recent myocardial infarction, aortic stenosis, poor ventricular function, and certain arrhythmias.

Since the appearance of the article by Goldman et al. in 1977, several noninvasive investigations have become available in routine practice, such as echocardiography and continuous ECG monitoring. These have enabled a more objective assessment to be made of the major prognostic factors whereas this had hitherto been possible only by clinical methods.

On the other hand, there are a number of factors with a poor perioperative prognosis that can be modified either by the passage of time (e.g., a recent myocardial infarction) or by specific treatment (e.g., certain types of cardiac insufficiency or arrhythmia).

Preoperative selection by the cardiologist must there-

Table 4.1. Scoring system of cardiac risk factors in relation to surgery

Factors		Points
Questionnaire:	age > 70 years	5
	MI < 6 months	10
	aortic stenosis	3
Clinical examination: B3, JVP, CCF		11
ECG: rhythm other than in sinus:		7
	VE 5/min	7
General assessment:	PO_2 < 60	3
	PCO_2 > 50	3
	K^+ < 3	3
	BUN > 50	3
	Creatinine > 30 mg/l	3
	Bedridden	3
Operative procedure:	emergency	4
	thoracic	3
	abdominal	3
	aortic	3
	Total	53
Classification CRIS:	I = 0- 5 points	
	II = 6-12 points	
	III = 13-25 points	
	IV = 26 points and over	

MI, Myocardial infarction; *BUN*, blood urea nitrogen; *B3*, gallop rhythm; *JVP*, raised jugular venous pressure; *VE*, ventricular extrasystoles; *CCF*, congestive cardiac failure; *CRIS*, cardiac risk index score

fore be strict. He must carry out additional investigations when necessary and must not turn down patients who may be able to benefit from surgery after special preparation. The cardiologist must have three objectives.

1. To identify definite contraindications, which are rare but include conditions that are not always markedly symptomatic but are potentially lethal, such as severe aortic stenosis and obstructive cardiomyopathy. There are also refractory conditions that could be accentuated by an increase in physical activity and include all cardiomyopathies bordering on permanent decompensation, refractory angina, certain abnormalities of ventricular rhythm, malignant hypertension, and peripheral arterial insufficiency of grades III and IV.

2. To recognize correctable contraindications and to carry out a later assessment following active treatment. In this category are: myocardial infarction within 6 months, coronary insufficiency as yet unrecognized and untreated, certain abnormalities of rhythm and conduction, and neglected or poorly controlled hypertension without major visceral repercussions.

3. To select those patients at cardiovascular risk but whose condition, if stabilized, could be improved favorably by a return to regular physical activity. This group includes patients with chronic angina and some forms of arteritis of the lower limbs.

4.3.2 Preoperative Diagnosis

Major surgery such as total hip replacement requires a strict and systematic cardiovascular assessment. These are the main conditions that must be detected:

Coronary Insufficiency

This is a constant worry in view of its frequency and potentially serious consequences. Positive diagnosis is based on a previous history of myocardial infarction or angina, on the presence of myocardial scarring on ECG, or on problems suggestive of ventricular repolarization.

Ischemic cardiomyopathy need not always manifest as angina, however, even in a quite disabled patient, and anomalies of repolarization are not always specific (isolated T-wave anomalies, in particular). One must be sure of the diagnosis, but as exercise testing is not possible, Holter monitoring, echocardiography, the isoproterenol test, or radioactive isotope investigation may be used.

An assessment of the progressive or nonprogressive nature of the coronary insufficiency is therefore essential.

Valvular Disease

The problem here is that a systolic murmur may be associated with a severe aortic stenosis or an obstructive cardiomyopathy which is being masked by the forced sedentary life of the patient.

An isolated systolic murmur is a very common finding in the elderly and is usually related to innocent valvular sclerosis. One must, however, be on one's guard and listen to the second heart sound with the subject lying down and standing after Valsalva's maneuver. In case of doubt, one can perform echocardiography.

In the presence of significant valvular disease it is important to know its effect on left ventricular function. One then relies not so much on clinical assessment (previous cardiac problems, dyspnea, gallop rhythm, or cardiomegaly) but more on echocardiography in order to assess cardiac competence.

Abnormalities of Rhythm and Conduction

Ventricular hyperexcitability must not be disregarded, and following preoperative discovery its significance must be determined by 24-h Holter monitoring and by looking for an underlying cardiomyopathy using echocardiography.
Abnormalities of supraventricular rhythm must also be taken into consideration, especially atrial fibrillation, which, regardless of its etiology, can predispose to acute cardiac failure or thromboembolism.
Problems of conduction and the attendant risks of syncope are assessed from the history and finally by complementary tests such as Holter monitoring and intracardiac investigations.

Hypertension

This is too often overlooked in elderly patients [1]. By definition, it is present when the systolic pressure is consistently above 160 mmHg or when the diastolic pressure is over 95 mmHg. Systolic blood pressure is characteristically labile in the geriatric age-group and is best assessed with the patient both standing and lying.
As well as measuring blood pressure at the beginning and end of the examination, in both arms and while the patient is lying and standing, one must look systematically for any arterial or cardiac sequelae, such as hypertensive or ischemic cardiomyopathy, cerebral atherosclerosis or involvement of the lower limbs, and aortic aneurysm.
In this respect, it is of interest to the anesthetist to know if there are problems with left ventricular compliance (suggested by left ventricular or atrial hypertrophy shown on ECG and confirmed by echocardiography) or any involvement of the carotids. Doppler investigation of the carotids should be routine in the hypertensive patient even in the absence of local signs, as the detection of a carotid bruit does not seem very sensitive or specific [3].
The cervical Doppler examination should also be routine in all atheromatous patients who already have involvement of the lower limbs or coronary insufficiency. If a narrow carotid stenosis is suspected then arteriography or angiography should be carried out.

Venous Thromboembolism

This remains one of the major complications of total hip replacements. The role of the cardiologist prior to surgery is to look for predisposing factors that are amenable to treatment (atrial fibrillation, obesity, extracellular dehydration). In patients with a previous history of phlebitis of the lower limbs, a Doppler examination of the veins will give a preoperative baseline.

4.3.3 Cardiovascular Preparation for Surgery

Following diagnosis, the cardiologist can advise going ahead with surgery, give reasons why it is inadvisable, or suggest a trial of treatment with a specific medical regime.
The main features of this preparation for surgery are now described in each case.

Treatment to Prevent Myocardial Ischemia

This is routinely given prior to surgery if there is sufficient evidence for ischemic cardiomyopathy, even in the absence of angina. It consists of the administration singly or in combination of:

1. *Beta-blockers.* These have a known anti-ischemic action in addition to antihypertensive and antiadrenergic effects and are given in the absence of the usual contraindications (i.e., cardiomegaly, certain conduction defects, and asthma). To cover the period of surgery, either a long-acting preparation is used or the drug is given just prior to the operation. A preparation that is cardioselective or has an intrinsic sympathomimetic action is chosen.

2. *Nitrates (i.e., Nitroglycerin or Isosorbide Dinitrate).* These not only have anti-ischemic activity but also reduce congestion by venous dilatation in high doses. Nitroglycerin can be administered intravenously during surgery.

3. *Calcium Antagonists.* These have antispasmodic and anti-ischemic action. Nifedipine is particularly interesting as an arterial vasodilator and it is a powerful hypotensive agent. However, it has a short half-life. Bepridil is useful in having a long half-life and in its antiarrhythmic action. These drugs have the disadvantage of causing "torsade de pointe" in cases where there is associated hypokalemia.

4. *Amiodarone.* This is of interest because of its anti-ischemic activity, its supraventricular and ventricular antiarrhythmic effects, and its long half-life.

Antihypertensive Treatment

The aim is to maintain the arterial pressure at a level below or equal to 160/95 mmHg for as long as there is any danger of significant cardiovascular repercussions. Several situations may be encountered.

1. Long-standing hypertension that is well controlled: The same treatment is continued, once it has been established that there is no hemoconcentration, renal insufficiency, hypokalemia, or hyperuricemia.
2. Poorly controlled or untreated hypertension: Beta-blockers or nifedipine are used because of their additional cardioprotective effects. In the case of resistant hypertension, captopril is used because it is effective and well tolerated, although renal function must be regularly monitored. This drug also has an anticongestive action.

The Treatment of Arrhythmias

Ventricular hyperexcitability is treated with quinidine, disopyramide, or amiodarone. Amiodarone is of interest because of its long half-life; on the other hand, its activity relies on previous impregnation of the myocardium.

Atrial hyperexcitability is treated with cardiac glycosides and also with quinidine, disopyramide, or amiodarone. Nadolol is of interest because it does not affect conduction.

Abnormalities of conduction at the sinoatrial, AV, or intraventricular level will require previous insertion of a pacemaker if they are symptomatic and therefore potentially dangerous.

Thromboembolism

This is a chapter in its own right [4]. Preoperative prophylaxis relies not so much on anticoagulant drugs and those reducing platelet aggregation, but also on the correction of obesity, elastic support stockings in the case of varices, the slowing down or controlling of atrial fibrillation, and the correction of hemoconcentration. Heparin therapy is used perioperatively in suitable doses.

4.3.4 In Conclusion

The role of the cardiologist is not solely "medicolegal". He must be a part of the medical and surgical team and must actively participate in the selection of patients and help in the preparation of those requiring his skills.

References

1. Forette F, de la Fuente X, Golmard JL, Henry JF, Hervy MP (1983) Risque d'accident vasculaire cérébral chez le sujet âgé hypertendu. Presse Med 12: 3036
2. Goldman L, Caldera DL, Nussbaum SR, Southwick RS, Krogstad D, Murray B, Burke D, O'Malley TA, Gorol AH, Caplan CH, Nolan J, Carabello B, Slater EE (1977) Multifactorial index of cardiac risk in noncardiac surgical procedures. N Engl J Med 297: 845
3. Ropper AH, Weschler LR, Wilson LS (1982) Carotid bruit and the risk of stroke in elective surgery. N Engl J Med 307: 1388
4. Salzman EW (1982) Program in preventing venous thromboembolism. N Engl J Med 309: 980
5. Wells PH, Kaplan JA (1981) Optimal management of patients with ischemic heart disease for noncardiac surgery by complementary anesthesiologist and cardiologist interaction. Am Heart J 102: 1029

4.4 Technical Preparation Prior to Total Hip Arthroplasty - The Choice of the Prosthesis

M. Kerboul

The aim of total hip arthroplasty is not solely to implant the two components of the prosthesis, but also to reconstruct an artificial hip which has the best possible mechanical function.

To achieve this involves restoring the architecture of the hip to a situation as near to normal as possible, with a centre of rotation at a selected point, and with a lateral lever arm and a femoral neck of sufficient length to restore maximal efficiency and balance to the periarticular muscles.

Restoration of limb length is also obtained if the following rules are adhered to and if the prosthesis has been chosen with care and the operative procedure has conformed to the preoperative plan.

Preoperative Study of the Roentgenogram. Tracings and transparencies of the two components that have been enlarged by 15% enable us to make a precise choice of prosthesis (Fig. 4.1).

If the lesion is unilateral (Fig. 4.2), then we have the healthy side for reference, and there is no excuse for any error which may result in a definitive inequality in length of the lower limbs.

Superimposition of transparencies on the femur and acetabulum on the healthy side enables us to choose the components that are best adapted to the features of the hip. The cup must be covered within the acetabulum. The femoral component must fill the medullary canal and the center of its head must be superimposed on that of the femoral head and the cup. The theoretical level of division of the femoral neck is then easily determined and its height above the lesser trochanter is measured.

The application of the transparencies to the side to be operated on is carried out as follows. The cup is first

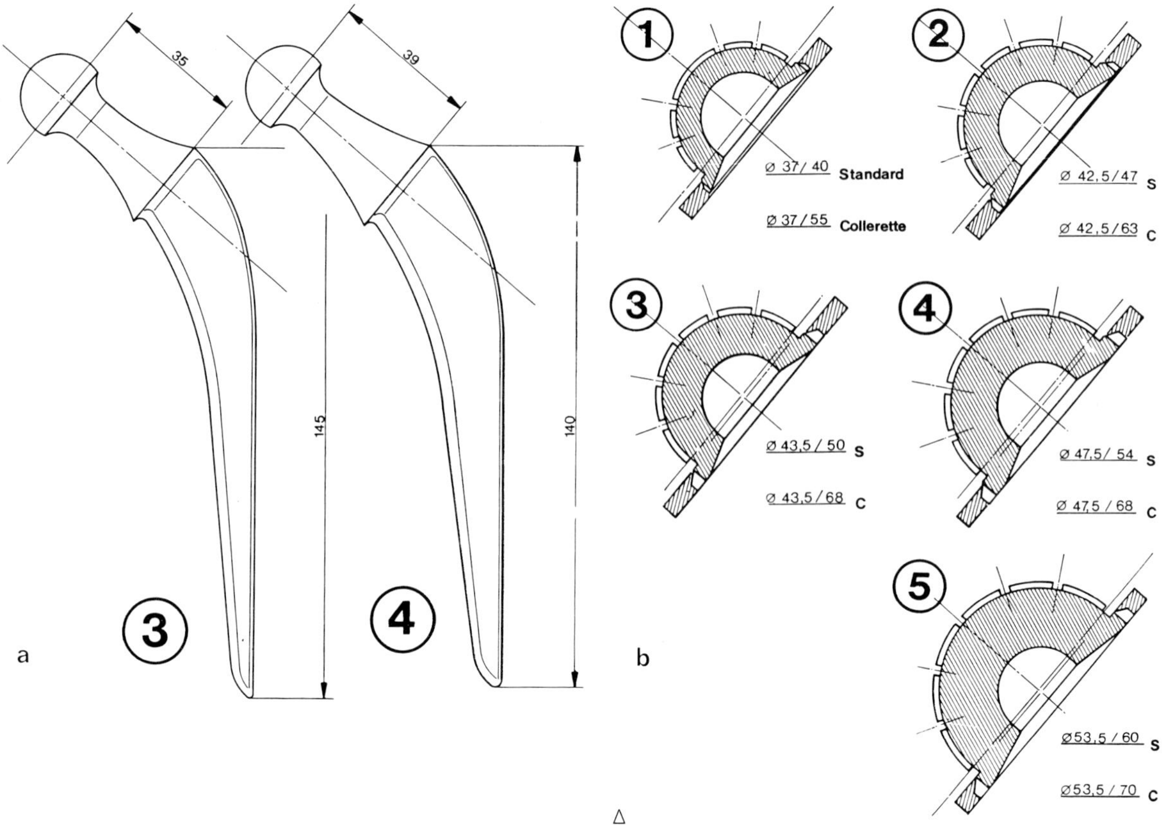

△

Fig. 4.1 a, b. Transparencies of the components, enlarged by 15%

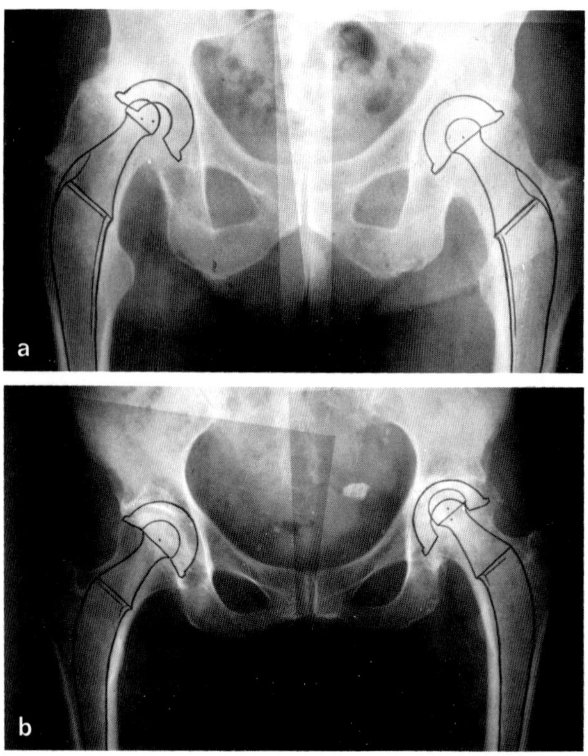

Fig. 4.2 a, b. Preoperative study and choice of prosthesis for a patient with a unilateral lesion

placed in the desired position. Having determined the theoretical level of the femoral cut taken from the healthy side, and having ensured that the femoral stem remains enclosed within the cortical margins of the diaphysis, we then superimpose the transparency of the femoral component on the roentgenogram of the femur. Superimposition of the centers of the two femoral heads is rarely obtained because of fixed external rotation, which gives a picture of false coxa valga. The distance between the center of the femoral prosthesis and the center of the cup then gives the exact amount of shortening that needs to be corrected.

If the lesion is bilateral, with significant destruction of each hip so that there is no healthy hip for reference, then there is room for error. Final correction is always possible when operating on the second side (Figs. 4.3, 4.4).

The principles remain unchanged. The cup is placed in the most suitable position and the femoral component is aligned so that it completely fills the medullary canal. The distance between the center of the femoral component and that of the cup then represents the

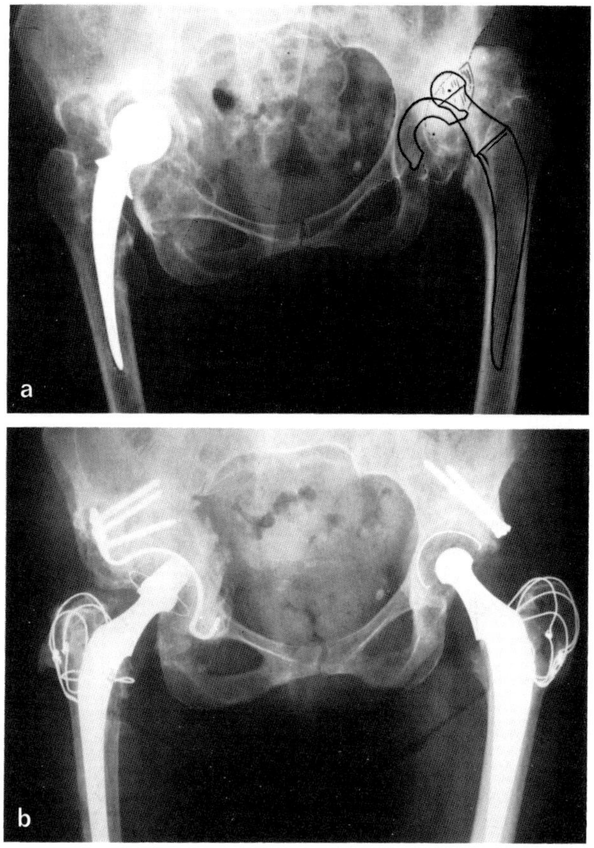

Fig. 4.3 a, b. Preoperative study and selection of prosthesis for a patient with bilateral disease involving marked bony destruction on both sides

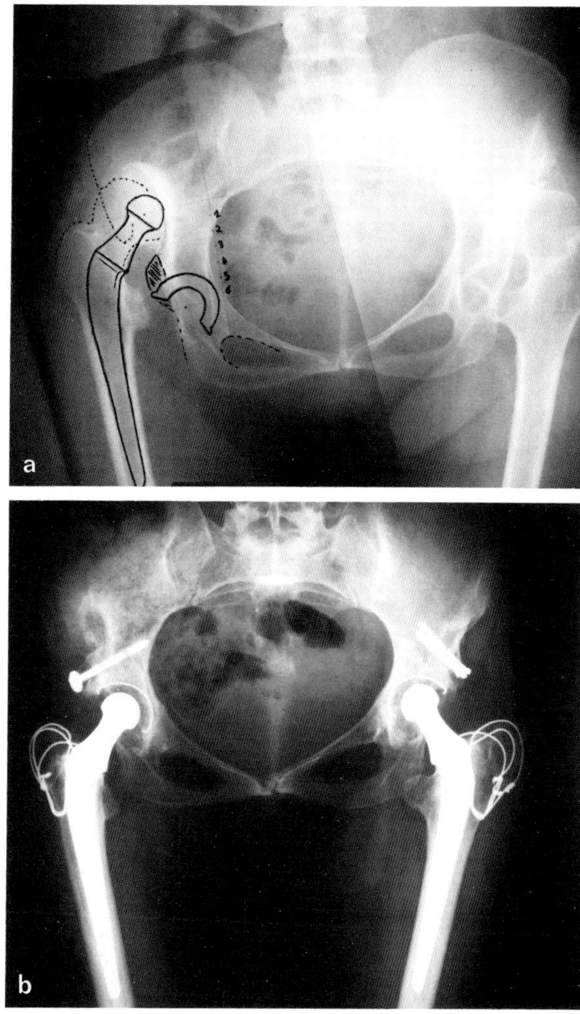

Fig. 4.4 a, b. Preoperative study of a grossly damaged hip. This patient has bilateral congenital dislocations

amount of lengthening that must be achieved during the operation.

In some cases of congenital dislocation there is a loss of substance in the anterosuperior part of the acetabulum, and this may need to be filled by screwing a graft into place.

This theoretical preoperative preparation is particularly valuable when the architecture of the hip is distorted, as may be the case in long-standing congenital dislocation. It provides a guide to the choice of the components, but it goes without saying that the definitive decision is made only during the operation.

The first decision to be made is the level of division of the femoral neck. Should there be doubt as to whether it will be possible to implant the component previously selected on the basis of the roentgenogram, then one must take a component of a smaller size in order not to risk cutting the neck too short, unless the series provides several stem sizes for one neck length. If the prosthesis selected on the basis of the roentgenogram proves to be the one of choice, then shortening the neck will enable the prosthesis to be seated at the correct height.

The second decision regards the cup. Its position determines the recentering of the hip. It must be placed as low as possible in the hollowed-out acetabulum at the expense of osteophytes of the fossa and of the posterior wall. The size of the cup selected is determined by the trial component, which must lie flush with the inferior border of the acetabulum after the osteophytes have been removed and must sit exactly within the cavity and the posterior wall.

In osteoarthrosis there is frequently wear anterosuperiorly, and after removal of the peripheral osteophytes a gap often remains between the cup and the worn acetabular wall. If this is extensive it must be filled with bone graft.

A common practice is to remodel the degenerated oval acetabulum into a sphere and then to take the largest diameter of the cavity, with the result that a very large cup has to be implanted. This is a mistake. It results in the useless sacrifice of bone and leads to displacement of the artificial hip upward, anteriorly, and outward, all of which have undesirable effects on the function of the new joint (Fig. 4.5 a, b).

4.5 Standard Technique for Total Hip Arthroplasty in Uncomplicated Osteoarthritis

M. Postel

Since 1952 we have used the so-called posterolateral approach for hip replacement; it is in fact a true lateral approach.

We have removed the greater trochanter routinely since 1969, after a period during which we divided the mm. glutei around the greater trochanter. Whether we were right to adopt such a rigid routine is open to debate. Some simple arthroplasties can be carried out with no difficulty by less extensive approaches, such as the Moore approach. However, we believe that the posterolateral approach with trochanterotomy gives us complete control over the correct positioning of the implant under all circumstances with all the precision that we require. It also preserves the external rotators, which is an important factor in preventing dislocation, and reduces the risk of fracture of the femoral shaft. It always gives good exposure from the outset, and we prefer this to the hazards of a more limited approach where extension of the incision in difficult cases results in unnecessary soft tissue damage. Finally, a simple dissection and the absence of any trauma from retractors are the best way of preserving the integrity of the musculature. For all these reasons, this approach has become routine in our department.

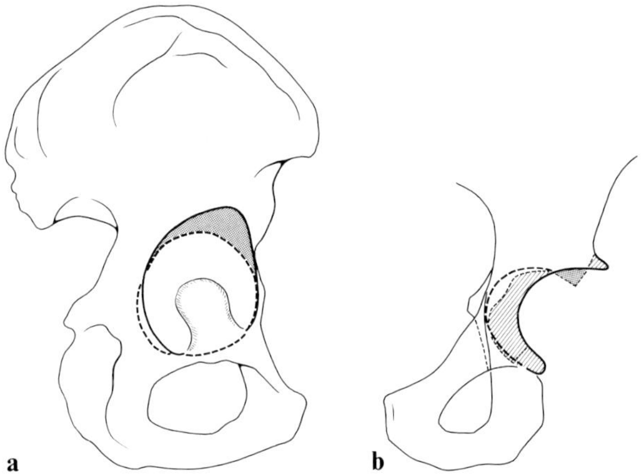

Fig. 4.5 a, b. The arthritic acetabulum, seen in the AP and lateral views *(solid line)*, has become oval following wear superiorly and anteriorly and filling-in by osteophytes inferiorly and medially. Recentering of the new hip is achieved by hollowing out a cavity in the chosen position *(broken line)*

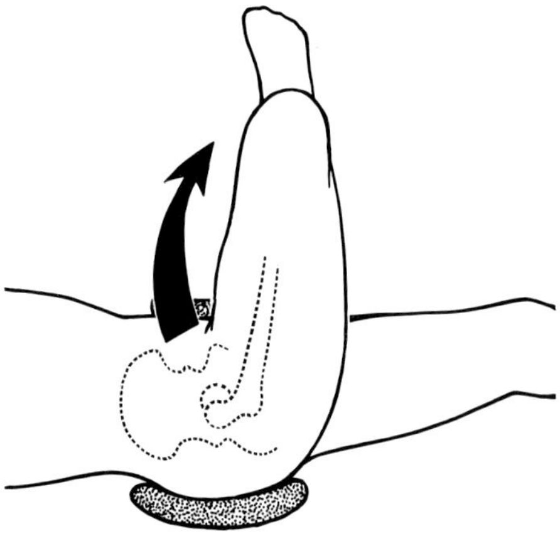

Fig. 4.7. The weight of the dislocated limb is liable to pull the pelvis anteriorly and result in cementing the cup in retroversion

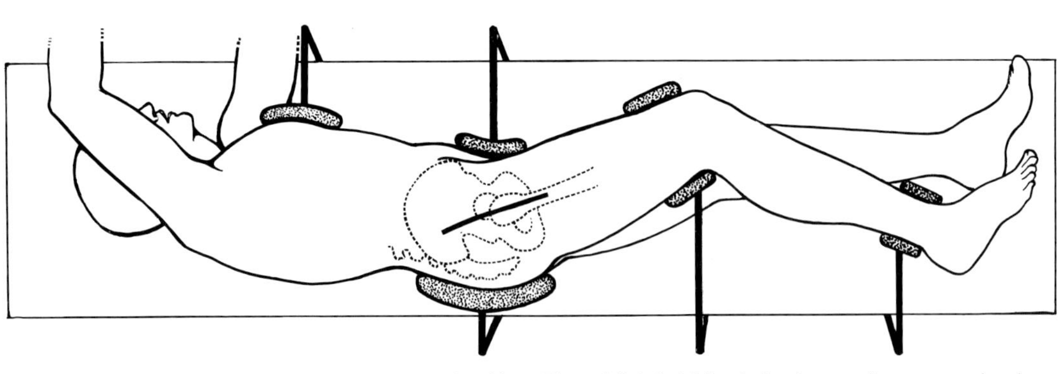

Fig. 4.6. The patient is positioned in strict lateral decubitus. The pelvis is held firmly in place against an anterior thoracic support

The technique described here is the routine procedure used in primary osteoarthritis with no significant deformity or anatomical anomaly.

4.5.1 Positioning of the Patient

It is necessary to have the patient in an exact and stable lateral decubitus position (Fig. 4.6). This is achieved by two special supports. Their positioning must be carefully supervised by the surgeon himself; otherwise, the dislocated limb may pull the pelvis anteriorly so that it will no longer remain in the vertical plane while the cup is being cemented in place (Fig. 4.7). There is then a risk of the cup being retroverted. Similarly, a fixed flexion deformity of the opposite hip may produce an accentuated lordosis during positioning, and this may lead to incorrect orientation of the cup.

4.5.2 Approach

The incision must be of sufficient length (20 cm) and centered over the greater trochanter. It must be exactly lateral to the femur and above all not displaced anteriorly, as this would cause the posterior margin of the wound to partly obscure the hip in the dislocated position (Fig. 4.8).

We routinely stitch a large, Betadine-soaked swab to the fascia lata, together with a waterproof drape.

We now replace all the instruments that may have been in contact with the skin with a clean set.

Anteriorly, we dissect the angle between the anterior margin of the mm. glutei and the m. vastus lateralis that covers them. A large Farabeuf retractor is inserted into the gap.

The sciatic nerve is identified if it is at the least risk, for instance when a subluxated hip has to be repositioned distally. However, it is not essential to visualize the sciatic nerve if one is sure that it will be away from the operative field. A large swab then protects the retractors that expose the posterior aspect of the joint.

Chisels are used to divide the greater trochanter (Figs. 4.9 and 4.10). We do not feel that the Gigli wire saw, as used by Charnley, gives a precise enough cut. It is better to use two large chisels placed 2–3 mm below the crest of the m. vastus lateralis and directed towards the junction of the neck and the trochanter. This V-shaped osteotomy ensures a more precise resection of the trochanter than a flat cut would. However, it prevents subsequent readjustment of orientation of the trochanter should one wish to adjust the balance of the external and internal rotators. The trochanter is gripped with a strong forceps and retracted proximally while the m. gluteus medius is separated from the capsule by sharp dissection up to the level of the acetabular rim. It is held back by a double-pointed retractor, or by two Steinmann pins. This can all be carried out with no damage to the mm. glutei (Fig. 4.11).

4.5.3 The Capsule

Once the capsule has beeen exposed superiorly, anteriorly, and posteriorly, it is divided along the axis of the neck from the acetabulum to the trochanter (Fig. 4.12). A further incision is carried around a semicircle along the acetabular rim. The hip can then be dislocated by lateral rotation in flexion followed by adduction. The femoral insertion of the capsule and the ligament of the head may be divided with a knife during this maneuver. Capsulectomy is completed only after division of the neck, because this allows the best view. The capsule and labrum can now be easily removed by passing a knife around the acetabular rim against the bone. If the point is kept within the cavity of the acetabulum the surrounding soft tissues are not at risk. Occasionally, it may suffice simply to split the inferior part of the capsule, so avoiding problems of hemostasis from the branch of the obturator artery that crosses the transverse ligament of the acetabulum. However, this is not possible if the capsule is contracted by a fixed adduction deformity or in the presence of periarticular ossification.

4.5.4 Osteotomy of the Femoral Neck

This can be carried out safely with a hand saw, as long as the point remains within the acetabulum. However, we prefer to use an oscillating power saw, which is more accurate, especially should the neck later have to be shortened by a few millimeters (Fig. 4.13). The plane and level of the cut are determined with the help of a trial femoral component whose head is centered over that of the head of the femur. The stem of the trial component is directed toward the center of the knee to achieve the correct orientation of the plane of the cut together with its normal slight anteversion. Superimposition of a transparency of the prosthesis over the roentgenogram may be helpful. If there is considerable destruction of the joint, the lesser trochanter is the only useful landmark in determining the level of the cut.

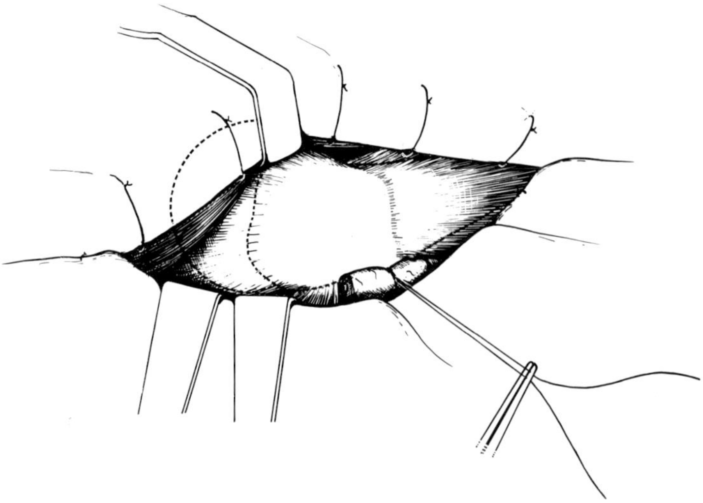

Fig. 4.8. The wound is closed. The trochanter is exposed. A swab placed behind the femur protects the sciatic nerve from the ends of the posterior retractors

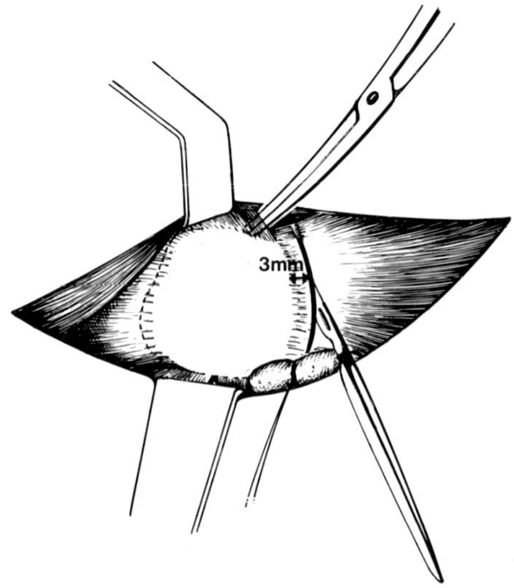

Fig. 4.9. Incision of the m. vastus lateralis 3 mm below the crest. Ligation of the artery that passes from the m. vastus lateralis to the anterior border of the mm. glutei

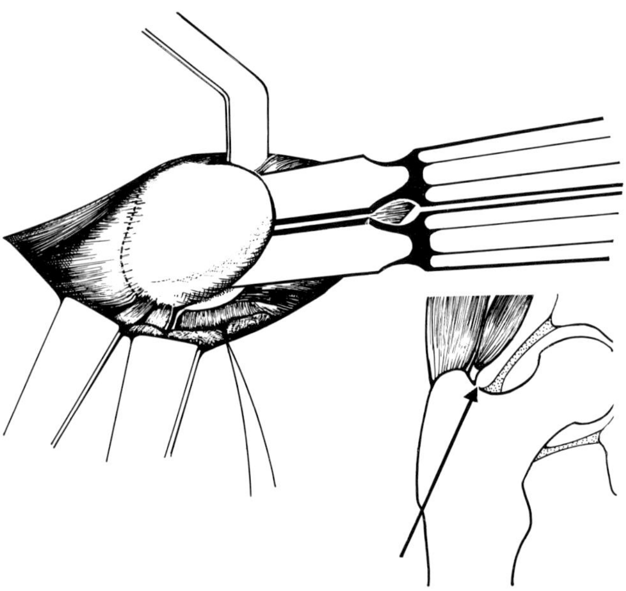

Fig. 4.10. Section of the trochanter with two large chisels, directed between the mm. glutei and the capsule

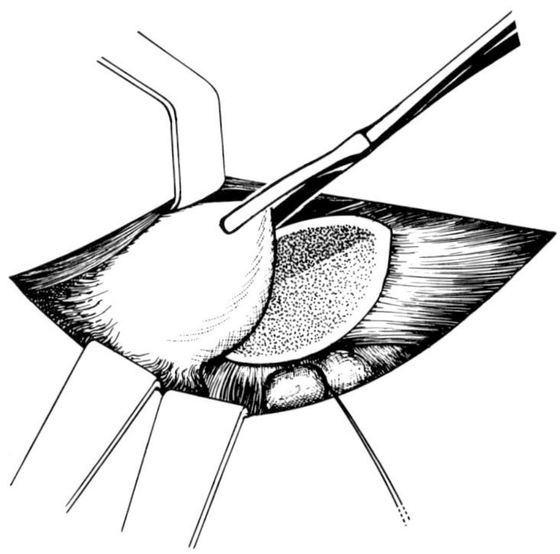

Fig. 4.11 *(right).* The trochanter is elevated and its surface deep to the mm. glutei is freed from the capsule by sharp dissection

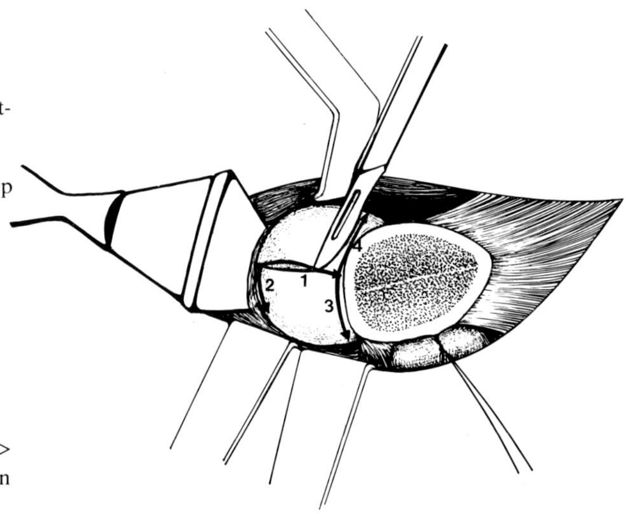

▷

Fig. 4.12. The capsule is opened longitudinally *(1)* and then along the acetabulum *(2)* and the base of the neck *(3)*

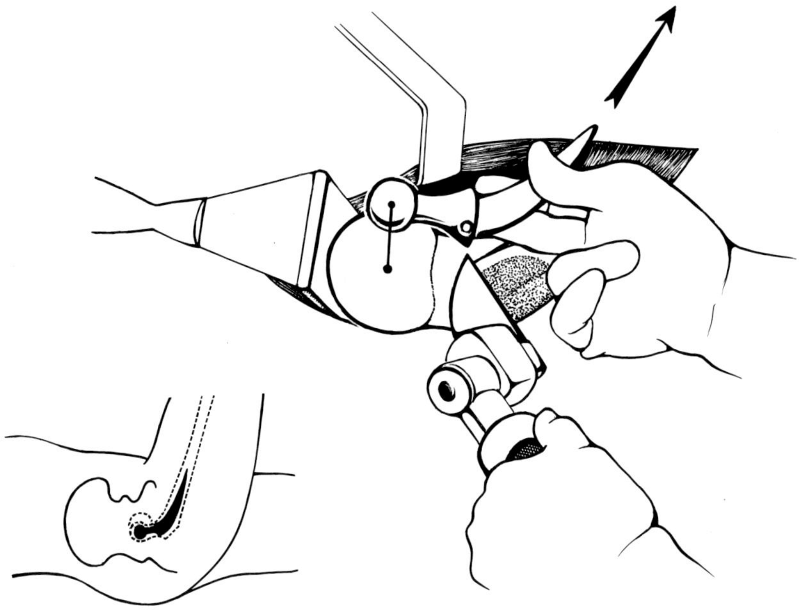

Fig. 4.13. The neck is divided with a saw. The orientation of the cup is given by positioning a trial prosthesis as if it were the definitive prosthesis. The level of the cup is determined by superimposing the center of the head on the center of the chosen prosthesis

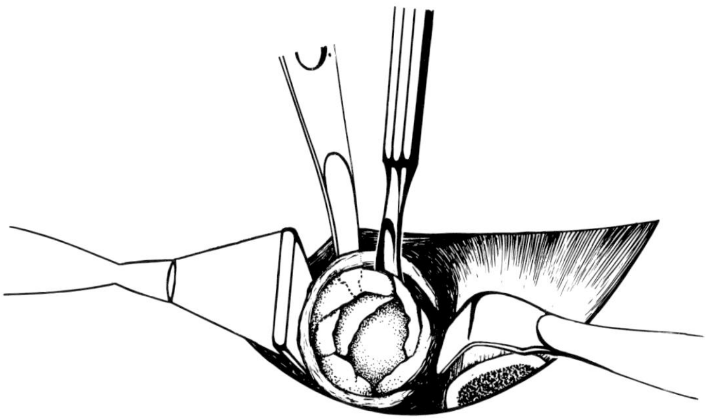

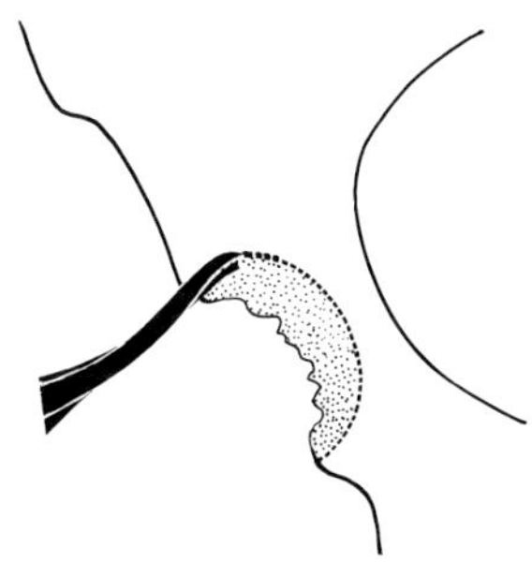

Fig. 4.14. The acetabulum is well exposed by a hooked retractor positioned in the obturator foramen inferior to the acetabulum and by a Homan retractor in front. The acetabulum is hollowed out with a concave/convex Smith-Petersen gouge and the acetabular rim is fashioned

4.5.5 Preparation of the Acetabulum

There are two important points. First, a well-centered hemispherical cavity must be prepared to a size which corresponds exactly to one of the cups. Its inferior border must be at the level of the superior margin of the obturator foramen. Medially, it must expose the quadrilateral plate, which must never be penetrated or damaged. Circular reamers are helpful, but they have the disadvantage of running on through soft bone and there is a tendency to displace the cup posteriorly. We prefer to prepare the cavity with two series of Smith-Petersen gouges, which are more precise if used skillfully. Final use of the reamer completes the preparation of the cavity and enables the exact positioning of the cup (Figs. 4.14 and 4.15).

Second, four key holes are made into the wall of the cavity, which now consists mainly of cancellous rather

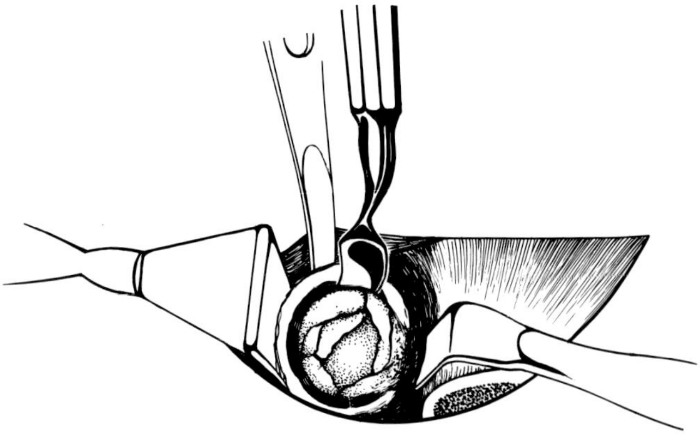

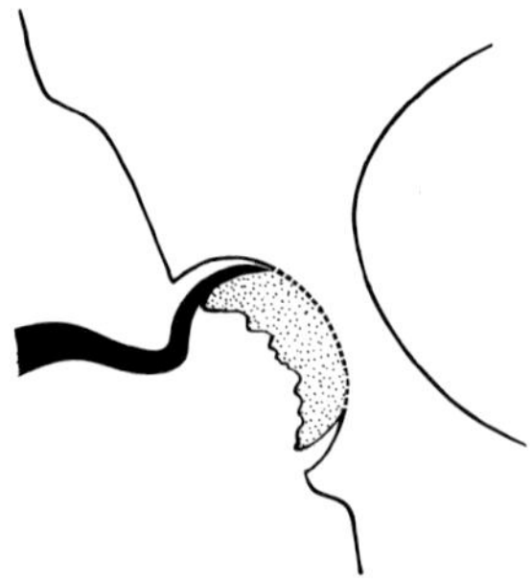

Fig. 4.15. Hollowing of the acetabulum is completed with Smith-Petersen gouges. It is taken just up to the medial cortex of the pelvic wall

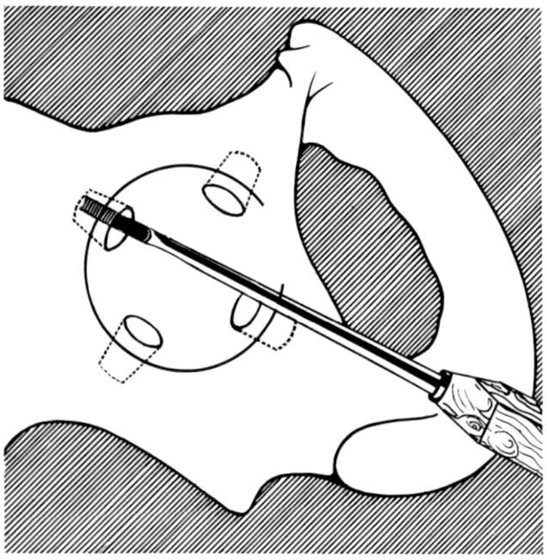

Fig. 4.16. The anchoring holes are begun with a long straight gouge

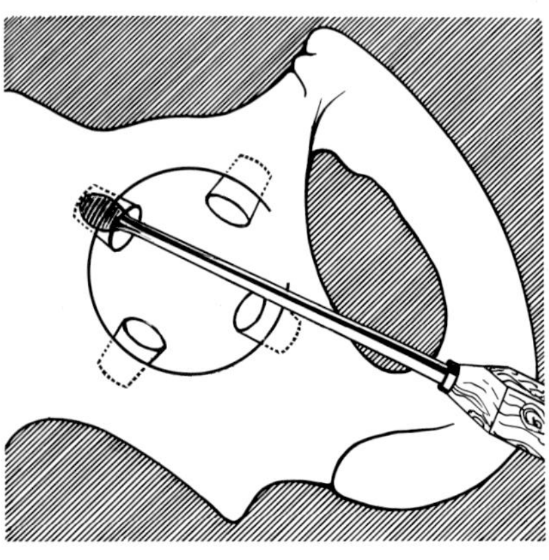

Fig. 4.17. The anchoring holes are enlarged with a curet

than cortical bone. One is placed in the pubis and one in the ischium, and two are placed superiorly. They must not penetrate into the pelvis (Figs. 4.16 and 4.17). In this way a cavity is fashioned that is well adapted to the cup and provides many anchoring points for the cement. Blood and clots are then removed by irrigation with a syringe and swabs.

4.5.6 *Cementing of the Cup*

We have used high-viscosity CMW acrylic cement since 1968. At present, we routinely add 80 mg gentamicin to each mix. The cement is introduced manually and pushed into each hole with a finger. The cup on its introducer is pushed into place, initially angled more horizontally than vertically, until it touches the quadrilateral plate. It is then repositioned until its inferior rim is flush with the superior margin of the obturator foramen and so that it lies in 10° of anteversion and is 45° open. Once the cup is in place, the excess cement is removed, care being taken not to disturb its orientation. At the same time we are careful to completely fill the space between the margin of the acetabulum and the rim of the cup (Fig. 4.18).

4.5.7 *Preparation of the Femur*

In the case of uncomplicated osteoarthrosis with an undeformed femur, the level of osteotomy of the femoral neck is determined by laying the femoral compo-

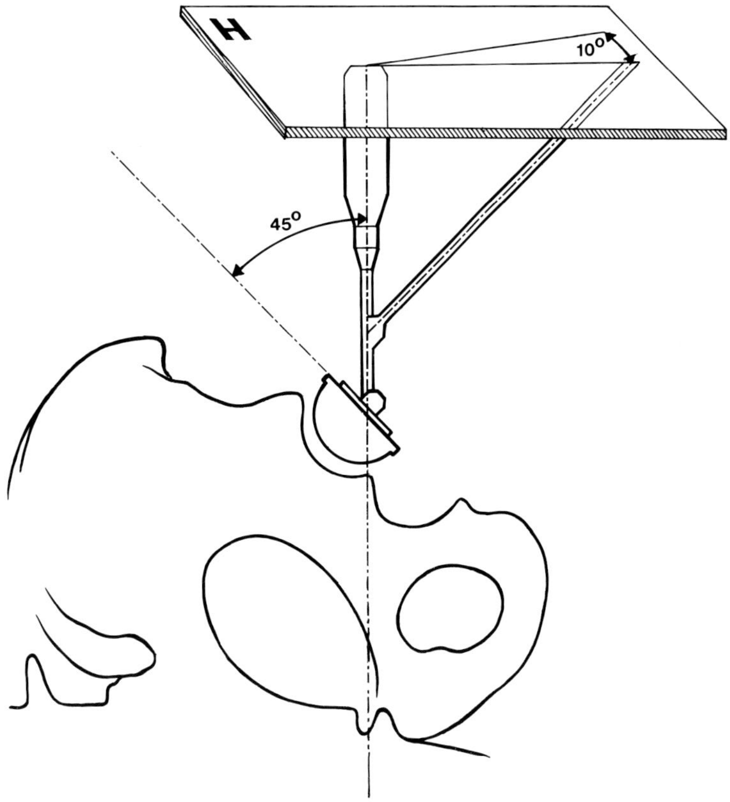

Fig. 4.18. The positioning of the cup must be very precise: angled 45° to the horizontal and with 10° of anteversion, with the help of a Y-shaped introducer

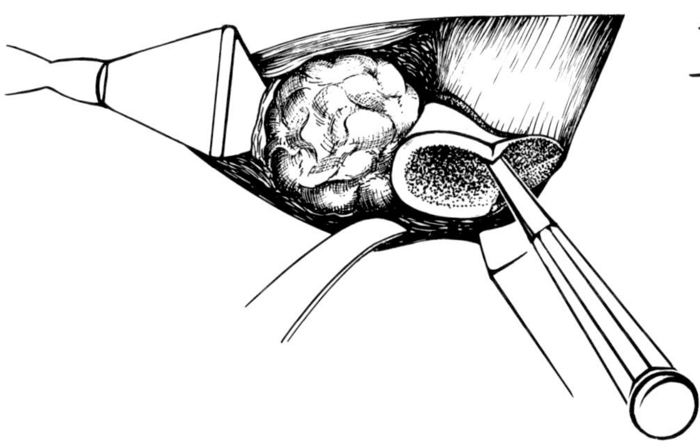

Fig. 4.19. Two blows with a straight chisel open the medullary canal

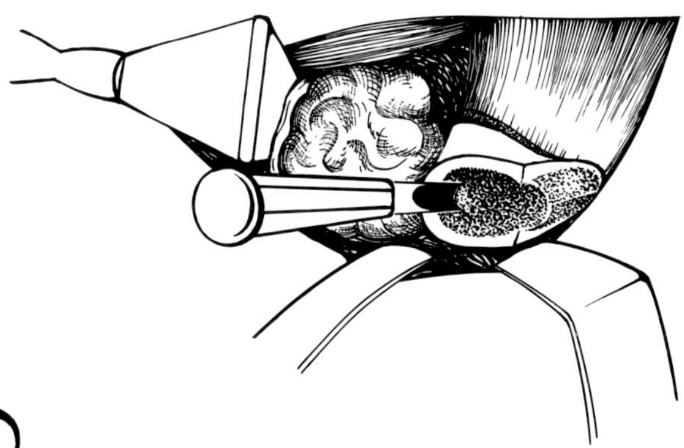

Fig. 4.20. Clearing the medullary canal is completed using a gouge

nent on the femur so that the centers of the two heads coincide. It is advisable to confirm this by reference to the lesser trochanter: cancellous bone is removed from the neck in one piece, encroaching as little as possible on that within the trochanter (Figs. 4.19 and 4.20). The medullary canal is easily identified with a curet and is then prepared with rasps (Fig. 4.21). The first rasp is one size smaller than that of the proposed prosthesis, and then a size larger is inserted. If the femoral component fits well, no further reaming is required; should it be freely mobile, a larger size is tried. This may necessitate shortening of the neck by a few millimeters, unless the range of prostheses available includes several stem sizes for the same length of neck. The medullary canal is then blocked with a piece of cancellous bone taken from the neck; it is trimmed to the size of the canal and pushed into place with a flexible introducer. This prevents the cement

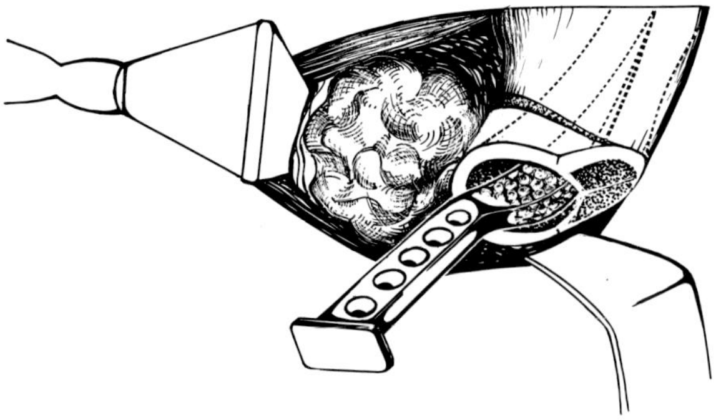

Fig. 4.21. The canal is prepared with a rasp, initially one a size smaller than the proposed prosthesis and then one of the same size

from extending too far distally, increases pressurization of the cement, and will not complicate any future revision. The wires to reattach the trochanter are now inserted. They pass through a hole in the lateral cortex of the femur, made with a sharp spike and situated 3 cm distal to the level of the trochanterotomy. They emerge through the femoral neck, two being anterior and two posterior (Fig. 4.22). Finally, the femur is thoroughly washed out with saline injected with a syringe.

4.5.8 Cementing of the Femoral Component

Cement is introduced by finger pressure after a cannula has been inserted to allow the escape of air and blood from the medullary canal. The femoral canal can be filled well if the cement is inserted in repeated small quantities. We do not feel that syringes or special pumps are needed. They involve unnecessary expense and require the cement to be very fluid. The prosthesis is held in an introducer and pushed into position. If the femur has been well filled, then considerable force is required, followed by a few blows with a hammer. Throughout the procedure the head of the prosthesis is carefully protected from any contact (Fig. 4.23).

4.5.9 Reduction

Reduction should be easy, without the use of force, following arthroplasty in uncomplicated osteoarthrosis. It is achieved by internal rotation of the limb held in extension and adduction. The head must not be scratched, and great care must be taken to avoid contact with any metal object.

The range of movement is tested and should be normal. It must be ensured that there is no abnormal contact at the extremes of movement that may later be the cause of dislocation. Before the trochanter is reattached, the posterior capsule is reconstituted if it has been preserved, and the external rotators are reopposed.

4.5.10 Reattachment of the Trochanter

The wires are passed through the mm. glutei at the level of the superior margin of the trochanter, which is then pulled down and held in place with a spike. The anterior and posterior wires which emerge medially from the neck and which hold down the trochanter most firmly are those which are tied first. The two others are tied afterwards. They must be pulled as tightly

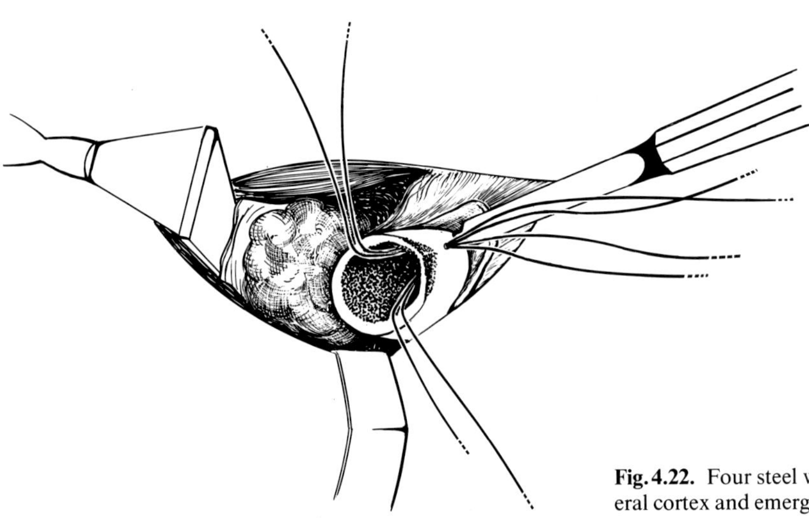

Fig. 4.22. Four steel wires size 12/10 are passed through the lateral cortex and emerge two in front, two behind the prosthesis

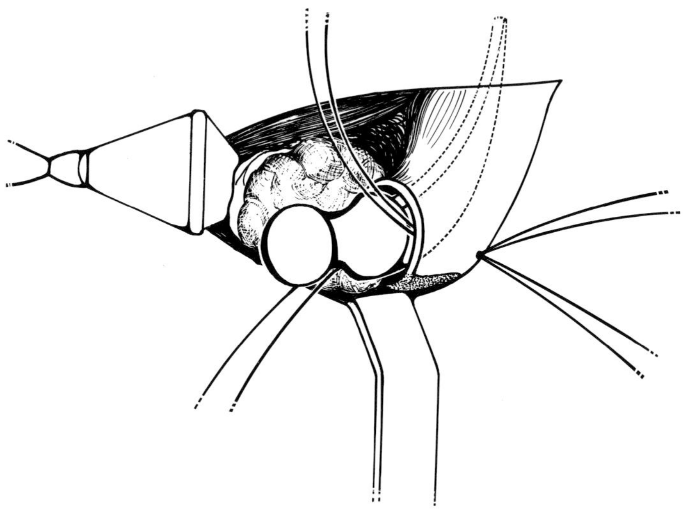

Fig. 4.23. The prosthesis in position

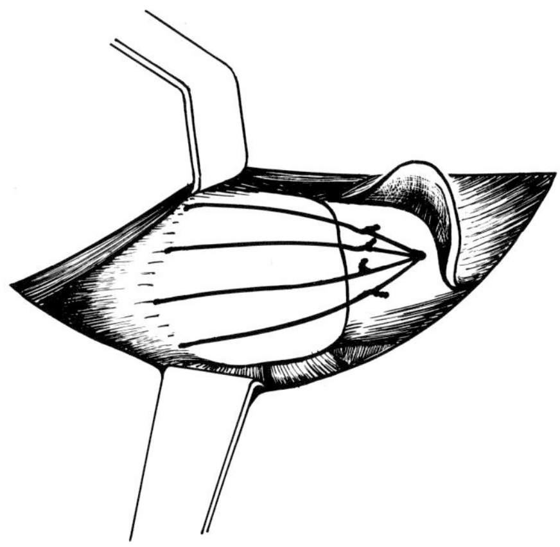

Fig. 4.24. The four wires have been passed just above the trochanter. They are tied on its lateral surface and the twisted ends are buried under the margin of the trochanter to prevent irritation of the fascia lata

and as evenly as possible. If not, there is a danger that the tightest one will break first, to be followed by the other three in succession (Fig. 4.24).

4.5.11 Closure

This is carried out over three suction drains. One is anterior and in contact with the prosthesis, the second is posterior, while the third is subcutaneous.

4.6 Postoperative Management and Follow-up

M. Postel and J. P. Lamas

The patients receive nursing care while lying in bed with no form of restraint, except in special circumstances. If the hip was very stiff prior to surgery, the limb may be suspended postoperatively to aid initial mobilization.

Foot exercises and static quadriceps contractions are begun on the first evening. This continues until the 4th day. On the 5th day the patient gets out of bed and can sit in a chair. Walking with crutches is begun on the following day.

Partial weight bearing and the use of crutches continue until the 30th day. It is not always easy to acquire a balanced gait throughout each step while carrying only 10% or 20% of the body weight on the operated leg. Bold young patients need to be slowed down, while elderly, unsteady patients need encouragement and guidance. This is the most important task of the physiotherapist following a routine total hip replacement, as the range of movement of the hip usually returns without any difficulty.

Free active flexion is restricted during this period. The stresses exerted on the greater trochanter are effectively as great during active hip flexion with the knee in extension as during walking with full weight bearing. Full weight bearing is begun only on the 30th day, after a control roentgenogram shows that consolidation of the greater trochanter has begun.

Intravenous antibiotics that were begun with the premedication are continued until the end of the 4th day. They are continued orally for a longer period if there is a persistent high pyrexia or if any of the routine peroperative bacteriology specimens are positive. After revisions, antibiotics are continued until all swabs are known to be negative, until the histology is seen to be normal, and until the erythrocyte sedimentation rate (ESR) is seen to be falling normally.

Prophylactic anticoagulation, consisting of subcutaneous heparin, is given during the first 4 days postoperatively, and also during the operation if there are high risk factors. We aim for normal coagulation during the operation, followed by slight anticoagulation postoperatively. From the 3rd or 4th postoperative day this is achieved by oral anticoagulants that are continued up to the point of full weight bearing.

In addition, elastic stockings are put on immediately postoperatively and worn until full weight bearing is achieved. Several hours after operation the patient is encouraged to move his foot as much as possible and to carry out static quadriceps and deep breathing exercises.

4.6.1 Progression of the Erythrocyte Sedimentation Rate

This has been studied in a consecutive series of 120 arthroplasties carried out by one surgeon from 1979 to 1980 and which, up to 1984, had not shown any evidence of infection. Three patients died over this period.

On average, and taking only the reading over the 1st h, a normal preoperative ESR rises to 90 toward the 10th day. It then falls to 20 after 1 month and has returned to the preoperative value by the 2nd month.

However, there are some variations. In fact, in 75% of the patients the ESR never exceeded 40 and returned to the preoperative value between the 30th and 60th day. For some patients without any obvious complications it rose much higher but returned to normal in 2 months.

In three patients who had large aseptic hematomas the ESR rose to 100 or 110 and returned to normal by 2 months. In four patients who had an infection unrelated to the hip (one case of sigmoiditis and three urinary tract infections) it rose to above 120, where it stayed for almost a month before descending rapidly to normal during the 2nd month.

Overall, the ESR seems to be of little value during the first few weeks, apart from providing a baseline. However, it should have returned to normal by 2 months postoperatively.

4.6.2 General Health of the Patient in Relation to the Postoperative Course

An in-depth review was carried out of the postoperative complications and preoperative problems in a series of 526 patients operated on in 1982 and involving 571 total arthroplasties. Twelve percent of these patients, therefore, had bilateral arthroplasties during 1 year. As well as their age, which was frequently over 70 years, they brought with them additional problems. One-third of the general population is hypertensive, the proportion reaching 60%-70% in the elderly, and this condition frequently remains untreated. In 22% of cases it is associated with cardiac pathology such as myocardial infarction, abnormalities of rhythm and conduction, and cardiac insufficiency. This requires a full preliminary examination, which is carried out during an anesthetic assessment 1 month prior to surgery. This time interval allows for a full assessment and the correction of the majority of problems. It ensures that only those patients who are ready for surgery are admitted. This simplifies administration and avoids having to tell a patient that the operation for which he has waited and psychologically prepared himself has had to be postponed. In spite of these precautions, 1% of patients had a myocardial infarction postoperatively, although without serious immediate problems.

Previous history of phlebitis (4%), pulmonary embolism (2%), and the presence of significant varicose veins (10%) require strict anticoagulant treatment. However, in our series 2% of the patients developed phlebitis and 1.5% pulmonary emboli postoperatively, with no fatalities.

Gastrointestinal problems are not uncommon and will affect the preparation for surgery in different ways. A hiatus hernia leads one to be conservative in anticoagulation. The presence of gallstones or cholecystitis may indicate preliminary surgery, but this is always a difficult problem. It would be unreasonable to remove all such doubtful gallbladders if they are asymptomatic. However, the prospect of hip arthroplasty is certainly a significant factor in deciding to operate upon a biliary tract for which there are already surgical indications. In spite of these precautions, 2% of the patients in this series suffered severe gastrointestinal problems. These were most frequently resolved by medical treatment but also occasionally resulted in emergency cholecystectomy or the removal of stones. Urinary tract infection presents a difficult problem and should be under control before the hip is operated on. It is rarely possible to cure such infection, and one must be satisfied with the prevention of bacteremia during the immediate postoperative period. It is also better to treat the prostate before the hip if there are significant prostatic symptoms and if eventual resection seems inevitable.

Thus, the morbidity associated with total hip replacement is not zero. There were no deaths in this series, possibly because the number of patients was small. The average mortality of this procedure seems to be 0.5%, although it is higher in some series. This is a figure that should be at the front of one's mind when the indications for hip replacement are being discussed.

4.6.3 Clinical and Radiological Follow-up

Regular clinical and radiological follow-up is begun once the immediate postoperative period has passed.

At 1 month a control roentgenogram is needed to confirm the solidity of the trochanter before full weight bearing can begin. The range of movement must be good and the hip painless.

At 3 or 4 months, the hip should be almost normal and the roentgenogram satisfactory. Clinical assessment should give a score of at least 6.5.5.

Progress is subsequently followed up by clinical examination, and an AP view of the pelvis, including the prosthesis, is taken at 1 year and at yearly intervals thereafter.

The range of movement will continue to improve up to the end of the 1st year. Stability will also improve over 2-3 months, or 6 months to 1 year in more difficult cases. The radiological features should not alter except for rounding off at the level of section of the neck. It is over successive examinations that signs of loosening or chronic infection may appear.

Clinical follow-up is straightforward. A good arthroplasty is completely painless, while a painful prosthesis is usually one which has problems. However, there are two provisos to this statement:

1. Some patients complain of pain in the region of the trochanter. It is not the prosthesis that is producing the pain, but the scarring of the fascia lata that rubs against the trochanter. This nearly always resolves eventually.
2. In rare cases the patient may experience aching, if not pain in the groin during active flexion. This seems most frequently to be related to the psoas rubbing against the anterior border of the cup. This pain is uncommon and improves with rest. However, it must be distinguished from inguinal pain, especially on starting to walk, which originates from the hip and is the first symptom of loosening in some cases.

Radiological follow-up is also straightforward. Nothing should alter in the appearance of the acetabulum or the femur. It is in these sequential roentgenograms that we look for the first signs of loosening or infection.

Let us recall that we have defined:

- *Definite acetabular loosening* as any alteration in the position or orientation of the cup, however small and whatever its effect on function.
- *Suspected loosening* as shown by a complete progressive lucent zone associated with functional symptoms.
- *Femoral loosening* as much more difficult to confirm on roentgenograms, which may remain unchanged for a long time.

The features of *chronic sepsis* must also be recognized. These may be:

1. *Clinical* - significant pain together with a collection of pus or a fistula
2. *Radiological* - periosteal reaction around the femur:
   - cysts between bone and cement,
   - osteolysis,
   - lucent zones.
3. *Pathology:*
   - increase in ESR,
   - positive cultures.

In addition to these features, we have classified the prostheses that we have reviewed as:

- *Definitely infected* if the bacteriology is positive and there is clinical and radiological confirmation, or if the histology following a revision leaves no doubt.
- *Probably infected* if the radiology and blood tests suggest chronic infection in spite of unconvincing histology or negative bacteriology.

5 Results with the Charnley-Kerboul Prosthesis

5.1 Introduction

M. Postel

What, then, are the functional and radiological results of this type of prosthesis, which has been the only one used at Cochin since the end of 1973, and which has been implanted using the same standardized technique throughout?

We shall now study the results obtained in several different conditions: (a) in uncomplicated osteoarthrosis, as this is the most common indication and will provide us with a baseline for further reference; (b) in other conditions which might be expected to give poorer results or which might present specific technical problems, e.g. rheumatoid arthritis, necrosis of the head, ankylosis, and congenital dislocation of the hip.

The first study concerns an uninterrupted series of 222 total arthroplasties for osteoarthrosis. This number may seem small in relation to the large number of arthroplasties carried out at Cochin over the last 15 years. Our aim was to obtain figures that approached reality as closely as possible. We therefore had to study an uninterrupted series with a follow-up that was sufficiently long to cover all the possible complications likely to appear. The study is based on the functional results and on a regular and painstaking radiological follow-up. The slightest anomaly was noted, in consideration of the possibility that each abnormal or progressive feature might later lead to more serious changes or may have repercussions on hip function. We believe that total hip arthroplasty should eventually become a "forgotten hip" as far as the patient is concerned, with a roentgenogram that remains unchanged.

The later studies are concerned with less common conditions and include all those patients since 1973 who have received this type of prosthesis for the indications described. These series deal with the specific problems arising from each individual condition in relation to technique and with the way in which the underlying disease process influences the result. We have therefore assembled the largest possible number of case files, all of which have, of course, been studied in the same detail as our baseline series.

5.2 Results in Osteoarthrosis

M. Postel, B. Coulondres, and J. P. Courpied

The series studied covers 222 total arthroplasties carried out for primary or secondary osteoarthrosis. The operations were carried out consecutively, during 1976 in the majority of cases, and the average age of the patients was 67.5 years at the time of surgery. Some hips (30) had already undergone previous extra-articular surgery, e.g., osteotomy, a shelf, or the Voss procedure.

5.2.1 Septic Complications

As the aim of this study is to assess the functional and mechanical results achieved with this prosthesis, we have excluded those that became infected. There were six definite infections (2.7%), but seven others were probably also septic, although no positive bacteriological culture was obtained. These figures are very worrying. Two explanations have been put forward: first, the fact that we work in a conventional operating room, and second, the fact that we do not routinely use prophylactic antibiotics. These factors will be studied in the chapter concerned with septic complications. We also noticed that the rate of infection was no higher in those hips undergoing a second operation than in fresh hips, an observation which contradicts currently held opinion. There are, then 209 non-infected total arthroplasties available for study.

5.2.2 Follow-up

In theory, the longest possible follow-up is 8 years, from the date of operation to the time when we began this review. Several patients were lost to follow-up, mainly during the first 2 years (29 at 3 years), and this figure now remains steady at 31. Nineteen patients died during the 8 years.

5.2.3 Functional Results

We studied the patients at 5 years postoperatively, because at this time there were still a sufficient number of usable case files, and because we found that the large majority of problems associated with the Charnley prosthesis had become apparent by this time. One hundred and twenty-nine cases were still available after 5 years. Pain was never scored below 5, and 92% of hips were rated at 6%; movement was 6 in 88% of hips; stability was never less than 4, and was 6 in 94% of cases.

In sum, 86% of hips were painless and stable (P6, S6), 80% scored a total P+M+S=18, and 16.5% had a PMS score or 16 of 17, so 96.5% of hips had a PMS score of 16, 17, or 18. It is of interest that the same figures are to be found if we review the files at the time of maximum follow-up instead of after 5 years.

These results are better still if we consider only patients with primary osteoarthritis who had not undergone previous surgery. Among these, 86% had a PMS score of 18 and 12% scored 16 or 17. Overall, 98% had a PMS score of 16, 17, or 18, and this represents very good results.

All these figures are in fact very close to those found with the Charnley prosthesis, if we exclude those with problems involving the femoral component. It is the radiological study that will show us where the difference lies.

5.2.4 Radiological Study

A follow-up of 5 years is certainly short. It does not allow us to consider wear of the components. On the other hand, our study of the Charnley prosthesis showed that the majority of radiological problems became apparent during the first 2 years. They can therefore be critically assessed at 5 years.

The progession of *acetabular fixation* did not reveal any significant features. We found 14 partially lucent areas (11%) that were always situated laterally. They were completely static with no sign of progression and had been present from the first postoperative roentgenogram (Figs. 5.1 and 5.2). There were two extensive lucent areas that did not seem to be progressive (1.5%) and did not represent loosening, but one wonders how

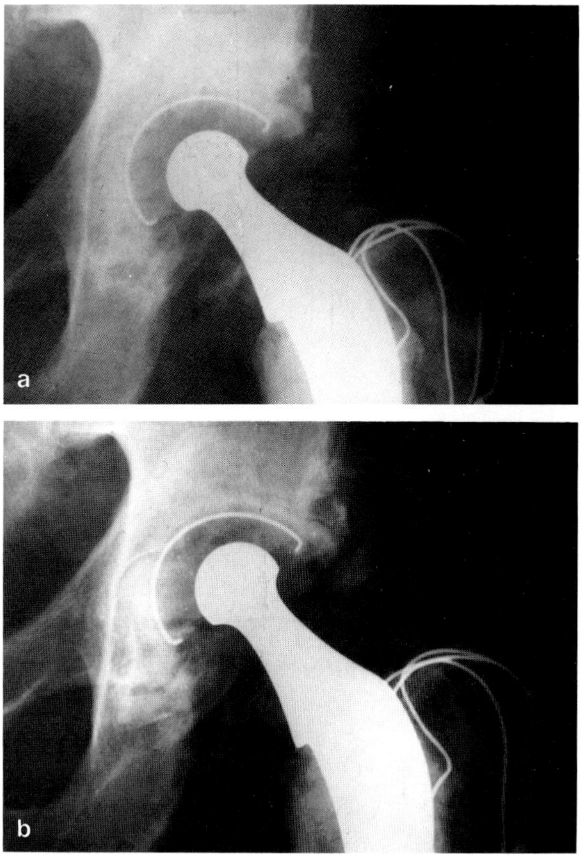

Fig. 5.1. a Partially lucent zone around the cup present several months after operation. **b** Unchanged 4 years later

they will develop in the long term. One lucent zone provoked concern and perhaps represents loosening that is still asymptomatic after 5 years.

Regarding *femoral fixation,* we noted five dorsal lucent zones between the cement and the prosthesis. This is only 2.4% and represents a very significant decrease compared with the incidence of 25% with the Charnley prosthesis. In addition, they were all very narrow, only 0.5-1 mm at maximum width, and were never extensive. None were associated with the slightest functional problem and none had increased in size by the end of the follow-up period.

There were six fractures at the distal end of the sheath of cement (2.9%). These also had a completely different appearance and the fracture line was very thin, always less than 1 mm. They were not seen on all views, and even a slight change in angle made them disappear. None have progressed. Those seen with the Charnley prosthesis were transverse and wide and gave the impression that the prosthesis had subsided 1 or 2 mm into the femur. Our findings seem to repre-

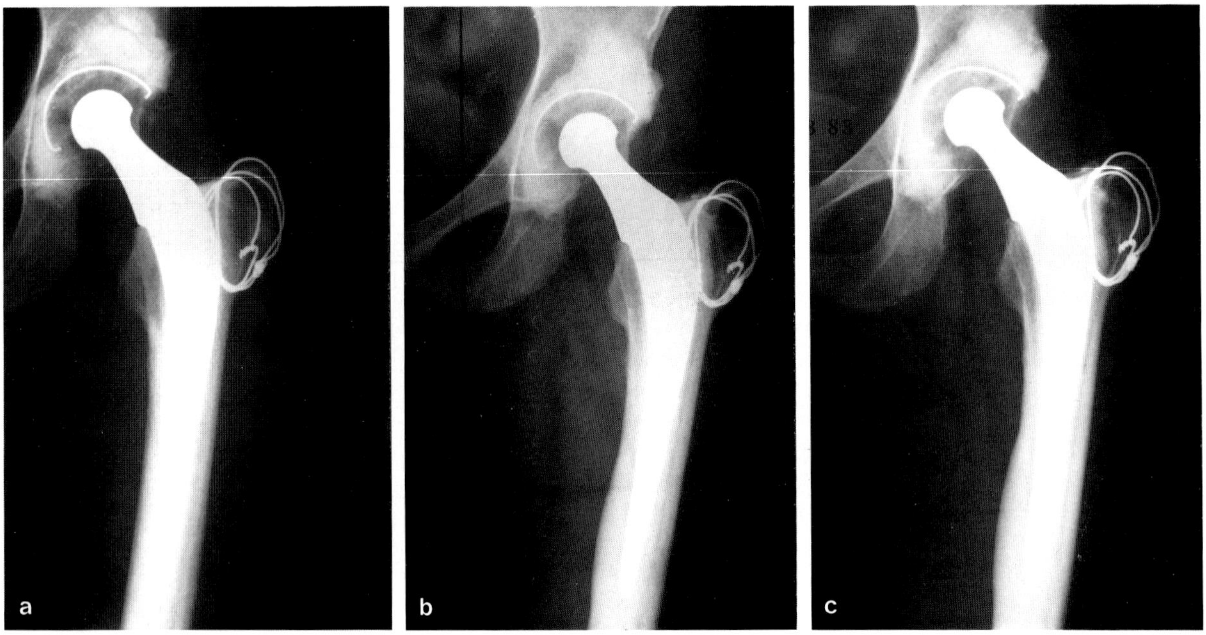

Fig. 5.2 a–c. Partially lucent zone around the cup (**a**). Unchanged (or disappeared) 6 years later (**b, c**). Note the cortical thickening medially

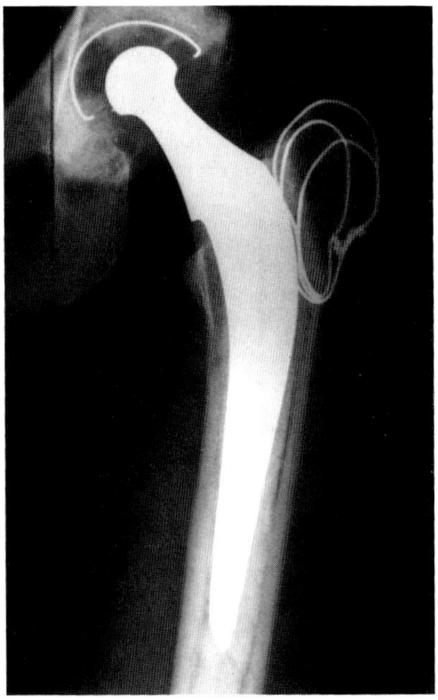

Fig. 5.3. Small oblique fissure within the cement sheath, beginning at apex of femoral stem

sent only an adjustment of stresses imparted to the distal end of the cement by the metal stem, and no true movement (Fig. 5.3).

There were two lucent areas between bone and cement. One of these was very extensive and seems to represent the only likely loosening in this series. The patient's death, however, prevented us from following its progression.

At the end of the study several features were noticed that suggested partial resorption of bone between the cortex and the cement. However, they were not taken to be significant. In fact, they were not found consistently in the same patient in sequential roentgenograms and were related to the degree of penetration of the X-ray. On closer inspection they did not represent a gap, but were filled with cancellous bone (Fig. 5.4).

Areas of cortical thickening were frequent but seemed to represent only a radiological finding with no functional significance (see Fig. 5.2). They appeared progressively, often after 2 or 3 years. They began with a feathery appearance, which to the untrained eye may suggest sepsis. They progressed slowly over 2 or 3 years and finally became static. They were noticed medially in 40 cases, laterally in eight, and bilaterally in 16. They were always very low on the diaphysis, at the level of the tip of the stem.

They did not seem to be related to the alignment of the

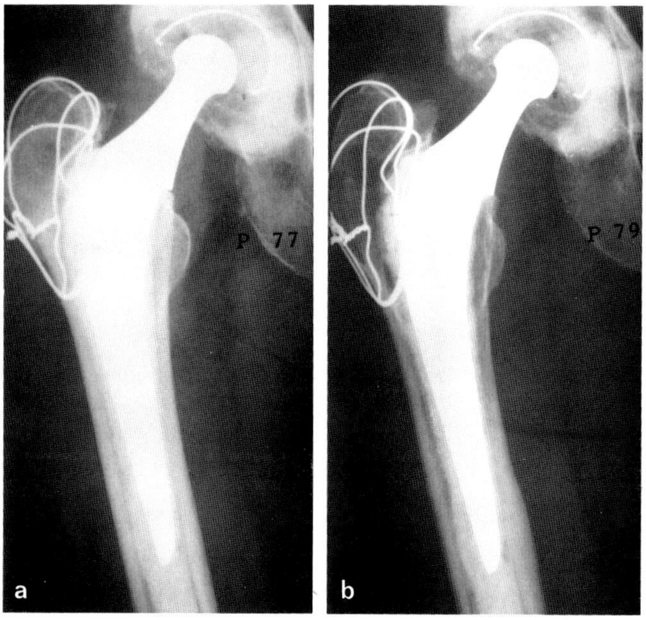

Fig. 5.4 a, b. The appearance of changes at the cement-stem interface is in reality a radiological artifact

prosthesis within the femur. Perhaps these reactions occur predominantly at the surface which happens to be in contact with the extremity of the stem. In fact, the stems were almost all completely centered. This seems to represent simply a mechanical response that is not significant and has no repercussions on function.

Thus, these are the figures that represent the results found in cases of primary osteoarthrosis, excluding sepsis: 86% perfect results, 98% excellent or perfect results. This provides a basis for comparison with other conditions that follow. It defines the remarkable quality of results which can be achieved with this type of prosthesis, which we believe should not be abandoned until one that is better has been found.

5.3 Necrosis of the Femoral Head

M. Mathieu and M. Postel

The outcome of total hip replacement as a treatment for femoral head necrosis has been studied in 77 patients. These hips with femoral necrosis of nontraumatic origin had not yet reached the stage of severe joint destruction at which they would have been classified among our cases of osteoarthrosis. One-third of the cases were related to steroid therapy and many to alcoholism. Fifty-five percent of patients were aged less than 50 years, and the predominant symptom was pain. Five hips had already undergone surgery, (two were cup arthroplasties and three had been drilled).

The rationale for performing total arthroplasty in cases of necrosis which had not yet progressed to arthrosis warrants further discussion, as there is a place for other procedures at this stage. We abandoned varus osteotomy because of the high incidence of subsequent degenerative change. However, the Sugioka rotation osteotomy is a possibility that we consider when there is a localized lesion that does not involve collapse of the head.

There are still good indications for interposition cup arthroplasty, even though the head may be considerably deformed by widespread necrosis. However, the number of very good results falls rapidly when there is any damage to the acetabulum, even if it involves only the articular cartilage. We believe that an interposition cup is still indicated in a young patient with a unilateral lesion, in spite of the lesser likelihood of obtaining a good result. In cases where the lesion is bilateral or the life expectancy short, or where heavy demands will be made on the hip, we move away from the interposition cup toward total arthroplasty (Fig. 5.5).

Operatively, this condition does not present any particular problems. The synovium is often inflamed and may be slightly hemorrhagic when it is excised. The acetabulum remains intact, and after the remaining articular cartilage is removed the quality of bone is generally good.

The postoperative course of these 77 arthroplasties

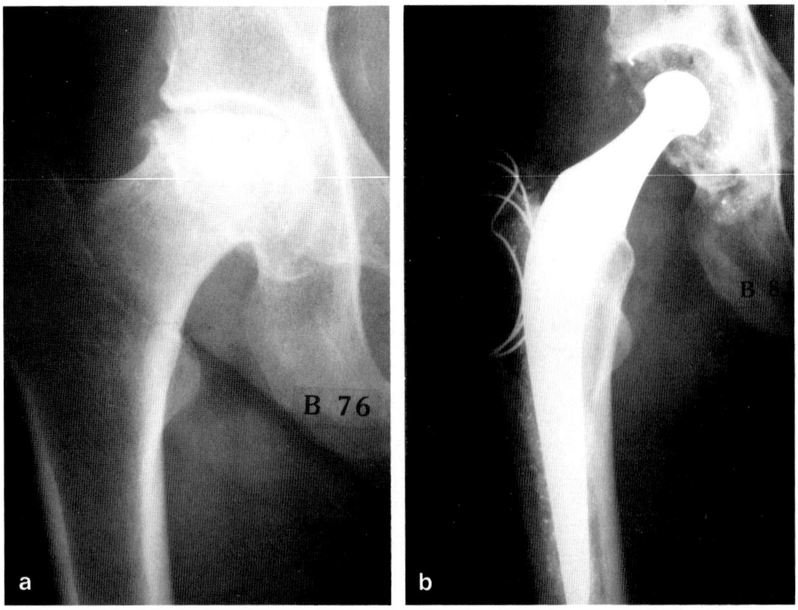

Fig. 5.5 a, b. Femoral necrosis in a 60-year-old man that has already led to collapse of the head and early degenerative changes in the acetabulum (**a**). Interposition cup arthroplasty has little chance of being effective (**b**)

was uneventful. The only complication was one unexplained popliteal nerve palsy that soon resolved spontaneously.

The functional results of these mechanically satisfactory hips, which have been implanted predominantly in young patients, are very good, as we expected. Ninety-five percent of hips scored over 16 at the end of 1 year, and 93% were rated at 18 after 3 years. The radiological results are excellent. No definite or suspected cup loosenings have been found during follow-up. We have seen three partially lucent zones and a fourth that is slightly more extensive, but this has not progressed and there is no functional disability. There are four femoral lucent zones that are not progressive.

For a long time it has been suggested that sepsis is more common in this condition. A thorough review at Cochin in 1979 of prostheses implanted between 1967 and 1974 produced figures showing a very large number of infections (13.5%). This figure was confirmed at a symposium in Bruges by J.O. Ramadier and J. Delcoulx. This led us to be very wary of total arthroplasty in femoral head necrosis.

However, our series, which is more recent and has an adequate follow-up, in no way confirms these results. There have been only two infections in 77 patients (2.6%), a number which falls within the accepted range during the period under consideration.

How can these different findings be explained? The first series is taken from 1967-1974 when the overall rate of infection was greater than subsequently (1974-1984). This reduction in infection is probably the result of stricter operating room discipline, the more frequent use of routine antibiotic prophylaxis, and, more recently, the addition of antibiotics to the cement.

In summary, total arthroplasty in femoral head necrosis has not presented any specific technical problems, and the results obtained fall within the spectrum of the wider series. It seems completely justified as a method of treatment when other procedures seem likely to give a poor result.

5.4 Total Hip Replacement in Ankylosing Spondylitis

D. Lance and B. Augereau

The hip is affected in one of three patients who suffer from ankylosing spondylitis. Often presenting during the first 5 years of the disease, the coxitis rapidly becomes incapacitating. It causes severe pain and limitation of movement that may progress to ankylosis.

Although interposition cup arthroplasty has given reasonable results, it is clear that the best results come from total hip arthroplasty. Of course, the patients are often very young, and total hip replacement cannot be carried out without a degree of apprehension. However, these young patients are frequently so badly afflicted that it seems reasonable to take long-term risks to enable them to regain an active life.

Seventy such patients have been operated upon in our

department from 1967 to 1980. Twenty-six of these have been given a Charnley-Kerboul prosthesis, and it is this smaller group that we shall now review.

5.4.1 The Patients

Between 1973 and 1980, 26 of these prostheses have been implanted into 21 patients whose average age is 43 years, with a range of 26–72 years.
All the patients fulfilled the diagnostic criteria for ankylosing spondylitis as defined by the Council for the International Organization of Medical Science. Sixteen patients had associated involvement of the dorsolumbar spine, and the knees were affected in three patients, one of whom had a Guépar arthroplasty.
One-third of the hips were ankylosed and the majority were fixed in an unsatisfactory position (flexion, abduction, and external rotation). The remainder retained a limited but painful range of movement and were often held in fixed flexion. Functional disability was severe in 21 patients; five of them used crutches with difficulty, while two were bedridden.

5.4.2 The Operation

This is always carried out using the lateral approach, with the patient under general anesthesia and in the lateral decubitus position. Difficulty with intubation is frequently encountered but it is usually overcome with the help of a fiberscope. Intubation was impossible in only one patient.
The mm. glutei were generally in a satisfactory condition, but there was a great difference between the muscles of patients who had continued to walk in spite of their pain and those of permanently bedridden patients, which were much less supple.
The subchondral bone is often porotic, but its consistency did not pose any serious problem in these cases.
In three patients a fixed flexion deformity remained at the end of the procedure, and the surgeon felt it necessary to tenotomize the mm. psoas and rectus femoris. Subsequent experience has shown that such fixed flexion corrects itself spontaneously during the postoperative period, and we no longer feel that tenotomy is necessary.

5.4.3 Complications

We regret that one death occurred on the 3rd postoperative day, from a massive pulmonary embolus without any obvious direct relation to the underlying condition.
There were three infections, giving a figure of 11.5%, though this is without statistical significance in this small series. However, of the 70 arthroplasties performed for ankylosing spondylitis in our department (grouping all the different prostheses together) there have been four infections (5.7%) which is a higher figure than that occurring in arthroplasty for other conditions. The risk of infection is probably not the same among all patients with ankylosing spondylitis. It is certainly higher in bedridden patients, whose skin is difficult to prepare preoperatively.
There is an increased incidence of periarticular ossification. Charnley [1] found that it was higher in ankylosing spondylitis than in rheumatoid arthritis and lowest in primary osteoarthrosis. Williams et al. [2] also report a 13% incidence of ossification in their series, where ankylosing spondylitis was treated by total arthroplasty as a primary procedure. On the basis of Brooker's classification, five fell into group I and one into group III. These numbers are small. On the other hand, ossification is frequent among our long-standing arthroplasties carried out for ankylosing spondylosis but using other types of prosthesis. One should look here more at the operative technique than at the type of prosthesis.
We could find no correlation between the onset of ossification and the stage of the disease, the range of movement of the hip before surgery, or the sedimentation rate at the time of operation.
The bad reputation of total arthroplasty in ankylosing spondylitis in relation to periarticular ossification therefore seems to be completely unjustified. Poor results are very rarely due to massive ossification.

5.4.4 Results

We shall now assess the results of the 21 arthroplasties, having excluded one death and three infections. The initial results are satisfactory, being excellent or good for 17 hips and passable or mediocre for four.
After 1 year, the beneficial effect of arthroplasty on pain relief was spectacular and all the hips were pain free (scoring 5 or 6). The effect on range of movement was less marked, in that one in five hips had flexion of less than 75°. Nevertheless, this represents a great improvement among a group of patients who frequently

suffered from a painful spine and two hips that were very stiff. Stability had been regained by this time.
These results are maintained in the long term. There has been no femoral or acetabular loosening in this series. The only radiological sign was early wear (after 2 years) of one polyethylene cup, and this was asymptomatic. Eight of the 21 arthroplasties were followed up for 10 years and all were assessed as good or very good (PMS > 15).
In conclusion, total arthroplasty can be of great benefit to patients with ankylosing spondylitis whose hips have become severely stiff. Troublesome secondary ossification is in fact uncommon, and even though the range of movement may occasionally be slightly limited, the increase in function remains significant.

References

1. Charnley J (1979) Low-friction arthroplasty of the hip. Springer, Berlin Heidelberg New York, pp 322-355
2. Williams E, Taylor AR, Arden GP, Edwards DH (1977) Arthroplasty of the hip in ankylosing spondylitis. J Bone Joint Surg [Br] 59/4: 393-397

5.5 Total Hip Replacement in Rheumatoid Arthritis

M. Kerboul, B. Coulondres, and M. Mathieu

Total hip replacement in rheumatoid arthritis introduces specific problems which deserve special emphasis. The majority of these arise from the disease itself, which is very variable and produces a wide-ranging clincial picture, from the involvement of one hip to all the joints of the body. Its progression can be extremely slow, even apparently burnt out, when its involvement of the hip is scarcely different from osteoarthrosis. On the other hand, there may be recurrent inflammatory exacerbation that can be only partially controlled by regular medication. The condition can be divided into adult and juvenile rheumatoid arthritis. They do not necessarily present a different clinical picture, but whereas the postoperative progress of hip arthroplasty is usually uncomplicated in the adult, it may take an unexpected turn in juvenile arthritis. We shall therefore consider the two conditions separately.

5.5.1 Adult Rheumatoid Arthritis

The problems raised by total hip arthroplasty in adult rheumatoid arthritis are due more to the extent of the disease than to the specific pathology found in the hip. A recent study enables us to appreciate the specific problems presented by hip arthroplasty in this condition.

The Patients

This study includes 39 patients with an average age of 50 years, ranging from 30 to 80 years. They received 48 total hip replacements between 1974 and 1980, using a modified Charnley prosthesis.

The Disease

There was considerable variation in severity from one patient to another, but the condition was more often advanced and diffuse than restricted to just a few joints. As well as frequently involving both hips, the disease often affected the knees, feet, and hands, and less commonly the shoulders, elbows, and cervical spine.
Among these 39 patients, two had been bedridden for some time prior to surgery. The majority (31) had received or were still receiving steroid therapy. Only two patients had undergone previous hip surgery (interposition cup).
Other joints, such as the knees, feet, hands, and occasionally the cervical spine had already been operated, or surgery was planned to follow the hip arthroplasty. Ten patients had already had one of their hips replaced by a total arthroplasty of a design different from that being studied here.

Indications for Surgery

Many of these patients therefore required several arthroplasties, and one of the most difficult problems is to know on which joint to operate first, when faced with a patient with multiple joint involvement who will obviously require many surgical procedures.
As a general rule, and after a thorough assessment of the patient and his disease in close collaboration with the rheumatologist, one embarks on a program involving a succession of procedures that usually begins with the lower limbs, as these are most frequently the worst affected. Occasionally, it is initially necessary to stabilize the atlanto-occipital joint should this be destroyed and when there are signs of medullary involvement.
With a bedridden patient in whom both knees and hips are destroyed, often in fixed flexion, the first aim is to get him or her standing on at least one limb. To achieve this, a hip and a knee prosthesis will be required in either one or two stages. Fixed equinus of the hindfoot may occasionally require correction by

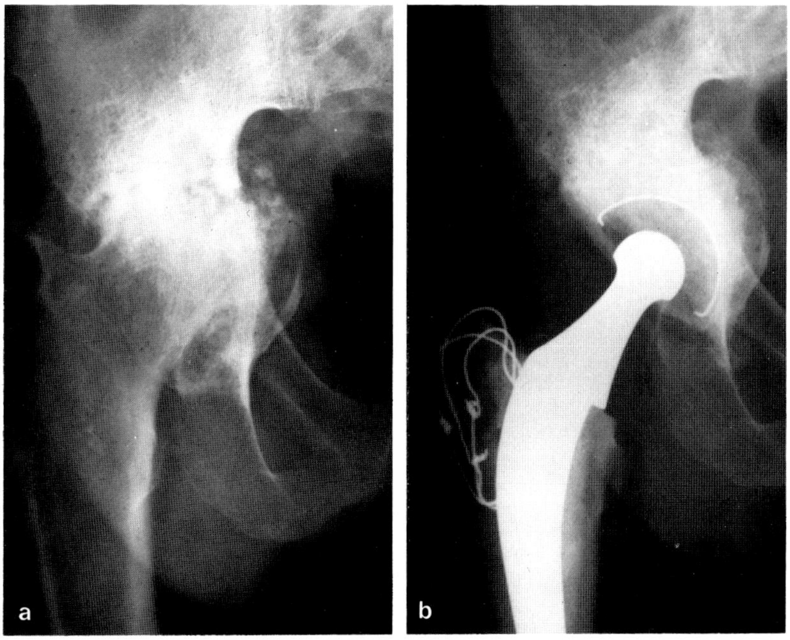

Fig. 5.6. **a** Protrusio with marked bony destruction of the acetabulum. **b** Bone graft and a cup with a large collar

arthrodesis. If the upper limbs are satisfactory, one may then hope to see the patient take a few steps on crutches. If not, the same procedures will be needed on the other side before walking can finally be achieved.

This is an arduous program that may be interrupted at any time by an intercurrent medical or surgical problem, and whose success can be threatened by the failure of any one procedure. Thus, every effort must be made to ensure that each operation proceeds in the best and most straightforward way. This long series of operations requires a very courageous patient with great determination that must not waver, even though the teams of surgeons and nurses may change.

When the joint involvement is less extensive, the surgical program may be limited to two hips, or to one knee and one hip. The likelihood of a good outcome thus increases, and the organization of the surgery requires less imagination. Two long-standing rules remain valuable:

1. When both a hip and a knee are involved, it is often advisable to begin with the hip, although this is not always absolutely essential.
2. Safety and care remain the best guarantees for eventual success, and the situation must non be compromised by undue haste.

Results

Careful study of total hip replacement in rheumatoid arthritis shows that it is an excellent operation in this condition, as in others. Of the 48 arthroplasties performed using the modified Charnley prosthesis, 17 involved considerably damaged hips, and there was protrusio acetabulae in 15 patients, while the anatomy was relatively well preserved in the remaining 16.

The procedure itself rarely presented special problems. There were occasional delays because of difficulty in intubation, even using a fiberscope, and it was occasionally necessary to use a bone graft or a cup with a large collar if the acetabulum had been completely destroyed. The postoperative course was usually remarkably straightforward (Fig. 5.6).

The complications in the series included one case of phlebitis, two early failures of wires holding the trochanter, and two short-lived dislocations. One case of infection proved to be a complete failure.

Analysis of the results is difficult for two reasons. First, when a long operative program is necessary, it is impossible to assess the hip arthroplasty objectively while the patient is unable to walk. Second, rheumatoid arthritis is essentially a medical condition. The patients are highly dependent on the rheumatologist, who will arrange for the hip to be operated upon by one surgeon, the knee by a second, the foot by a third, and occasionally the hand by a fourth. Surgical follow-up is therefore difficult, as the patient is under-

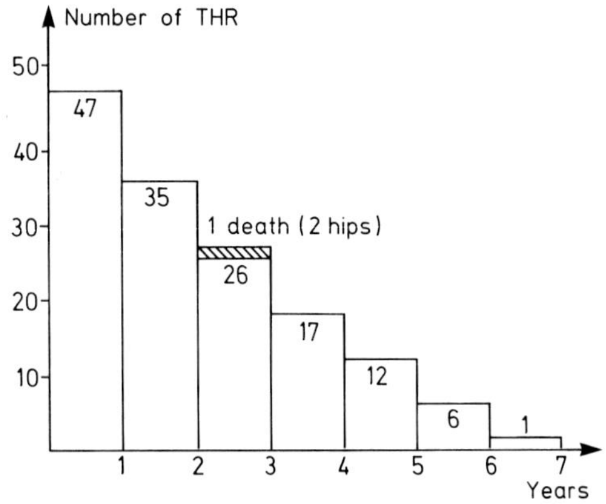

Fig. 5.7. Postoperative follow-up

standably reluctant to make the rounds of three or four surgeons. Working from the surgical files becomes fragmented and virtually impossible. This explains why our period of postoperative follow-up in no way reflects the time that had elapsed since surgery, which was a minimum of 3 years (Fig. 5.7).

By this stage, half of the patients operated upon had already been lost to follow-up and one patient had died. Be that as it may, we can say that:

1. Clinically, having excluded the one case of sepsis, which was a failure, all patients were doing very well at 1 year, and at 3 years, 26 of the 48 patients reviewed were very good. This held true at 5 years (Table. 5.1).
2. Radiological changes were uncommon postoperatively, and without any obvious clinical significance. These consisted of minor ossification in two cases, one partially lucent area around the cup, one lucent zone between the cement and the prosthesis, and three thickenings of the femoral cortex.

There was no wear of the cup and no aseptic loosening, which dispelled the frequently expressed fears over the security of the fixation of the components in bone of such poor quality.

5.5.2 *Juvenile Rheumatoid Arthritis*

By definition, this disease begins before 16 years of age and often in infancy. No matter how the condition may have begun, joint involvement is widespread and the patients are often severely disabled by the time they come to us.

Here, as in adult rheumatoid arthritis, it is difficult to compile a complete set of records. Only 25 of 38 were really usable in our series. Each patient had undergone an average of three operations, the majority of which involved the hip (43) and included 32 total arthroplasties, 28 using the Charnley prosthesis, original or modified.

Table 5.1. Postoperative assessment of hip function

	No. of hips at (years)			
P+M+S	1	3	5	7
15	1			
16 or 17	6	2		
18	40	24	12	1

The problems encountered are similar to those with adults; they are related to indications for surgery and anesthesia because of the extent and severity of the lesions. But, as the patients are young and generally in good health, there is less risk involved in carrying out two or even three surgical procedures during one operation.

Cortisone dwarfs present a separate problem because of their slender skeletons that require especially small components.

Results

These can be assessed objectively only when the surgical program has been completed, that is to say after two, three, or four arthroplasties and several additional operations on the feet. The greater the number of surgical procedures, the greater the risk of failure.

Of the 19 total hip arthroplasties with follow-up of more than 4 years, 17 have excellent results clinically and two could not be used.

Study of the postoperative roentgenograms produced some unexpected results. There was no true loosening and usually very little alteration of femoral fixation, even though osteolysis of the calcar, which was rare elsewhere, was seen here. In particular, a lucent zone around the cup was common, and early wear of the cup was not unusual.

The roentgenograms in the majority of patients were very satisfactory and after 4–6 years were still almost identical to the immediate postoperative films. However, at least three patients will need further surgery sooner or later. One patient with bilateral arthroplasty showed significant wear of the cup (2 mm) at 6 years postoperatively (she weighs only 28 kg; Fig. 5.8).

The second patient has bilateral lucent zones around the cups with wear of 1 mm at 4 years postoperatively (Fig. 5.9).

The third has a lucent zone around the cup with wear

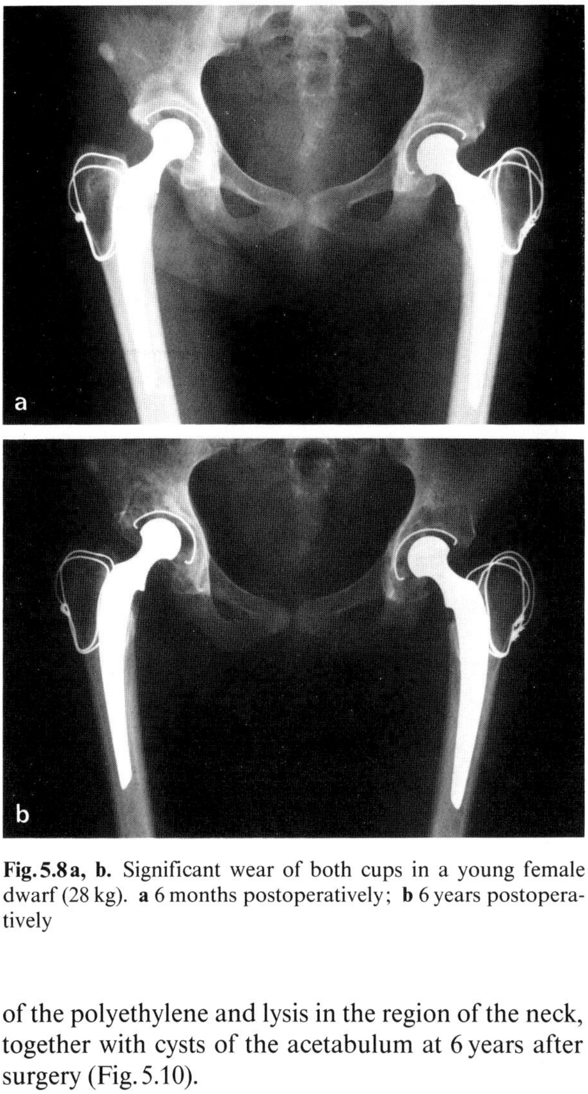

Fig. 5.8 a, b. Significant wear of both cups in a young female dwarf (28 kg). **a** 6 months postoperatively; **b** 6 years postoperatively

of the polyethylene and lysis in the region of the neck, together with cysts of the acetabulum at 6 years after surgery (Fig. 5.10).

In spite of these disturbing radiological features, these patients have normal hip function at present, although it is highly likely that they will deteriorate and require further surgery. Another patient has already reached this stage: A young woman with an ectopic bladder and aplasia of the pubis suffered from juvenile arthritis that had destroyed one hip by the time she was 20 and the second by the time she was 24. Total hip replacement (the right in 1970 and the left in 1974) enabled her to lead a normal life. However, 14 years after her first arthroplasty there is a lucent area surrounding the cup on the right, together with a fatigue fracture of the acetabulum and severe wear of the cup. There is a similar lucent area on the left but with no obvious wear of the cup. Although her function remains good, we have decided to revise the right hip before bony damage makes repair of the acetabulum too hazardous (Fig. 5.11).

Discussion

What is the cause of these lucent zones that are not seen in other conditions, not even in adult rheumatoid arthritis? The lysis is not the result of rheumatoid pannus or low-level sepsis. Perhaps it is a mechanical problem arising from a difference between the young, elastic bone and the rigid mass formed by the cement and the cup.

Why do these cups become worn so quickly? Is it because they are often small (37–40 mm in diameter) and relatively thin, making them susceptible to early wear? Cups of the same size are often used in congenital dislocation in relatively young women who are more active and altogether heavier than the dwarfs, and these do not become worn prematurely. On the other hand, cups which are of normal size also show early wear in juvenile rheumatoid arthritis. This is not caused by the prosthesis itself, as these features occur only in this specific condition. The fact that other types of prostheses suffer even more damage does not reassure us or begin to provide an explanation.

5.6 Total Hip Replacement in Ankylosis

B. Loty and J. P. Courpied

In this chapter we will consider replacement of hips which have fused either following arthrodesis or spontaneously, excluding the condition of ankylosing spondylitis. Sixty total arthroplasties were carried out on such hips at Cochin Hospital between 1967 and 1983. Here we shall study arthroplasties using the Charnley-Kerboul prosthesis, introduced in 1973, and will consider only patients operated on prior to 1980 in order to allow for sufficient follow-up.

This series of patients operated upon between 1973 and 1980 consists of 23 total arthroplasties, two of which were bilateral.

5.6.1 Patients

The etiology of the ankylosis was septic arthritis in 16 cases, with equal numbers of tuberculous and nontuberculous infection. Five cases resulted from osteoarthrosis in dysplastic hips. The other two cases involved arthrodesis for primary osteoarthrosis and ankylosis following spondyloepiphyseal dysplasia. In 12 patients, the ankylosis occurred during childhood. The number of spontaneous ankyloses (11) and that of arthrodesis (12) are comparable. All arthrodeses except one were intra-articular.

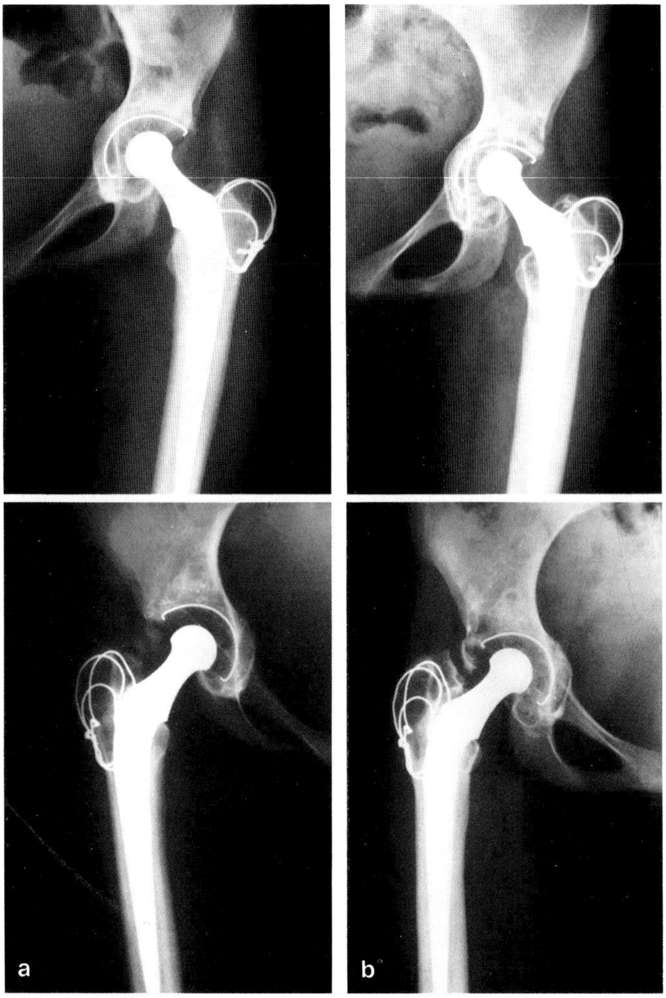

◁ **Fig. 5.9 a, b.** Wear and lucent area around the cup already present at 4 years postoperatively. **a** After 2 months; **b** after 4 years

Fig. 5.10. a. Rheumatoid arthritis of the left hip in a young girl. **b** This was treated by total arthroplasty in 1978. **c** Five years later, there was a lucent area around the cup with cysts of the acetabulum and femur. The cup is clearly worn

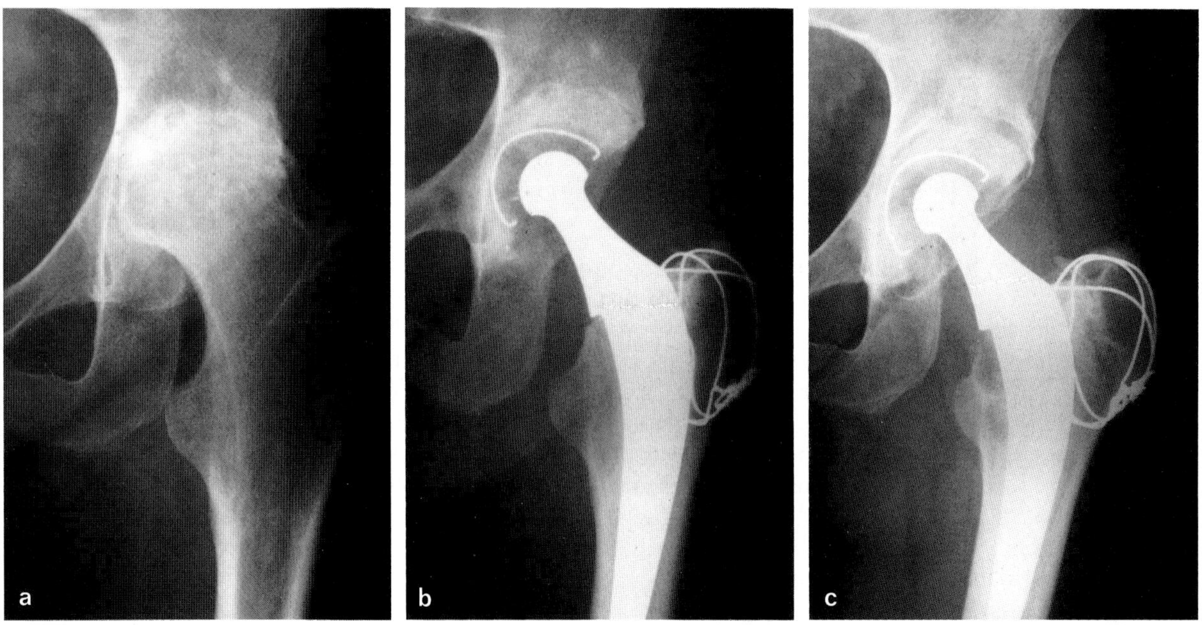

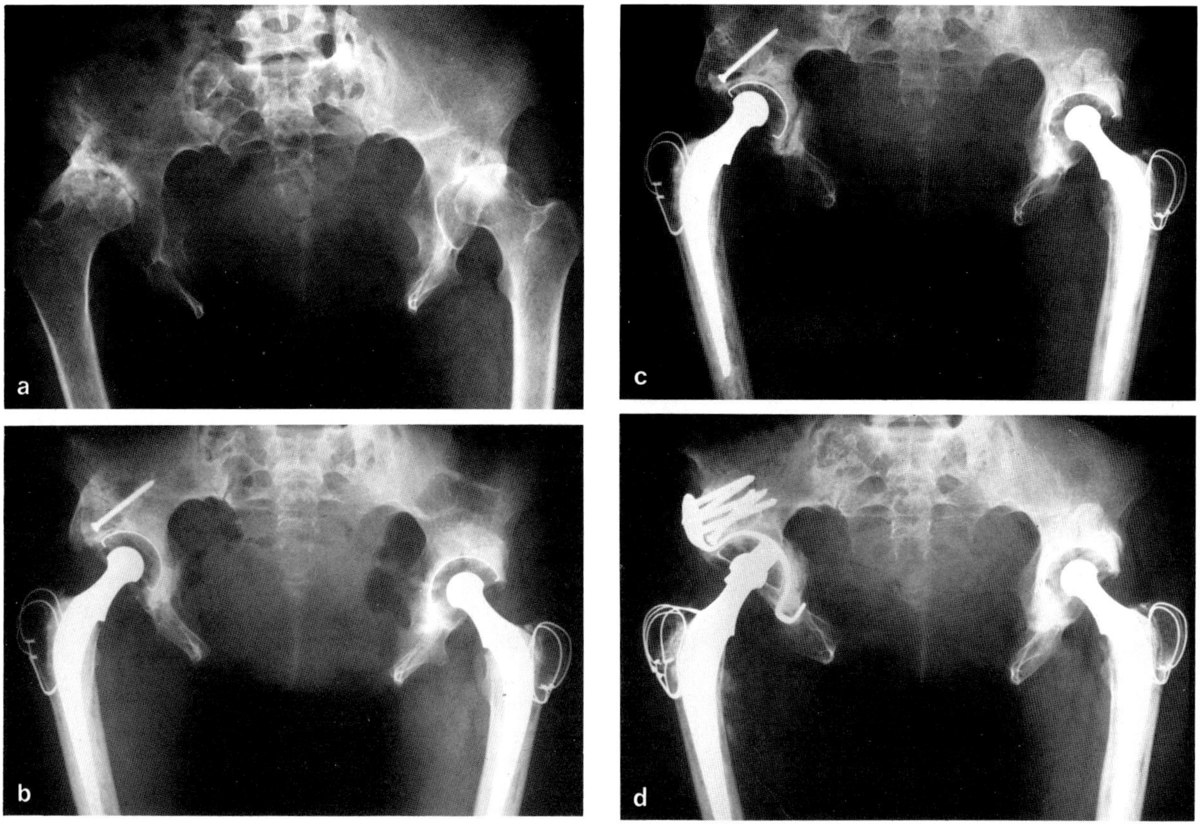

Fig. 5.11. **a** Severe juvenile arthritis in a young girl presenting with an ectopic bladder and aplasia of the pubis. **b** Bilateral total arthroplasty was carried out, on the right in 1970 and on the left in 1974. **c** Fourteen years after the first operation and 10 years after the second, there are lucent areas around both cups with a fissure across the right acetabulum and wear of the polyethylene cup. **d** Revision was carried out on the right to reconstruct the acetabulum and change the prosthesis

The position of the ankylosis was considered to be good when fixed flexion did not exceed 20°, when adduction was between 0 and 10°, and when external rotation was between 0 and 20°. Based on this criterion, 21 were ankylosed in unsatisfactory postures, fixed flexion and abduction being the most common problems. Two ankyloses were in good positions but were unfortunately bilateral.

The average duration of the ankylosis was 29 years at the time of the arthroplasty, and in half of the cases it was more than 30 years. The average age of the patients was 56 years, and half of them were over 60 years old.

5.6.2 Indications

The indication for hip arthroplasty was degeneration in an adjacent joint in 17 of the 21 patients. In this group of patients, 16 complained of back pain, with or without sciatica, while 7 suffered from knee pain, which in one case was bilateral; therefore, eight knees were involved.

Further analysis of the patients with spinal symptoms showed that they all had ankylosis of the hip in an unsatisfactory position, which nearly always consisted in fixed flexion (13 of 16).

Among the patients with knee pain, the knee involved was on the *same side* as the ankylosed hip in five cases. In two cases the hip was in abduction, producing stress on the lateral compartment of the knee, and the knees were in slight valgus (less than 10°). In three cases, the hip was in adduction causing stress on the medial compartment of the knee, one of these knees being in slight varus (2°). Two other patients complained of pain in the knee *contralateral* to the ankylosed hip; their hips were in marked fixed flexion and there was significant genu valgum (15°–20°). Finally, one patient with knee pain had degenerative changes and malalignment of the knee with marked valgus, although both hips were ankylosed in a good position.

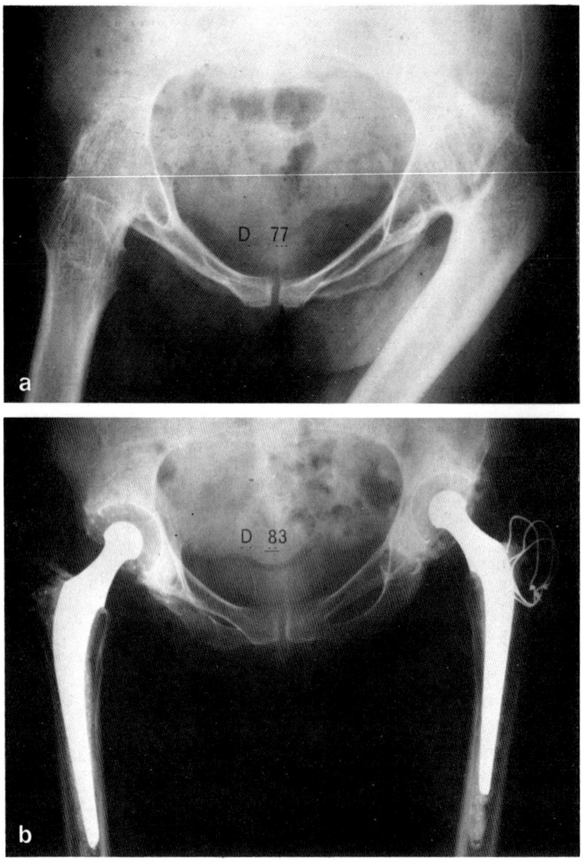

Fig. 5.12. **a** Bilateral ankylosis following streptococcal arthritis. **b** Bilateral hip replacements

Four patients were operated upon for other reasons. Three had considerable functional impairment with difficulty in walking as a result of limited abduction; the hip was ankylosed in a poor position and there was also involvement of the contralateral hip. One patient had nonunion of the femoral neck below an ankylosed hip.

Thus, our indications for mobilizing an ankylosed hip arose predominantly from symptoms in adjacent joints such as the knee and the spine. It is very rare that the function of the ankylosed hip itself justifies its mobilization. Up to now we have almost always resisted the request of patients who were otherwise well but wanted to be rid of the inconvenience of an ankylosed hip.

5.6.3 *Technique*

Although ankylosis requires certain modifications of technique, we try to follow our routine procedure as closely as possible. Positioning of the patient is made difficult by the ankylosis, the more so if it is in adduction. It is also difficult to disinfect and adequately shut off the perineum. Deformity of the hip can lead to an abnormal position of the pelvis on the table, which must be avoided if at all possible but should be taken into account while cementing the cup. The condition of the mm. glutei is poor in one case in two. They are always fragile and must be treated with the greatest care. It is not always easy to identify the crest of the m. vastus lateralis or the medial surface of the trochanter when looking for the best place to divide the ankylosis.

Very careful preliminary dissection is necessary to free the anterior and posterior margins of the m. gluteus medius. Once the trochanter has been elevated, the mass of the bony ankylosis must be carefully dissected out and all fibrous tissue surrounding it must be removed. This is done with a knife and not a rasp in order to reduce the risk of leaving behind fragments of bone that could lead to ossification. The ankylosis is most frequently divided on the old joint line, using the same set of gouges as that employed in the routine preparation of the acetabulum. The cavity that will receive the cup can be prepared at the same time and the position of the rim of the old acetabulum is identified (Fig. 5.12).

When the ankylosis is situated higher than normal, or when no landmarks can be identified, it is divided flush with the iliac bone and the new acetabulum is hollowed out with a gouge. Any extra-articular bony bridges related to the arthrodesis are resected, after they have been carefully separated from surrounding muscle. A shelf was constructed over the acetabulum in six cases where the iliac crest was atrophic or preparation with the gouge was inadequate (Fig. 5.13). Five atrophic femora had to be reamed in ankyloses that had been present since childhood.

Additional treatment comprised routine antibiotic therapy, as in total hip replacement, and pre- and postoperative antituberculosis treatment if tuberculosis was known to have been the etiology of the ankylosis. Suspended traction was set up in 12 cases for 12 days to aid initial mobilization.

5.6.4 *Results*

The length of follow-up ranged from 2 to 7 years, and more than half of the patients were followed up for more than 5 years.

We have had no postoperative sepsis, loosening, dislocation, or neurological complications. Major ossifica-

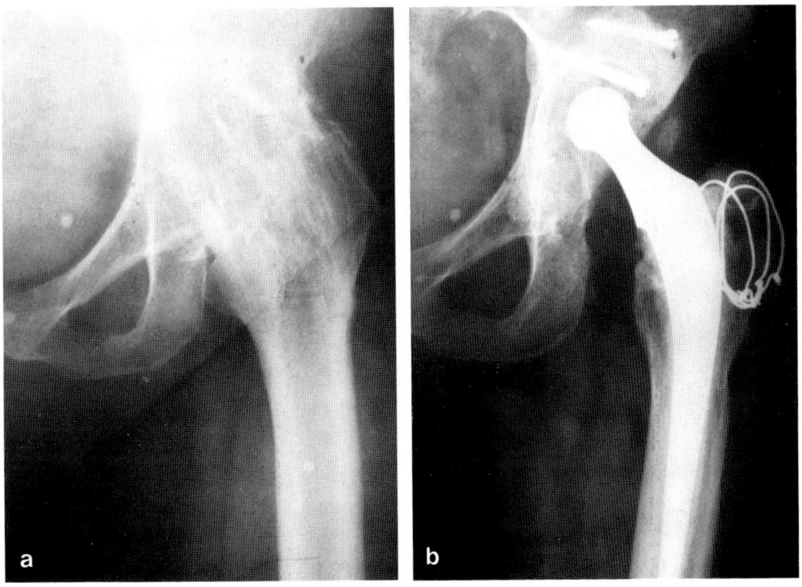

Fig. 5.13 a, b. The ankylosis of the left hip has been freed through the joint line (**a**). The integrity of the acetabulum has been restored by a shelf, but the high position of the cup on the postoperative roentgenograms (**b**) demonstrates the difficulties in identifying landmarks

tion appeared in two patients and ossification of a lesser extent in three others. There was a recrudesence of tuberculosis in one patient who had not received prophylactic antituberculosis treatment.

The 23 arthroplasties have been assessed according to the Merle d'Aubigné and Postel scoring system and the results are presented in Table 5.2. Twenty-two hips are almost or completely pain free. Only 15 have flexion greater than 75°, but there is no residual deformity apart from slight fixed flexion in three cases. There is no significant correlation between the range of movement achieved and the etiology or duration of the ankylosis. Neither did we find any significant correlation between stability and the origin or duration of the ankylosis or the age of the patients. Complete stability was often achieved only after 1 year and sometimes 3 or even 4 years. This emphasizes the importance of postoperative physiotherapy.

Finally, 11 hips had a perfect or almost perfect result

Table 5.2. Results of hip function following arthroplasty (23 hips with longest follow-up)

Pain	No. of hips	Range of movement	No. of hips	Stability	No. of hips
:6	18	:6	11	:6	16
:5	4	:5	4	:5	3
:4	1	:4	5	:4	2
:3		:3	1	:3	2
:2		:2	2	:2	
:1		:1		:1	
:0		:0		:0	

(17 and 18). Seven hips had a satisfactory result (15 and 16) with very little or no pain, with flexion greater than 70°, with no residual deformity, and with perfect or good stability. Five results were less satisfactory, with two cases of major ossification, but there was no significant pain, no fixed deformity, and no marked instability.

Back pain disappeared in ten of the 16 cases. There was marked improvement in five other cases; one patient did not improve significantly, but none become worse. We were not able to demonstrate a definite association between the progression of back pain and the presence of lumbar spondylosis (eight cases) or scoliosis (five cases), but our series did not include any severe case of fixed scoliosis resulting from a fixed pelvis.

Knee pain disappeared completely in two and almost completely in three of the five patients with knee pathology below an ipsilateral unsatisfactorily ankylosed hip. However, the condition of one patient with genu varum of 2° has deteriorated after 3 years of initial significant improvement, and this patient is now awaiting knee surgery. The three other patients with knee pain on the contralateral side to the ankylosis who had severe valgus deformities have been completely relieved of their symptoms by a supracondylar femoral osteotomy after hip arthroplasty.

What, then, are the overall results in terms of the quality of the arthroplasty and its effect on each patient? Among the 17 patients with back and/or knee pain, 13 had a good result in relation to the spine, the knee, and the hip. Three had good relief of back and knee

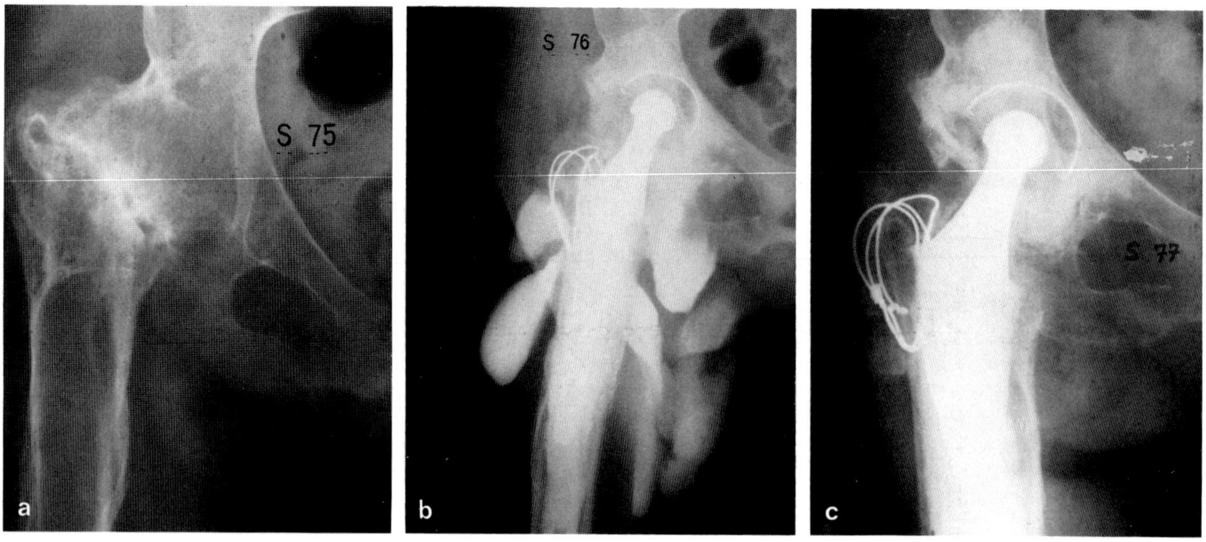

Fig. 5.14. **a** Recurrence of an old tuberculous infection in a hip with an ununited fracture of the femoral neck beneath an ankylosis. **b** A cure was achieved using systemic and local antibiotic therapy, together with intra-articular injections. **c** Outline of the abscess cavity 1 year after hip replacement

pain, but hip function was only fair. The daily life of these three patients was transformed by the relief of their knee and back symptoms, and even though their hips had only an average range of movement, they were pain free and stable, having lost the fixed deformity. Thus, even though these hips were scored as only fair, one cannot talk of failure in these cases, as we are concerned with a good subjective result. Finally, one patient whose indication for surgery was back pain did not improve, and the operation is classed as a failure, in spite of good hip function.

The arthroplasties performed on the three patients with functional disability relating to the unsatisfactory ankylosis produced one good result and two failures caused by massive ossification, although without pain or fixed deformity. The patient with a nonunion of the femoral neck below an ankylosed hip had a good result in spite of a recurrence of tuberculosis (Fig. 5.14).

From a total of 21 patients, 18 were satisfied with the result (85%), 15 of whom scored a good result (70%). There were three failures; one patient had persistent back pain and two developed ossification postoperatively.

5.6.5 *Conclusion*

Arthroplasty and the mobilization of a hip that is ankylosed in an unsatisfactory position are indicated if the condition is producing symptoms in a neighboring joint. However, a good result can be expected only if the adjacent involved joint is still in reasonable condition, and if the musculature around the hip is sufficient to stabilize the arthroplasty. Back pain can be tolerated for a long period, but a recent increase in symptoms and recurrent acute episodes are good indications for dearthrodesis of the hip, as long as the spine is mobile and there are only minimal or no degenerative changes.

If the pelvis is tilted and fixed in relation to the lumbar spine, this constitutes a contraindication to mobilization of the ankylosis. Pain in the knee is tolerated much better than back pain, but it must be carefully assessed to determine how much is due to malalignment and how much to fixity of the hip. An osteotomy to realign a poor ankylosis into a good position often remains a good operation. However, arthroplasty is vital when the patellofemoral joint is affected or where proximal migration of the femur is the origin of the pelvic tilt, especially in association with severe back pain. If, in addition, the knee is malaligned, surgery of the knee will be fruitless if it is not preceded by mobilization of the ankylosed hip.

Before the decision is made to mobilize a long-standing ankylosis, the question of the functional strength of the mm. glutei must be addressed. We have tried to assess this by electromyography but have not found the results very convincing. There are always some motor units that function, and their detection depends on the areas explored. In practice, there are two lines of approach which we have found will provide us with adequate information. Palpation of the mm. glutei during walking or on active abduction allows one to feel their contraction. Careful study or roentgenograms (noting any iliofemoral grafts or ossification within the muscle) and clinical examination of any scars and related fibrosis will give an idea of previous damage to muscles. Gluteal weakness is more closely related to previous surgery than to the duration of the ankylosis. Disuse atrophy is always associated with long-standing ankylosis that has not undergone surgery, but this responds to reactivation.

Overall, this type of procedure is very often beneficial, in spite of a longer postoperative course than with uncomplicated arthroplasty. However, it involves a heavy program that may include surgery of the knee after surgery of the hip.

5.7 Total Hip Replacement for Congenital Dislocation of the Hip

M. Kerboul, M. Mathieu, and Ph. Sauzières

Total hip replacement for congenital dislocation of the hip is set apart in the spectrum of hip arthroplasties by virtue of the technical problems frequently encountered and by the type of patient on whom it is carried out.

Whether treated in childhood or not, congenital dislocation of the hip (uni- or bilateral) will sooner or later result in a combination of deformities in the adult, many of which are irreversible. The function of the hip will also deteriorate as a result of osteoarthrosis and the increasing inadequacy of the periarticular muscles. The lateral displacement of the joint and the long-standing severe instability of the hip subject the spine to excessive lateral and anteroposterior forces at every step. Although the condition is well tolerated for a long time, the spine eventually becomes irreversibly deformed, once the spondylosis has become sufficiently advanced to make it rigid and painful.

The ipsilateral knee also functions under adverse mechanical conditions and this excessive load leads to pain and arthrosis. This occurs earlier and is more common if orthopedic or surgical treatment of the hip in childhood has disturbed growth, and the resulting knee in the adult is then deformed, malaligned, lax, and degenerate.

Finally, the frequent asymmetry of the lesions, the inequality of leg length, and abnormalities of rotation of different segments of the limb complete this tiered combination of deformities, each of which compensates to a greater or lesser extent for the malformation of the hip, which is the underlying causative factor. However, late correction of the hip will not lead to improvement of these other components once deformities, postures, and habits have become irreversibly fixed.

To carry out a total hip arthroplasty in such a complex situation requires a careful study of all those features which, although secondary, may become of primary importance in the indications for surgery and in determining the quality of the result.

5.7.1 Patients

A series of 90 patients were operated upon between 1968 and 1980. The majority were women (84 women and six men), and the average age was 55 years, ranging from 31 to 75 years. Total hip replacement became necessary sooner if the hip had been operated on in childhood (53 years) and if the residual dislocation was low (52 years).

5.7.2 The Condition

These 90 patients had 118 dislocated hips among them, 107 of which were treated by total hip replacement; 11 have not yet been operated on or have been operated on using procedures other than THR. The dislocated hips were classified as anterior, intermediate, or posterior, as this related best to the pathological anatomy of the condition (Fig. 5.15).

Of these 118 congenitally dislocated hips, 28 were bilateral. Of the 62 contralateral hips that were not dislocated, two-thirds showed osteoarthritic changes while one-third did not. Thirty-one of these had already been operated upon, on one or more occasions, and 26 had been replaced by a total prosthesis. The hips in this study receiving a total arthroplasty included 14 anterior, 52 intermediate, and 31 posterior dislocations.

The 107 prostheses were implanted into 67 virgin hips and into 40 hips which had already been operated on. The most common previous procedure (17) was an osteomy, the main effect of which was to aggravate the shortening of the dislocated limb. This shortening was 4.75 mm on average, ranging from 2 to 8 cm and being greatest when the dislocation was more posterior. As the lesions were usually asymmetric, the lower limbs were rarely of equal length (18 cases). The difference in length was on average 2.6 cm, maximum 8 cm.

In order to compensate for the inequality of leg length the pelvis tilts to the short side, thus increasing the lat-

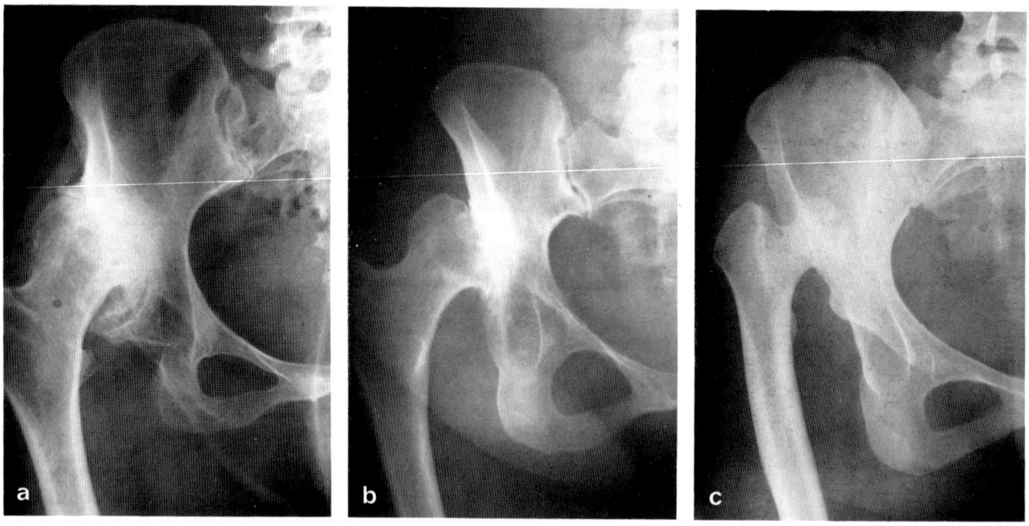

Fig. 5.15 a–c. Long-standing congenitally dislocated hips can be classified into groups according to the anteroposterior position of the new articulation. Posterior dislocations are situated higher than anterior dislocations. On the AP views one can easily recognize an anterior dislocation (**a**), an intermediate dislocation (**b**), and a posterior dislocation (**c**)

eral stress acting on the valgus knee below. The lumbar spine curves laterally to redress the obliquity of the pelvis, and this may even result in a true scoliosis. Spondylosis develops rapidly, stiffening the lumbar segment, and this deformity soon becomes irreducible and perpetuates the pelvic obliquity on weight bearing. The pelvic tilt is nearly always related to the short side, thus accentuating the functional shortening. This must be taken into account during both the preoperative calculations and the operative procedure, in order to have the greatest chance of equalizing the length of the lower limbs.

In one of two cases, and usually when one of the two hips is stable and not dislocated, the lateral spinal curve and pelvic tilt are still reducible and disappear on sitting or lying. One can therefore hope to achieve a level pelvis and a straight spine postoperatively. However, this must be taken into account in calculating the equalization of leg lengths if an unpleasant surprise is to be avoided postoperatively.

Finally, lumbar lordosis may compensate for the anterior rotation of the pelvis that is especially common in bilateral posterior dislocations. For a long while this remains reducible. When one of the hips is normal, this lordosis is less marked and may even be absent, but in this situation, an abnormal rotation of the spine may appear there in order to compensate for the anteroposterior asymmetry of the hips. This rapidly becomes fixed and leads to a permanent anteroposterior tilt of the pelvis, even after reconstruction of the new hip in the elected position and after correction of excessive femoral anteversion.

For these different reasons, backache is common (65 cases) and is often the most severe cause of pain. Together with pain from degenerative changes in the ipsilateral knee, back pain is one of the patient's main symptoms.

The knee below the dislocation is often almost normal or only malaligned into slight valgus in patients where the congenital dislocation has not been treated previously. This was so in 47 cases of this series. When the knee is malaligned, the deformity is nearly always into valgus and 12 of our patients already had advanced osteoarthrosis.

5.7.3 Preoperative Hip Function

Instability of the hip is the most common feature: patients with a low, weight-bearing dislocation walk with a Duchenne-type limp, while those with a high dislocation have a Trendelenburg gait. Pain is almost always present, at a varying level of intensity. Good mobility of the hip is maintained; it was more than 80° in one in three of our patients.

5.7.4 Length of Follow-up

Follow-up averaged 3.5 years at the time of this study in 1981. It is now 6 years. Very few patients have been lost to follow-up. One died after 2 years, four failed to keep appointments after 1 year, and three did not attend after 4 years. Nearly all patients returned religiously for their annual assessment; 103 patients have been followed up for over 1 year.

5.7.5 The Operation

As always, the procedure is carried out in the lateral decubitus position on a conventional operating table using the lateral approach and trochanterotomy.
The hip is dislocated and the neck is divided. A careful and complete excision of the joint capsule is carried out, together with all fibrous scar tissue and any shelf or osteophytes that overhang the new acetabulum. The acetabular cavity was most frequently hollowed out at the site of the old acetabulum in this series (70 cases), and in 75% of cases a graft was fashioned and screwed into place. The cups used were almost always small Charnley components (45 no. 1 and 48 no. 2). The six McKee's that were used in 1968 were not well adapted to a pelvis of such small dimensions.
Preparation of the femur nearly always requires reaming and occasionally correction of any angulation below the level of the trochanter. The femoral component is selected according to the size of the medullary canal (usually a small one: 11 no. 1, 59 no. 2, 27 no. 3). The femoral neck is divided at a level determined by the position of the prosthetic cup and by the degree of lengthening required, being limited only by the need to achieve reduction. In this series, 89 of the femoral components were seated at the level of the lesser trochanter, while ten were above and eight were below. Reduction is occasionally difficult, especially if the lengthening exceeds 5 cm. However, bringing down the trochanter is usually easy, and its reattachment is very rarely a problem.

5.7.6 Complications

Postoperative management is little different from that of a routine arthroplasty. Weight bearing is delayed only if the roof of the acetabulum has been almost completely replaced by a graft.
Sixty-seven hips were completely uncomplicated while 40 provided a few problems; fortunately, the majority were only minor and there were no fatalities.

Operative complications included three false passages during reaming, nine fractures of the acetabulum, and five fissures of the femur. In two cases the head of the femoral component was scratched because it impinged on the screws holding a shelf in place, and the components were immediately changed.

Systemic complications included one serious urinary tract infection, one myocardial infarction, three episodes of phlebitis, and one pulmonary embolism, all of which were treated and resolved uneventfully. In two cases over-anticoagulation produced large hematomas; one of these was evacuated in time, while the other resulted in a sciatic nerve palsy which recovered very slowly. This was the only significant neurological complication in this series.
One partial sciatic palsy occurred after overzealous lengthening of a limb. This was noticed when the patient awoke from the anesthetic, and it resolved after a few minutes once the knee had been put into flexion.

Local complications included five dislocations that occurred in the immediate postoperative period, two of which required open reduction. One became recurrent as a result of a retroverted cup and initial multiple tenotomies. After several revisions the prosthesis was eventually removed.
Of four nonunions of the trochanter, three were not explored, and one consolidated after further surgery.
Periarticular ossification occurred in seven cases (three of type II and four of type III) but had no deleterious effects on the mobility of the joints.
Five prostheses became loose, two of which were infected. One septic infection dried up after further surgery and the prosthesis remains in place; the other prosthesis was removed. The three loose aseptic prostheses involved both components of a McKee arthroplasty and the cups of two Charnley hips implanted in a high position.
Abnormal radiological signs consisted of lucent areas around five cups (three McKee and two high Charnley cups) which for the moment have produced no clinical symptoms, but which remain as probable or potential loosenings.
Following two revisions, one patient suffered a fatigue fracture of the acetabulum which consolidated spontaneously without loosening.

5.7.7 Results

There were seven *failures* resulting from mechanical or infectious complications. In three cases the function was classed as only poor (one aseptic loosening, reoperated upon after 13 years, and two probable loosenings) and in four cases it was clearly bad (in

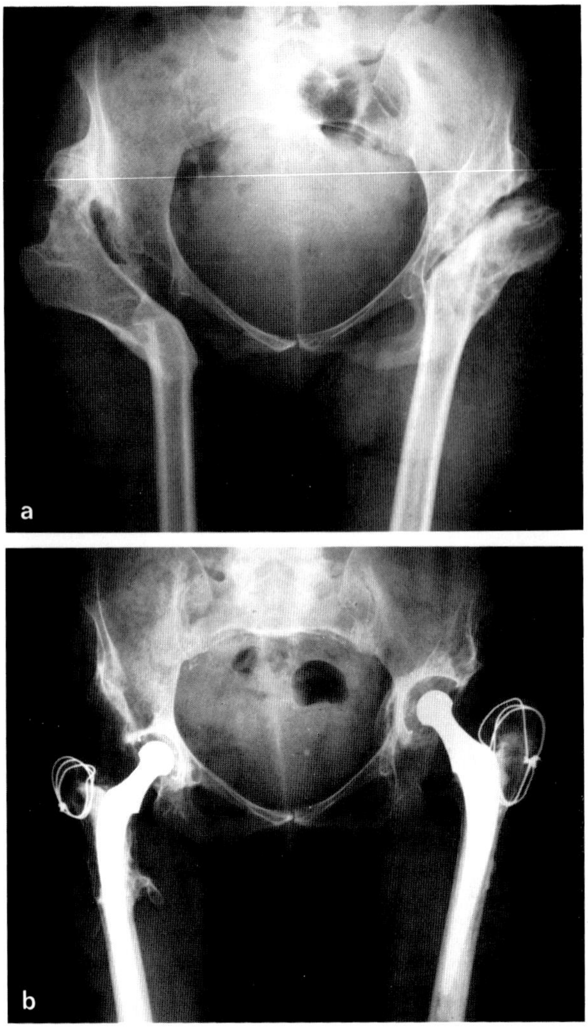

Fig. 5.16 a, b. Bilateral intermediate dislocations. After a wedge resection in the left and a low osteotomy on the right (**a**), both hips were unstable, stiff, and painful and the lumbar spine and knees were equally symptomatic. Following bilateral total hip replacement (**b**), with correction of the osteotomy on the right but not on the left, (the cup being placed high) both hips are now mobile and painless but unstable. A marked residual limp led to this being classified as an average result

three of these the prosthesis has since been removed).

There were 21 *fair results*. Two factors were responsible for inadequate function: residual instability was the most important cause and the second, less common, cause was persistent stiffness. Inadequate results may be attributed to the use of a prosthesis that is not well suited to this type of hip problem, such as the McKee (one good result out of six) and also to technical difficulties encountered during surgery. The latter may arise in the case of previous osteotomies which often require correction before the prosthesis can be implanted (13 good results out of 17).

Reoperation on a previously failed total arthroplasty has a high risk of complications, and the associated bony and muscular damage naturally does not help a good return to function (one good result in two). In fact, a number of poor results are associated simply with a mistake or with inadequate technique (Figs. 5.16–5.19).

There were 75 *good results*, and 57 hips among these functioned perfectly, scoring 18. The roentgenograms showed that the joints had been exactly reconstructed in all cases (Figs. 5.20–5.25).

5.7.8 Analysis

A closer analysis of the results shows that in this series, as in all total hip arthroplasties, complete relief of pain is usually achieved (95% of cases) and that although mobility is most often improved, it is not always perfect (61% were scored at 6). Significant preoperative stiffness remains a problem that cannot always be overcome. Stability on weight bearing and on walking was perfect in only two out of three cases. This residual limb, which was marked in 20% of the patients, is undoubtedly largely responsible for the poor results.

The more normal the hip that is undergoing surgery, the greater the chance of obtaining a good overall result. A perfect result was achieved in 80% of cases when the dislocation was anterior, in 56% when it was intermediate, and in 44% when it was posterior. It is the presence of a limb that usually alters the quality of the result, and there was a significant limb in one of 15 anterior dislocations, in nine of 54 intermediate dislocations, and in nine of 31 posterior dislocations. These findings might lead one to think that the major cause of a postoperative limb is the preoperative height of the dislocation. This is not so; what most determines the quality of support of the operated limb is the precision with which the joint has been reconstructed and, most importantly, the position of the cup. The closer the cup to its ideal position (the old acetabulum), the greater the likelihood of the hip being perfectly stable. If the cup is more than 2 cm from this position it is almost impossible to achieve excellent stability when weight is put on the prosthetic hip. On the other hand, excellent stability nearly always results when the cup has been placed in the old acetabulum, whatever the preoperative height of the dislocation. This recentering of the joint is equally beneficial for the range of postoperative movement. Lengthen-

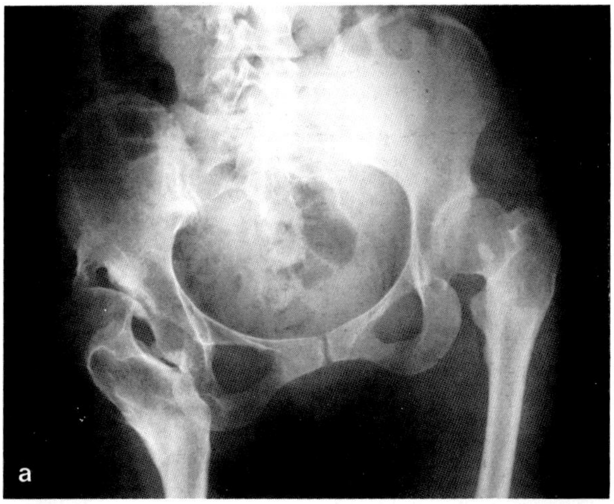

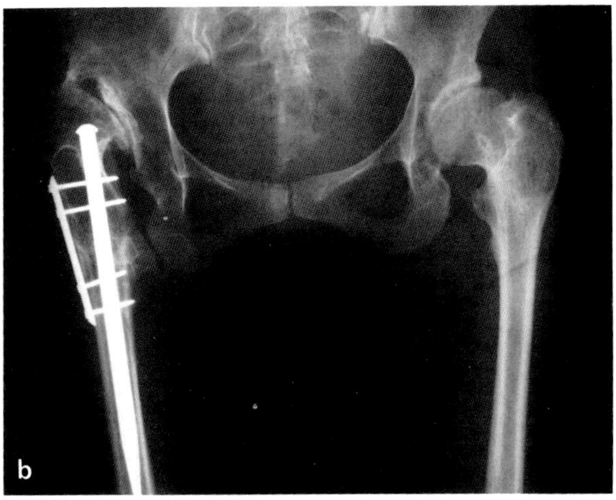

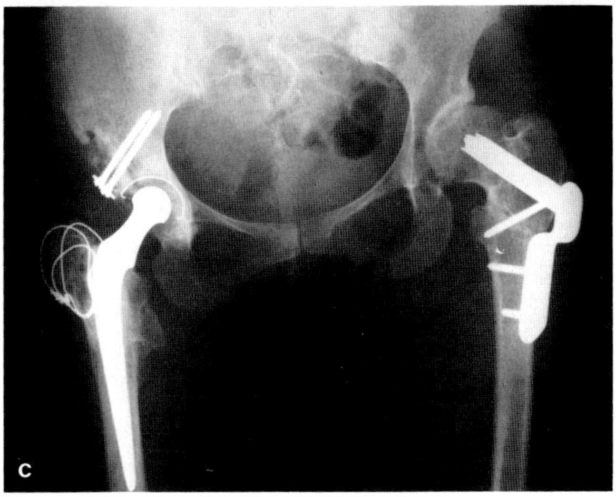

Fig. 5.17. **a** Intermediate dislocation on the right, treated by a shelf and osteotomy. A simple dysplasia on the left was treated by osteotomy (residual anteversion in excess of 50°). Both hips are slightly painful, but the spine and a left valgus knee are more symptomatic due to the tilt of the pelvis. **b** A simple deosteotomy on the right greatly improved the functional situation and relieved the knee and spine sufficiently for arthroplasty of the right hip to be deferred for 7 years. **c** Three years after total hip replacement and 1 year after a further osteotomy on the left (to correct irreducible internal rotation of the left lower limb). The back pain has now practically disappeared and the right hip is painless, stable, and mobile, but the valgus right knee will need a corrective osteotomy

ing of the limb and the tension that it creates within the periarticular muscles have never been found to alter the range of joint movement. On the contrary, muscles which are returned to a more normal tension and orientation will act more efficiently. Sixty of 70 hips that were exactly recentered retained or completely regained satisfactory movement. This contrasts with nine of 17 hips in which the acetabulum remained 2 cm or more from the ideal position and which had a poor range of movement.

Significant lengthening of the limb was often achieved, average 3.5 cm, maximum 7 cm. Half of the very mobile hips had undergone 4-6 cm of lengthening, while 11 of the 16 limbs that had been lengthened by less than 2 cm remained with hips that were stiff to a varying degree. A gain of 3-5 points often occurred in association with 3-5 cm of lengthening and was more common in these cases than in those where less than 2 cm of lengthening was achieved (22 cases compared with 14). Finally, although we had feared that such a large increase in length would lead to postoperative complications and a poor result, this never proved to be a problem. On the contrary, all but two of the limbs with bad or poor results had undergone only minor lengthening, under 3 cm in all cases.

Overall, preoperative shortening was remarkably well corrected, being exactly achieved in 29 cases and to within 1 cm in 37 others. It was inequality of leg length that was nearly always improved upon. Only 18 patients had lower limbs of equal length preoperatively, compared with 52 patients after surgery. When inequality persisted it was never great (1 cm in 16 cases and 2 cm in 14 cases). However, eight patients had an inequality of 3-5 cm postoperatively, and four of these had had lower limbs of equal length prior to surgery.

In certain cases, this equalization of leg length can be a difficult problem to resolve. It is one of the main aims of the procedure and must not be neglected.

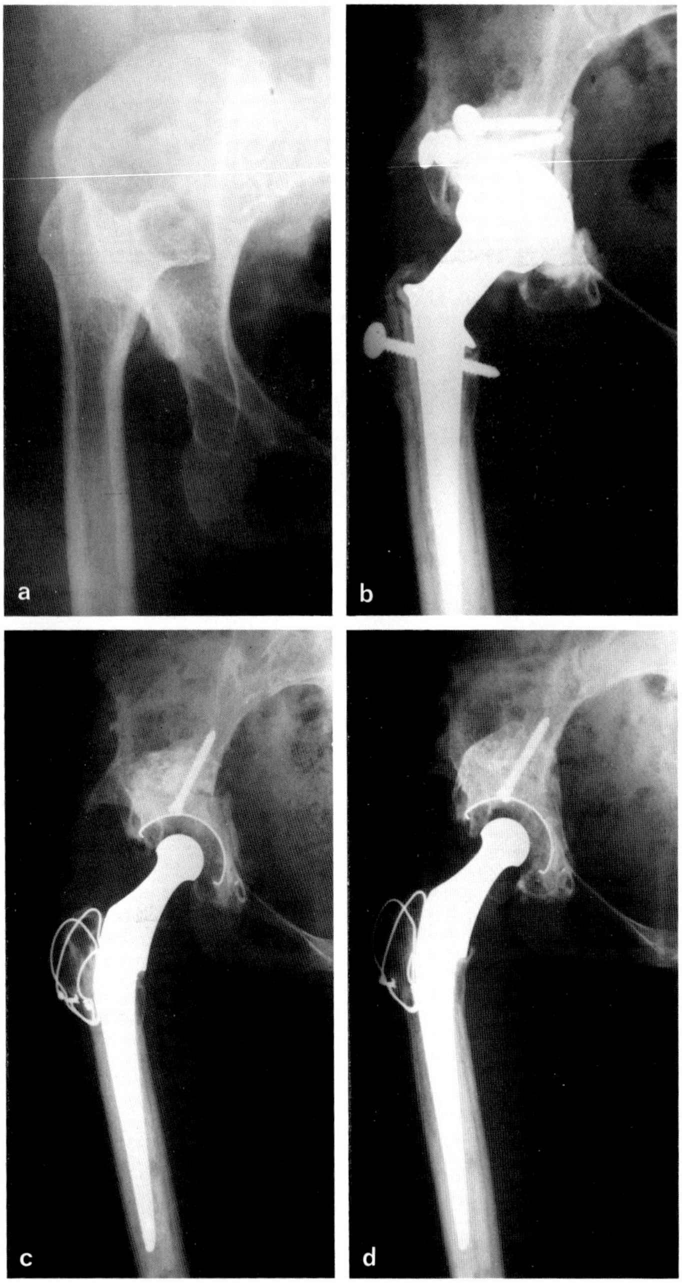

Fig. 5.18. a Unilateral posterior dislocation on the right. **b** A metal-to-metal total hip replacement has a loose cup, and there is considerable bony destruction. **c** Reconstruction of the acetabulum by autograft and a new total arthroplasty. **d** An excellent functional result 5 years later with excellent consolidation of the graft

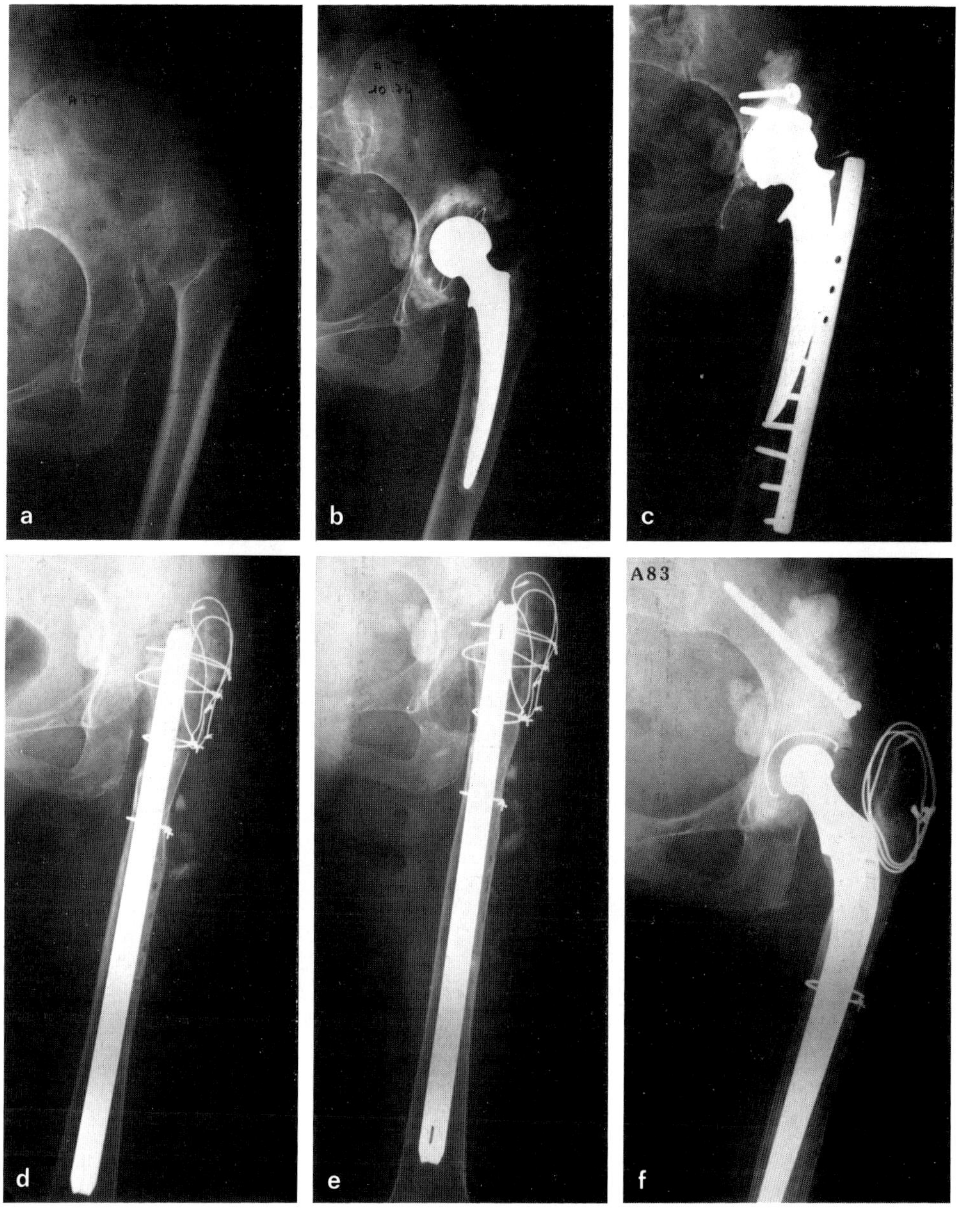

Fig. 5.19 a–f. Unilateral intermediate dislocation on the left (**a**) treated by a total hip replacement, whose stem rapidly loosened (**b**). Revision by a new prosthesis, both of whose components rapidly became loose and produced significant destruction of bone in the femur and acetabulum (**c**). Reconstruction of the missing proximal 12 cm of the femur, using iliac autografts around a Küntscher nail (**d**). Following consolidation of the femur (**e**), a new total hip replacement with reconstruction of the acetabular roof by homograft, held by screws (**f**). Four years later the hip is painless and mobile, but a persisting limp has led to a poor result

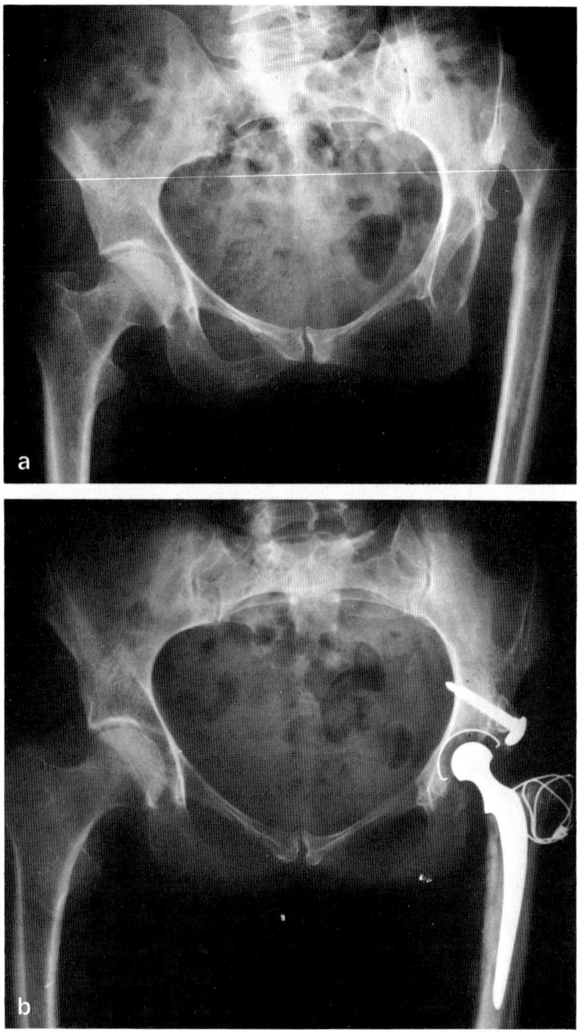

Fig. 5.20. **a** Very high unilateral posterior dislocation on the left with a 7 cm inequality in length. Total hip replacement on the left with 6.5 cm of lengthening. **b** An excellent result at 4 years

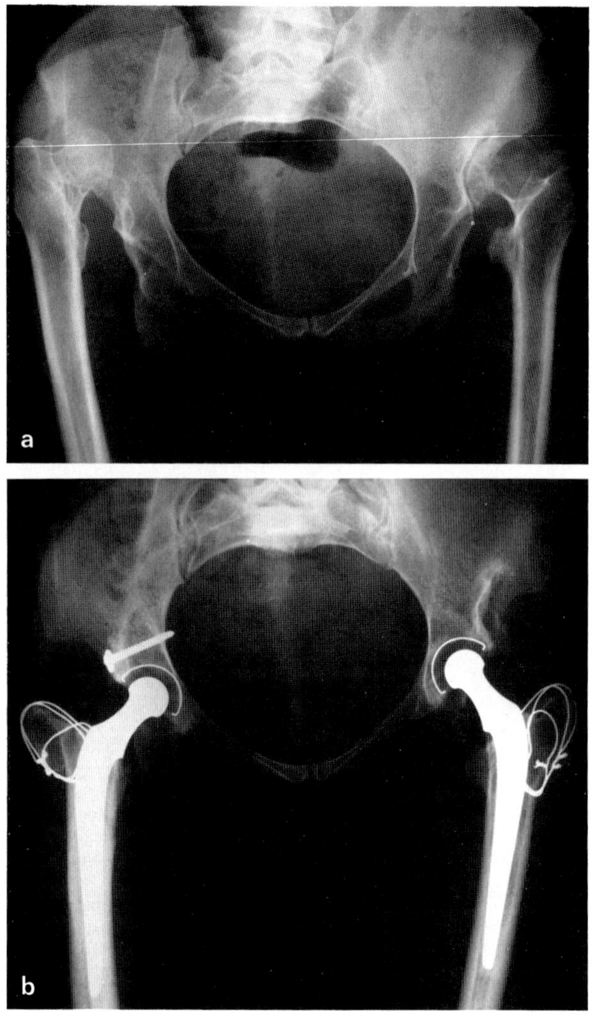

Fig. 5.21. **a** Bilateral dislocation, posterior on the right and intermediate on the left. **b** Excellent functional result after 4 years, with lengthening of 6 cm on the right and 5 cm on the left. Final equalization of leg length

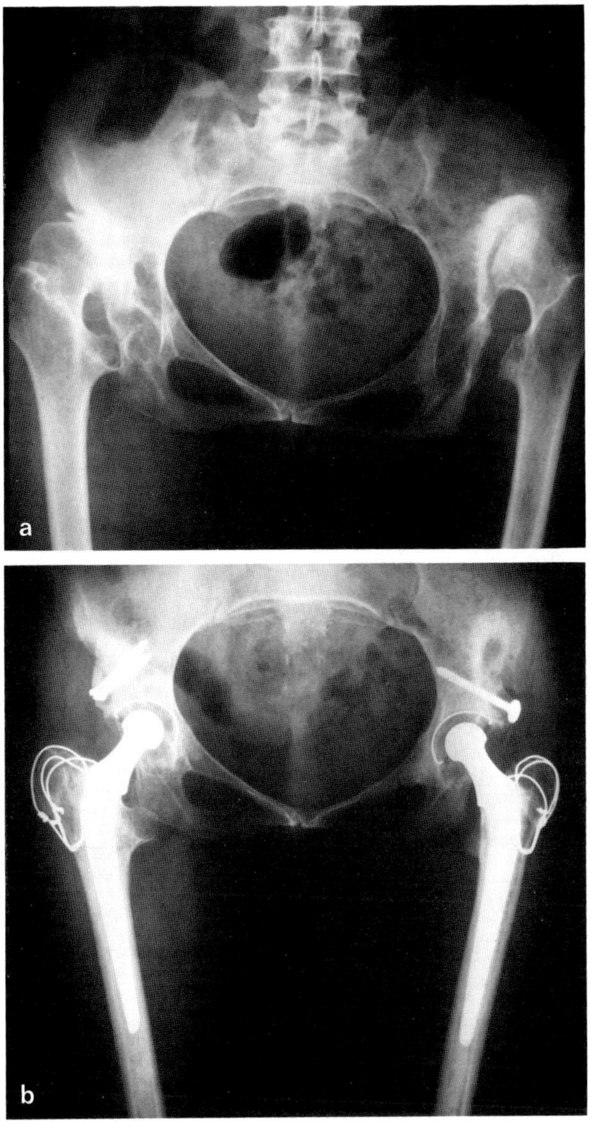

Fig. 5.22. **a** Bilateral intermediate dislocation. **b** Good clinical and radiological result at 5 years

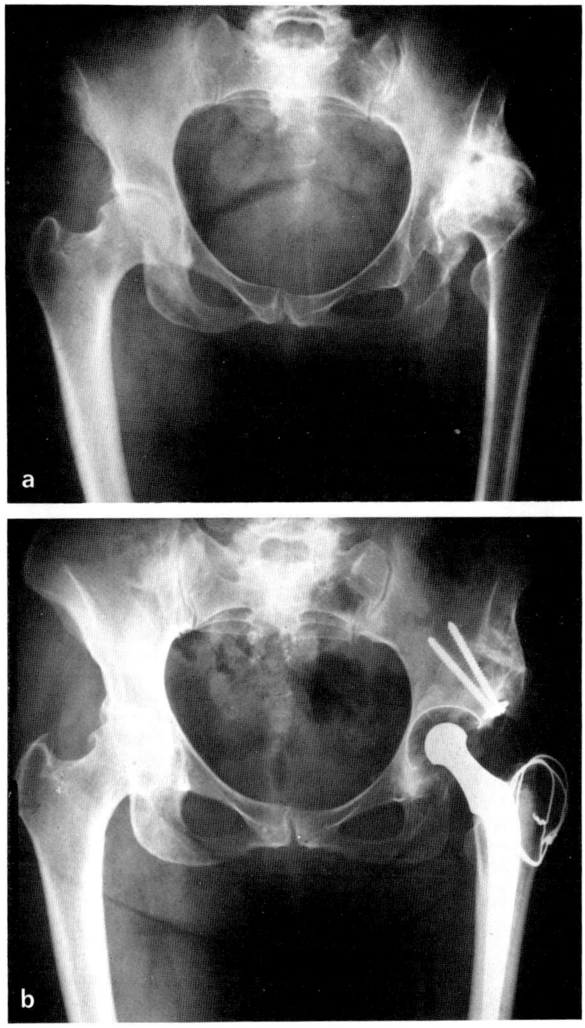

Fig. 5.23. **a** Anterior dislocation on the left. **b** Excellent clinical and radiological result at 11 years

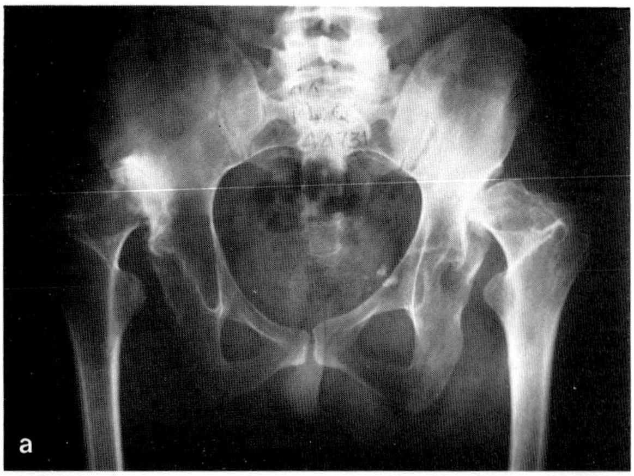

Fig. 5.24. a Bilateral intermediate dislocation. **b** Roentgenogram 1 year after bilateral total hip replacement. **c** Excellent clinical and radiological result 12 years later

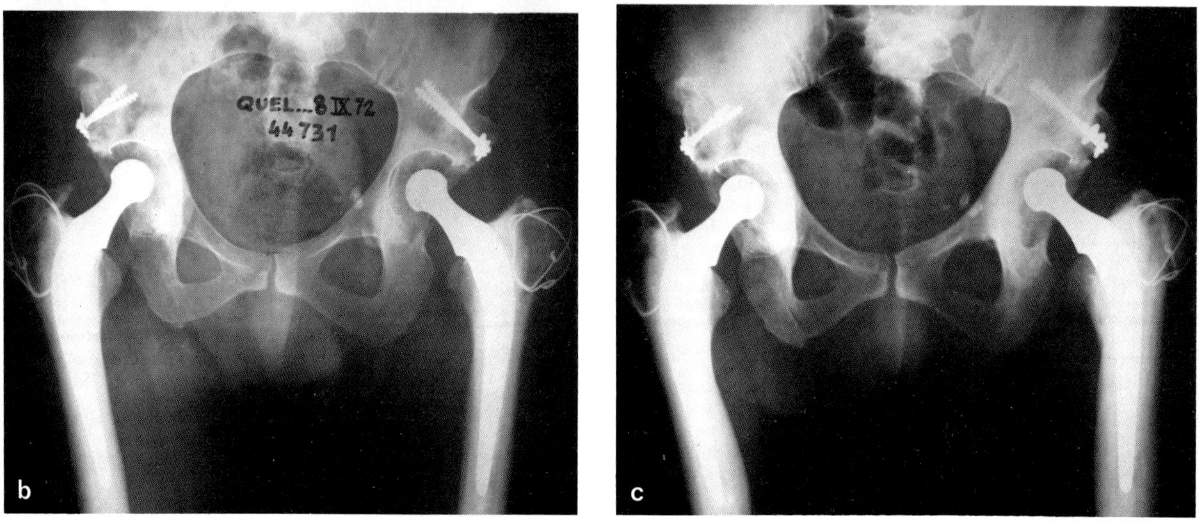

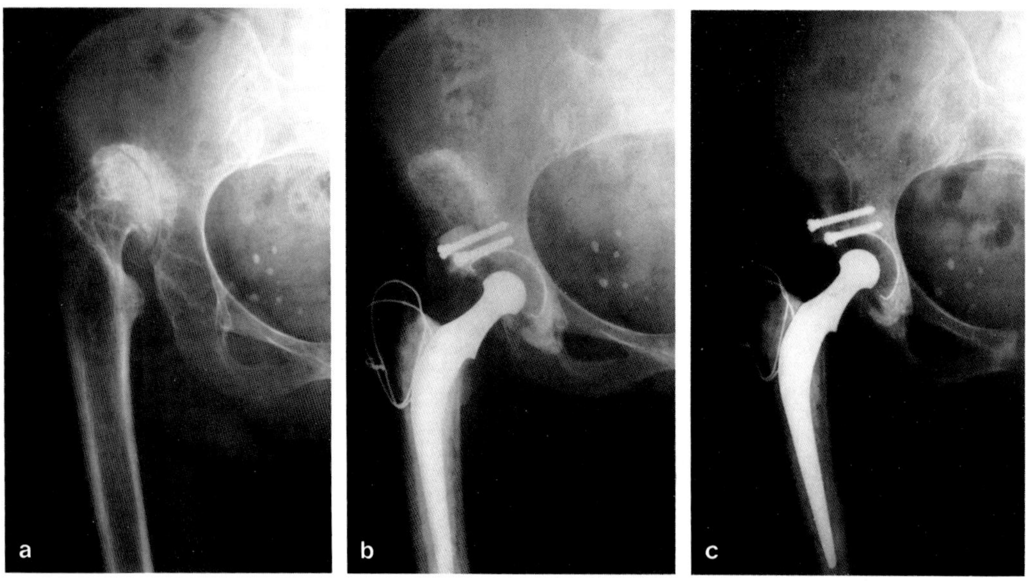

Fig. 5.25. a Intermediate unilateral dislocation on the right. **b** The postoperative roentgenogram. **c** Excellent clinical and radiological result after 14 years

Residual or increased inequality may lead to continuing back pain and can contribute to a poor functional result. A marked, but temporary inequality is not serious, as it can be corrected during the operation on the second hip. However, permanent shortening after two or three complex operations is poorly tolerated by the patient, especially if it was present before surgery. It reflects badly on the surgeon, especially when the only logical and embarrassing solution is a large orthopedic shoe. This situation must be avoided, and the equalization of leg length must form part of the planning of the operation from the outset. It is often preferable to begin with the shorter and most difficult side. Subsequent adjustments will be easier on the simpler hip, and it is exceptional to have to resort to shortening of the femoral diaphysis to achieve equality of length of the lower limbs (Figs. 5.26 and 5.27).
The lateral curvature of the lumbar spine is often fixed as a result of advanced osteoarthritis, and this should also be taken into account. This explains why a pelvis that is oblique before surgery often remains so afterwards, why back pain is rarely relieved, and why the lateral stress on a valgus knee below may not be reduced sufficiently to avoid later corrections by osteotomy. Whether a tilted pelvis remains fixed or not can add confusion to the problem of equalizing the limbs. A persistent tilt toward the short side can add 1-2 cm of functional lengthening to the anatomical length, while a tilt to the long side results in functional inequality even though the anatomical length is exact. Reducing the pelvic tilt more often aggravates than compensates for inadequate lengthening (see Figs. 5.28-5.30).

5.7.9 **Conclusion**

Detailed preoperative study is essential to ensure the best chance of a successful result in total hip replacement for congenital dislocation of the hip. These patients have very distorted anatomy, and there are many pitfalls to be avoided if one is to reconstruct an artificial hip with as good a function as is possible. However, one must remain reasonable in the choice of indications. A few simple rules may help in finding a solution to this sometimes difficult problem.

1. An exact assessment must be made of the shape and size of the femur. One must beware of a roentgenogram of the pelvis taken with the hip in flexion, as this enlarges the femur. Anteroposterior and lateral roentgenograms must be taken with the femur in contact with the plate, as a small angulation on the anteroposterior view may present as a large spur on the lateral if the femur has been curved or deformed by a previous osteotomy. A range of small prostheses must be available, together with the means to ream the femur and to revise an osteotomy.

2. Painstaking excision of the whole of the capsule, of fibrous tissue, and of osteophytes or an old shelf must be carried out, but extensive tenotomies must not be made (adductors, m. rectus femoris, m. gluteus maximus and fascia lata). Such tenotomies are not helpful and can be dangerous, making the hip unstable and allowing too great an increase in length that could put the sciatic nerve at risk.

3. The hip must be reconstructed at the level of the old acetabulum. Dissection of the capsule will reveal the old acetabulum, the landmark being the superior margin of the obturator foramen. This is the only site at which a proper bony cavity can be hollowed out in spongy bone of good quality. This cavity can be carved out at the expense of the bone of the ischium, which is always extensive.
This is the only mechanically satisfactory position capable of guaranteeing a stable hip on weight bearing. When the center of rotation of the hip is lowered and medially displaced, the correct lever arms are restored and the periarticular muscles are returned to their normal orientation and length. All these factors lead to greater efficiency.
All gain in length is made by lowering the acetabulum and this allows the neck to be cut at the level of the lesser trochanter, thus overcoming problems caused by exaggerated anteversion. Also, one can then ream across an angled osteotomy, if it is not too low, and avoid the necessity of revising it.

4. Reduction. It must be confirmed that the hip can be reduced before the femoral component is cemented in place. The use of traction on the limb will not enable the head to enter the cup even if there is only a moderate degree of lengthening, because traction has the effect of tilting the pelvis into abduction. Reduction is achieved by direct pressure on the head and the trochanter while the limb is held in adduction and extension, with the knee slightly flexed to relax the sciatic nerve. Once reduced, the hip will usually lie in a position of flexion and abduction, and its movements are reduced because of the strong tension in the periarticular muscles. Occasionally, tension of the m. rectus femoris even prevents flexion of the knee with the hip in extension. More rarely, tension within the hamstrings prevents any extension at the knee.

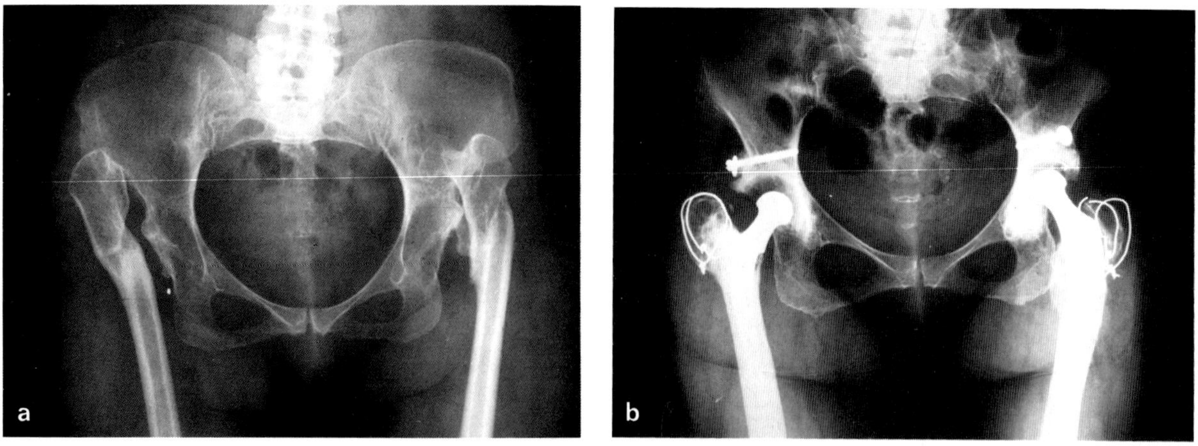

Fig. 5.26. **a** Bilateral posterior dislocations, with previous bilateral osteotomies. **b** Bilateral arthroplasties short-circuiting the osteotomies, which were not greatly angulated, with moderate lengthening on the right and greater lengthening on the left. The ▷ lower limbs, which were of equal length before bilateral arthroplasty (**c**) had a subsequent difference in length of 5 cm (**d**)

Fig. 5.27 and 5.28 *see pp. 64, 65*

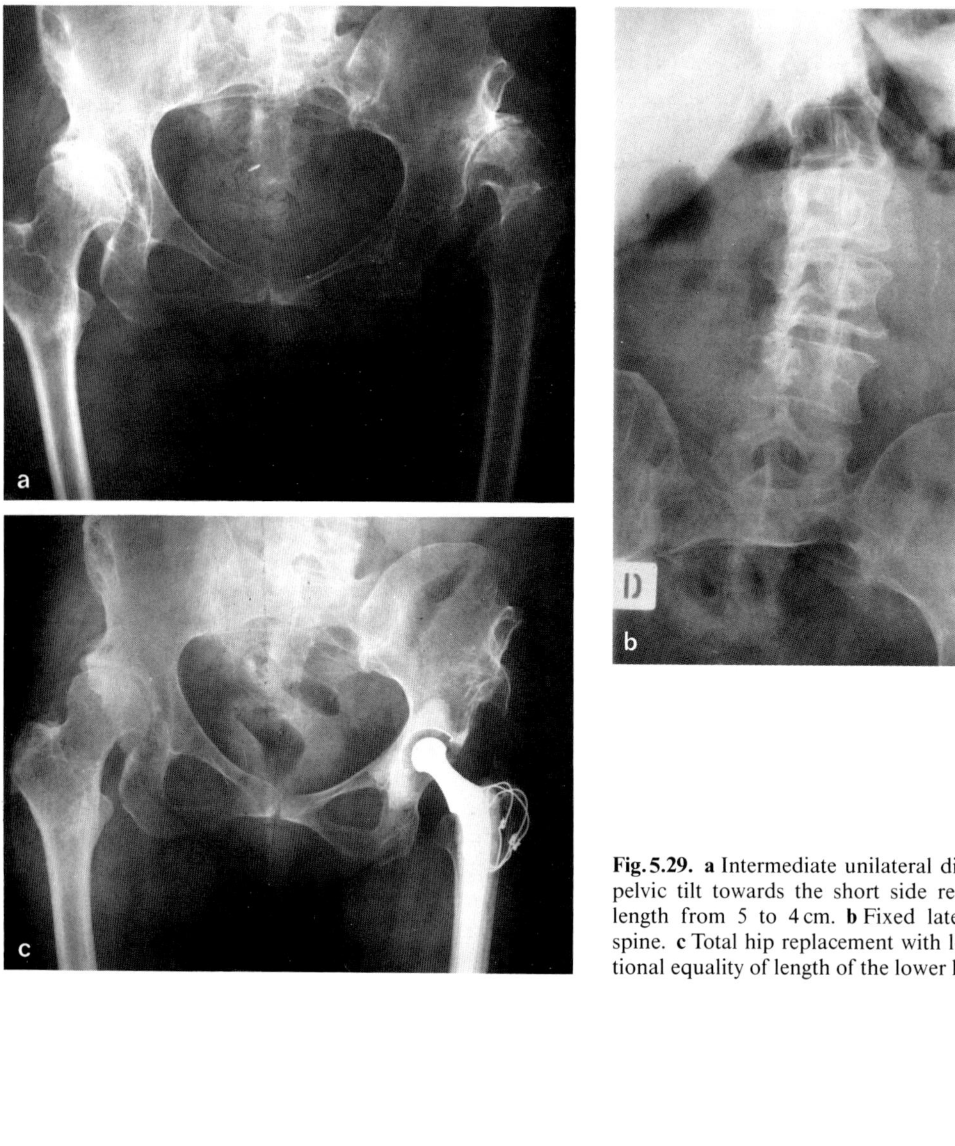

Fig. 5.29. **a** Intermediate unilateral dislocation on the left. The pelvic tilt towards the short side reduces the discrepancy in length from 5 to 4 cm. **b** Fixed lateral curve of the lumbar spine. **c** Total hip replacement with lengthening of 4 cm; functional equality of length of the lower limbs

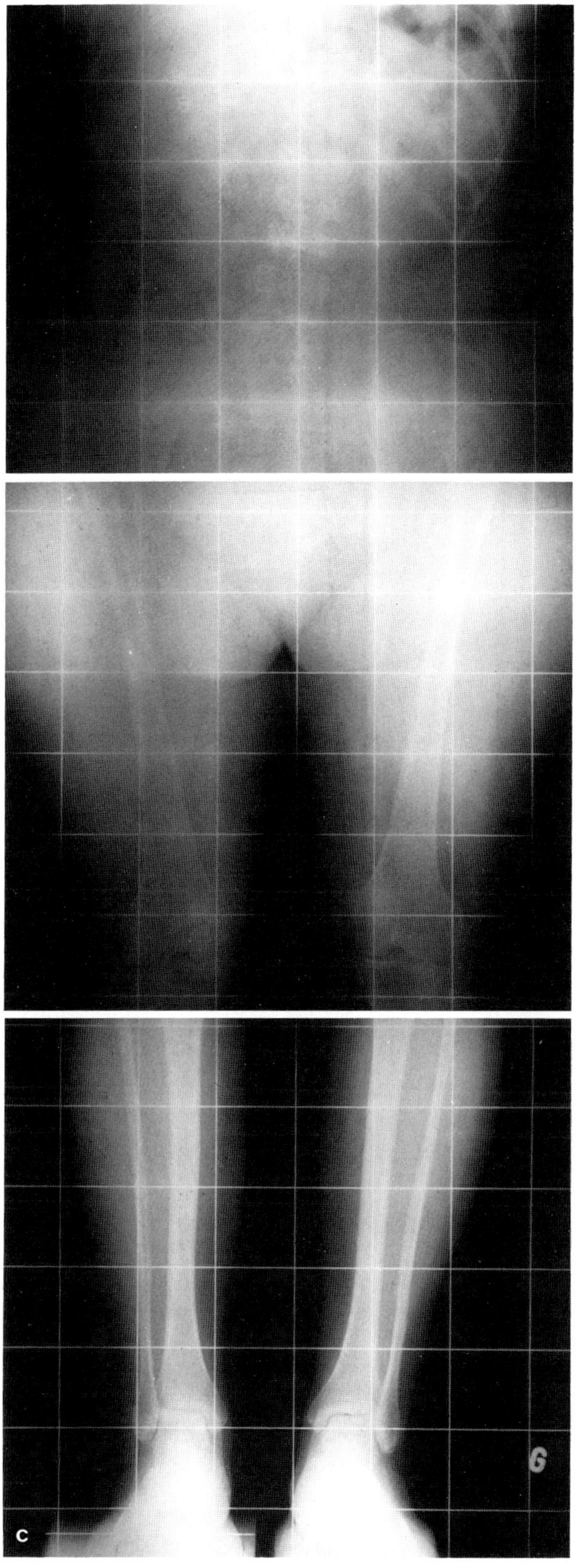

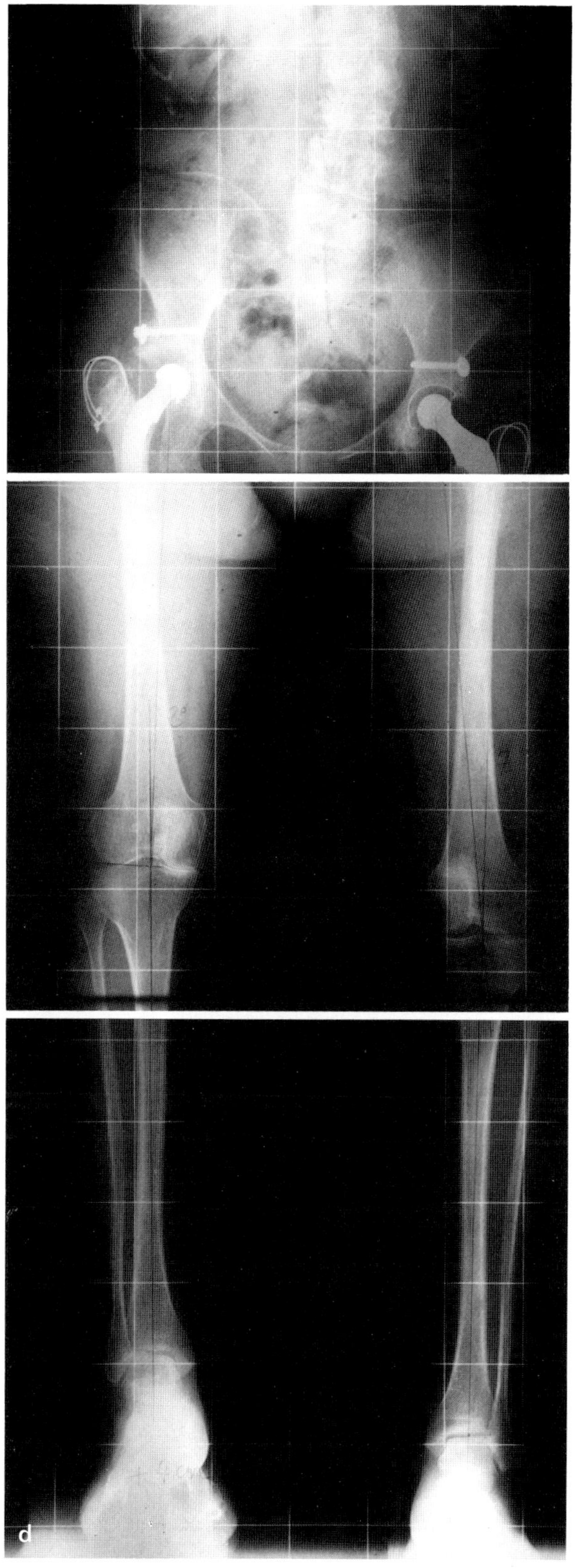

Fig. 5.26 c, d

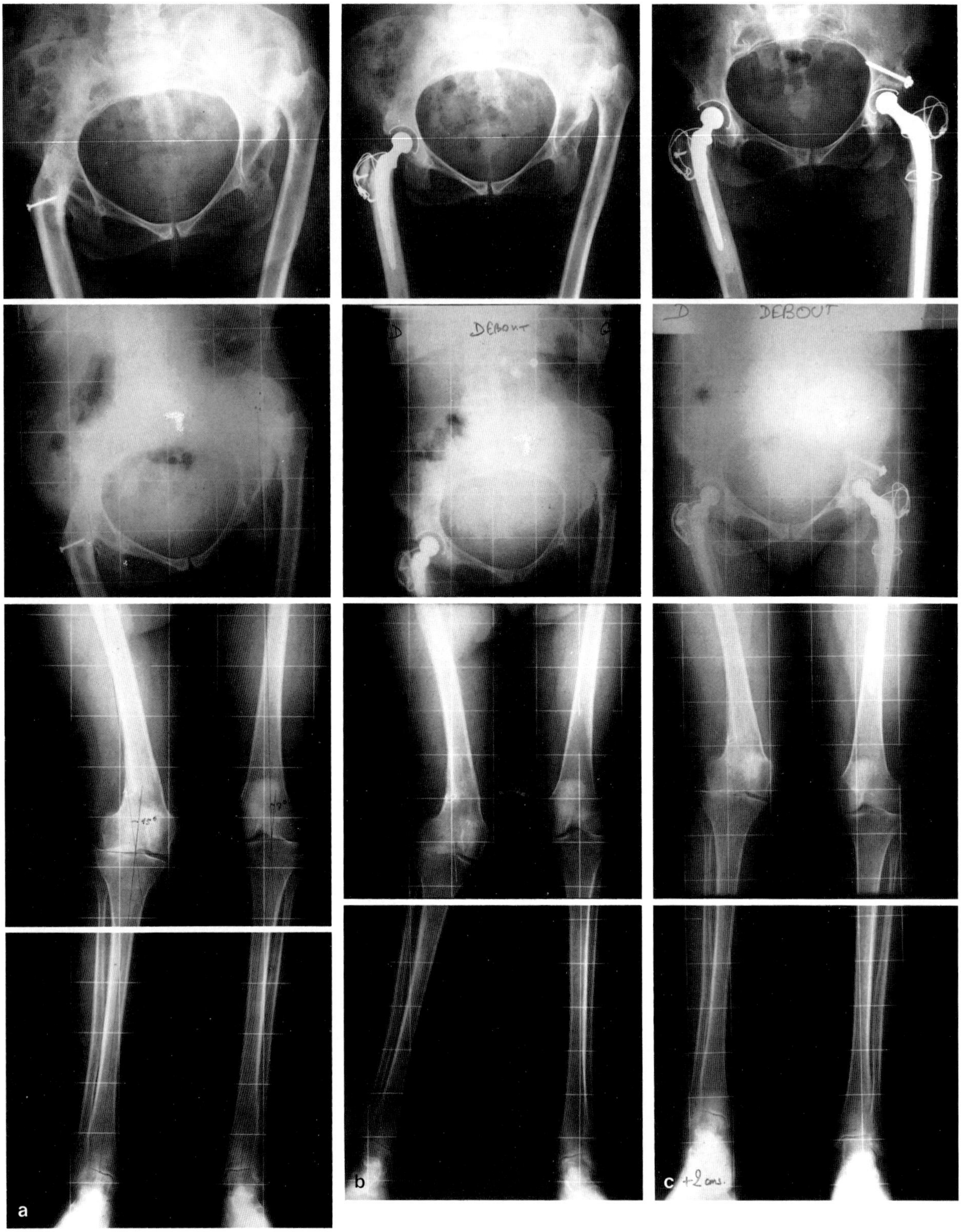
DEBOUT
D
DEBOUT
a
b
c +2 cms.

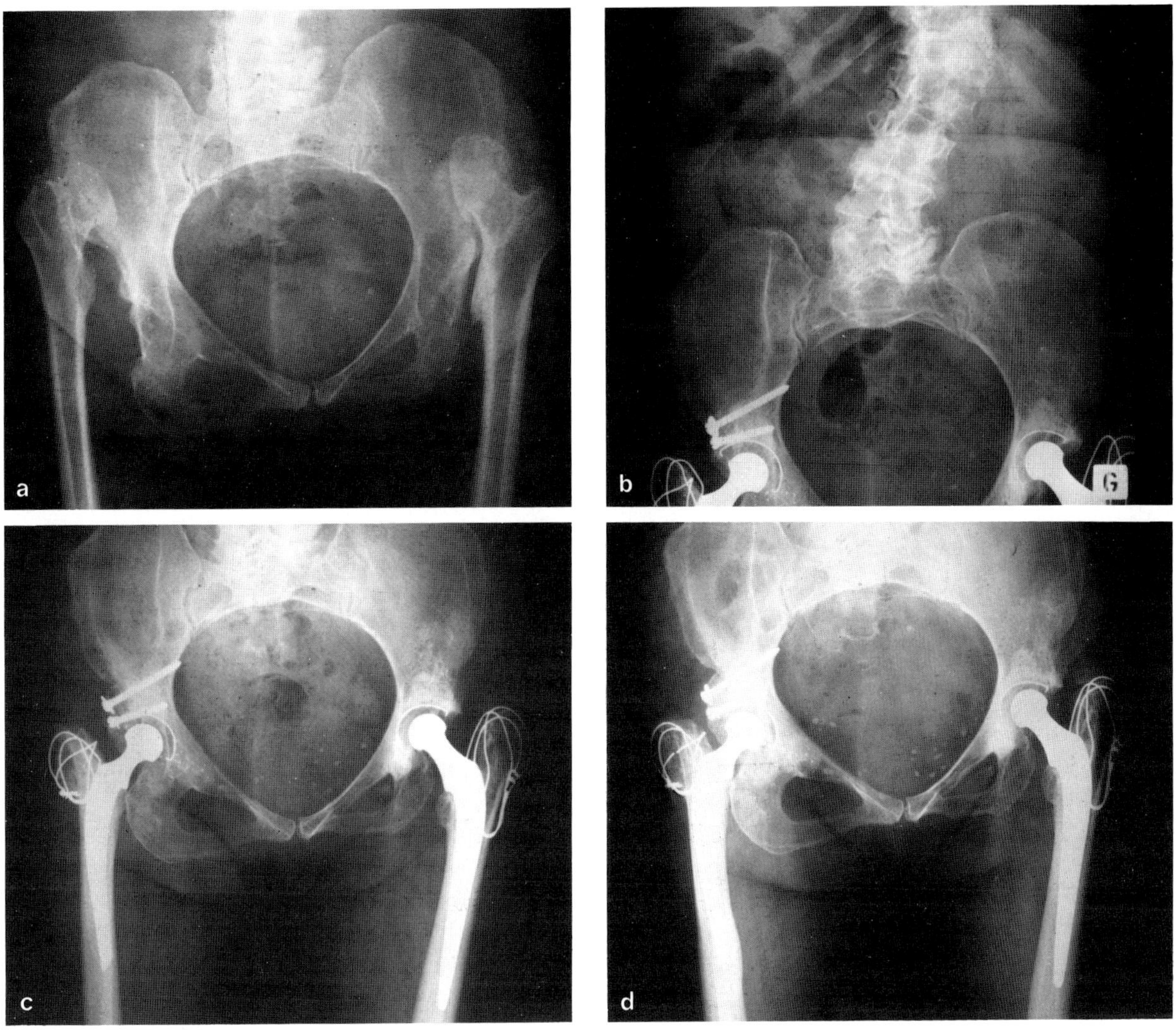

Fig. 5.28. **a** Bilateral posterior dislocation, higher on the right than the left. Pelvic tilt to the short side. **b** Dorsolumbar scoliosis with arthrosis above. **c** Bilateral total hip replacement. Persistent pelvic tilt caused by fixed lateral curve of the lumbar spine. **d** Excellent function of both hips 6 years after surgery, but back pain scarcely improved

Fig. 29 *see p. 62*

◁ **Fig. 5.27.** **a** Gross inequality of leg length beneath congenital bilateral dislocations arthrodesed in abduction on the right and remaining posteriorly dislocated on the left. In spite of the inevitable pelvic tilt, the lumbar spine remains mobile. **b** Total hip replacement on the right, in a very sclerotic hip, allowed only 2 cm of lengthening, which was cancelled out by the partial leveling of the pelvis. **c** The length of the left femur is such that it is necessary to shorten the diaphysis by 5 cm at the same time a left total arthroplasty is implanted, in the hope of equalizing the length of the lower limbs. This will be achieved after a lower femoral varus osteotomy on the right

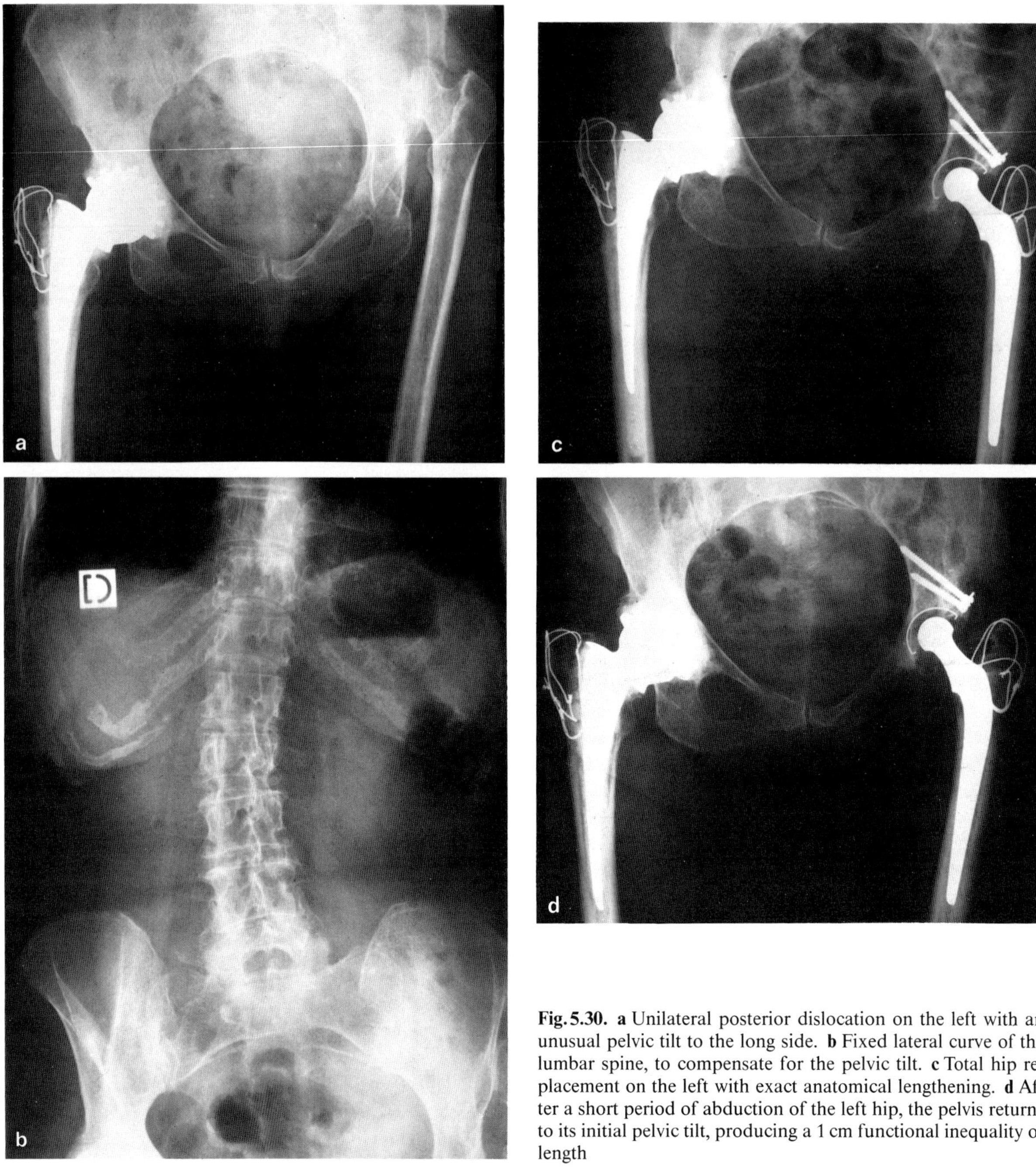

Fig. 5.30. **a** Unilateral posterior dislocation on the left with an unusual pelvic tilt to the long side. **b** Fixed lateral curve of the lumbar spine, to compensate for the pelvic tilt. **c** Total hip replacement on the left with exact anatomical lengthening. **d** After a short period of abduction of the left hip, the pelvis returns to its initial pelvic tilt, producing a 1 cm functional inequality of length

This is not a matter of concern, as it settles down in a few days or months. If the sciatic nerve is tightly stretched at the end of the operation, the knee should be kept in flexion for a while.

5. It is advisable to *exclude from surgery* those patients who are too old, especially if they have bilateral posterior dislocations or a very degenerate spine. The functional benefit is then likely to be poor. One must know how to limit one's ambition when the undertaking is too dangerous. But when all goes well, the patient is radically transformed both physically and psychologically, to his great satisfaction and that of the surgeon.

6 Aseptic Complications Following Total Hip Replacement

6.1 Ossification

T. Arama, J. P. Courpied, and M. Postel

The significance of periarticular ossification following total hip replacement varies according to its size and extent. Such ossification may be divided into three types on the basis of the Brooker classification, the last two groups of which have here been combined:

Type I: Ossification limited to islands or spurs situated between the femur and the pelvis (Fig. 6.1)

Type II: Ossification that occupies more than half of the joint space, but with no continuity of bone between the femur and the pelvis (Fig. 6.2)

Type III: Ossification leaving a gap of less than 1 cm and occasionally forming a continuous bridge of bone (Fig. 6.3)

As we shall see, there is a correlation between the amount of ossification and the clinical presentation.

Our study consists of a computer analysis of 956 total hip replacements that were implanted into previously unoperated hips as a primary procedure.

Ossification appears early in the postoperative period and is seen in the first few weeks or up to 18 months following surgery. It becomes stable radiologically around 12 months postoperatively. However, maturation of the new bone continues over a longer period, as shown by repeated scans.

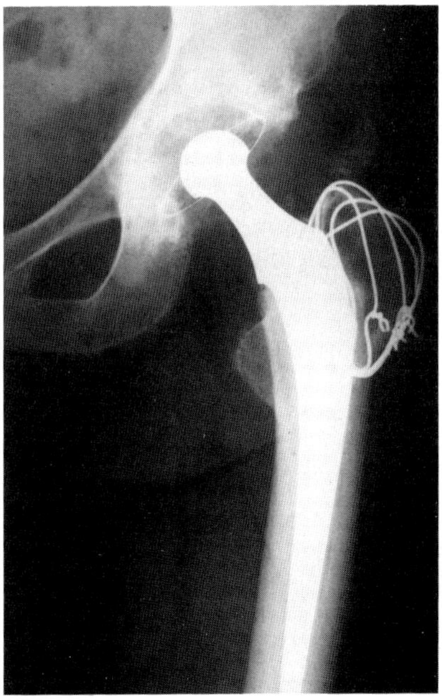

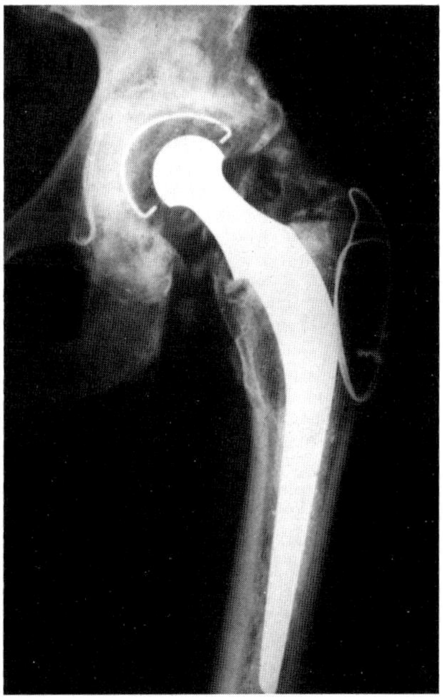

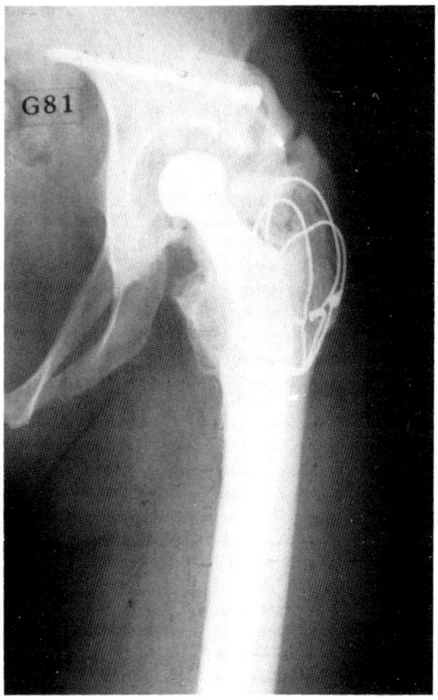

Fig. 6.1 *(left)*. Type-I ossification, 1 year after total hip replacement

Fig. 6.2 *(middle)*. Type-II ossification, 3 years after total hip replacement

Fig. 6.3 *(right)*. Type-III ossification, 1 year after total hip replacement for ankylosis

The 956 patients can be classified as follows: 163 of type I, 42 of type II, and three of type III. Only types II and III had any effect on function (4.4% and 0.3% respectively). Systematic analysis of the case files showed that certain factors were implicated in the formation of new bone.

6.1.1 Predisposing Factors

The Patient

Age has a slight influence, in that the incidence of type-II ossification was 2.7% in patients below 60 years of age and 4.2% in those over 60 years. *Sex* certainly has an influence, as 24 of the 42 type-II patients were male, although only 38% of the overall population studied were men. All three of the type-III ossifications occurred in men.

The *underlying pathology* of the diseased hip does not seem to influence the appearance of ossification of types I and II. On the other hand, type-III ossification always appears in hips that were very stiff or ankylosed prior to hip replacement. Ossification following total hip replacement in ankylosed hips has been discussed in Sect. 5.5. Hips with large marginal osteophytes have a greater tendency to develop ossification around the prosthesis. This is the productive type of arthropathy characterized by Forestier's disease (hyperostotic vertebral ankylosis). Among 28 such hips, three developed ossification of type II and two of type III. This gives an incidence of 10.7% and 7.1% respectively, compared with a 4.4% and 0.3% incidence in the series overall, and it is statistically significant.

Surgical Technique

Several observations have led us to believe that surgical technique plays a very important part in the development of ossification.

The Year of Operation. If we divide the work of the orthopedic department at Cochin into two groups - before and after 1974 - it becomes apparent that the incidence of significant ossification decreased from 5.9% during the first period to 2.3% during the second. As the operative procedure became less traumatic and more routine, there was a reduction in the incidence of ossification.

The Approach. This seems to be a significant factor, as the division of the mm. glutei carried out early in the series produced a much higher rate of ossification than occurred in the later approach, using trochanterotomy with reflection of the mm. glutei (Table 6.1). The posterior approach with division of the external rotators produced at least as much if not more ossification than the lateral approach through muscle. We therefore abandoned the posterior approach completely.

The Experience of the Surgeon. We compared 472 total arthroplasties that had been implanted by two very experienced surgeons with 484 performed by surgeons of varying experience. The incidence of type-II ossification was 1.3% and 5.2% respectively, which suggests that surgical technique is a significant factor.

The Influence of Blood Loss. It was reasonable to suspect that marked hemorrhage occurring during surgery and the initial postoperative period would be a factor that could lead to new bone formation. If blood loss exceeds 1.5 l during surgery and the first 24 h postoperatively then there is a definite increase in ossification. It is difficult to evaluate the influence of large postoperative hematomas. Eight postoperative hematomas required surgical drainage. In one instance this was followed by type-II ossification, but this is not statistically significant.

Thus, technical considerations seem to play an important role during the procedure of hip arthoplasty. However, there is some overlapping of all the above factors. The posterior approach with division of the mm. glutei was used early on, and surgeons can acquire experience only gradually. We remain convinced that the best way to prevent ossification is to use a gentle technique that reduces muscle trauma to a minimum. This is one of the many advantages of trochanterotomy. However, there are still many as yet unknown factors, probably related to the constitution of the individual patient.

Table 6.1. Incidence of postoperative ossification according to surgical approach

Approach through muscle (103 THRs)	11 Type-II (10.6%)
	2 Type-III (1.9%)
Trochanterotomy (795 THRs)	29 Type-II (3.6%)
	1 Type-III (0.12%)

THR, Total hip replacement

Table 6.2. Function of 37 total arthroplasties with type-II ossification 3 years after surgery

Pain	No. of hips	Range of movement	No. of hips	P/M/S	No. of hips
6	32	6	16	18	12
5	2	5	7	16–17	14
4	2	4	8	15	4
3		3	4	12–14	7
2		2	2		
1		1		0–11	
0		0			

6.1.2 Effect on Function

Type-I ossification is of no functional significance in either the short or the long term. However, this does not hold true for types II and III; 30% of type II had an average or poor result, while all those of type III were classified as bad (Table 6.2).
The bad function of hips with type-II ossification is caused by an inadequate range of movement. Of 37 such patients followed up for more than 3 years, 14 had a range of movement scoring only 4 or less. It is said that hips affected by ossification are painful. Of the 37 hips with type-II ossification, two became increasingly painful. One had a McKee prosthesis with a loose cup and the other had a Charnley with a loose femoral component. The remainder continued to be pain free. The bad results among the type-III patients are also caused by stiffness or ankylosis without any pain. When there is late onset of pain in a hip with surrounding ossification, one must be suspicious of a new complication.

6.1.3 Infection

It has long been said that infected hips are often the site of ossification. This seems to be confirmed by our overall study. Of the 1312 prostheses reviewed, 73 were infected. Among these, 12.3% had ossification of type II; this is almost three times greater than in the series as a whole.
Ossification is, therefore, a relatively common radiological feature of infected prostheses, although it does not occur frequently enough to be of diagnostic significance in its own right. Ossification progresses more slowly in infected than in aseptic prostheses, but continues over a longer period. It is only in infected cases that ossification progresses from type II to type III in the long term.

6.1.4 Treatment

Surgery is the only effective treatment and requires painstaking dissection of all the new bone, using a knife rather than a rasp.
Should surgery be used in combination with other treatments? We have used diphosphonates in a few cases but to no great effect. Radiotherapy as suggested by Coventry [1] may be considered (20 Gy in 12 sessions, beginning on the 2nd or 3rd postoperative day). The one case in which we used radiotherapy was not successful, but treatment did not commence until the 12th day because of practical problems.
In this series three operations were carried out for stiffness or ankylosis but were not successful. However, on reviewing all our patients over the past 15 years, we found six cases with ossification not included in this series which had undergone surgery, and three of these were successful.
We believe that there are few indications for further surgery. Surgery is not justified solely to improve an existing but reduced range of movement. On the other hand, it is justified in the rare cases of bilateral ankylosis, or where the hip is ankylosed in an unsatisfactory and disabling position. The ossification must also be old and completely mature – there should be a minimum delay of at least 2–3 years after the original procedure. If surgery is contemplated, it is probably advantageous to combine it with preoperative diphosphonate treatment and early postoperative radiotherapy.

6.1.5 Conclusion

There are several types of ossification which have a serious adverse effect on hip arthroplasty. Their origin remains a mystery and their prevention uncertain. This is a difficult problem when considering surgery on a painful hip and there is periarticular ossification in the contralateral hip.

Reference

1. Coventry MB, Scanlon PW (1981) The use of radiotion to discourage ectopic bone. J Bone Joint Surg [Am] 63: 201

6.2 Complications of Trochanterotomy

T. Arama, J. P. Courpied, and M. Postel

We use the lateral approach with trochanterotomy for all arthroplasties, for reasons described elsewhere.

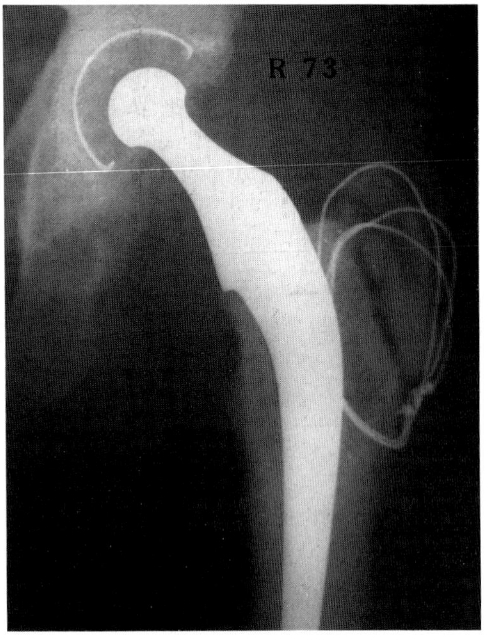

Fig. 6.4. Gap between trochanter and femur resulting from poor attachment of the greater trochanter

However, this has its own complication: failure of fixation of the greater trochanter. The circumstances in which this occurred have been studied in 1100 patients operated upon between 1969 and 1980.

This series includes 31 nonunions of the trochanter among 27 patients (four were bilateral), which is an overall incidence of 2.8%. This is an early complication; it occurred before 30 days in 23 cases and between 30 and 90 days in the remaining eight cases.

Adherence to rigorous operative technique will reduce the incidence of nonunion. We originally used only two anterior wires, but then increased this to three, and finally to four steel wires (12/10). This did not completly resolve the problem, but at the same time we stopped our regimen of postoperative traction and mobilized our patients on the 4th postoperative day. The point of entry of the wires must be such that they are not only supported by bone, with the subsequent risk of cutting out, but also surrounded by cement over an adequate distance. The point of entry must therefore be at least 2 cm below the crest of the m. vastus lateralis, although it could be placed more distally with no adverse effect. The position of reattachment of the greater trochanter has very little effect on the incidence of nonunion and is of less importance than the quality of the bone surfaces in apposition. However, excessive tension can put unwanted stress on the fixation.

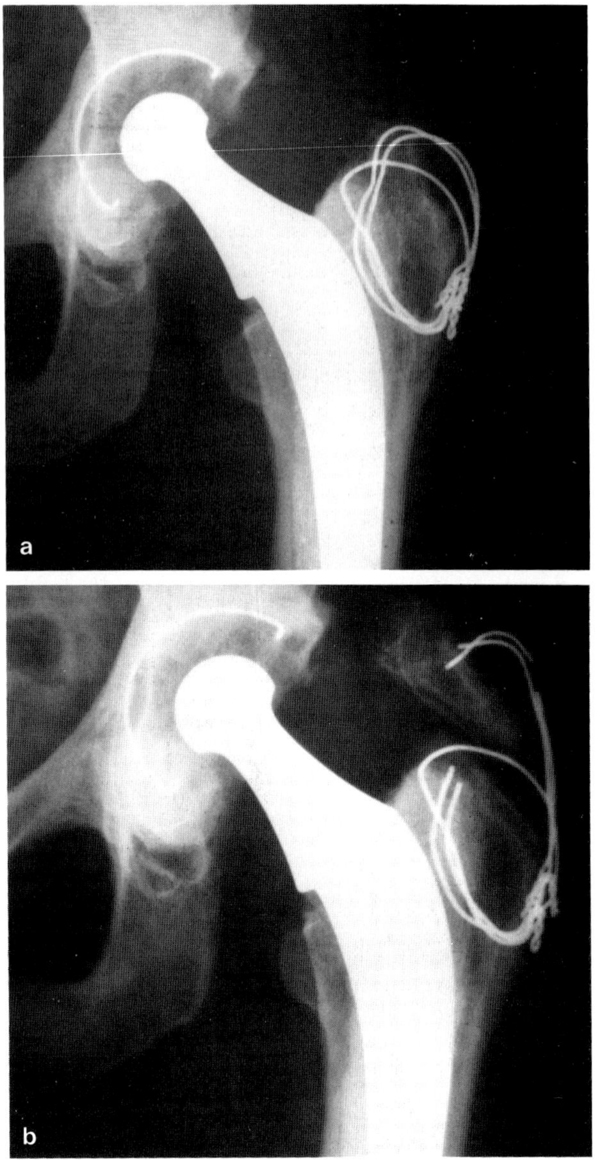

Fig. 6.5. **a** The metal wires have not been adequately tightened and are not well attached to the lateral surface of the greater trochanter. **b** Failure of fixation, one of the wires remaining intact

6.2.1 Causes of Nonunion

Technical faults are the most important factors. The only roentgenogram available for analysis is the routine AP view of the pelvis. Nevertheless, on this view we can detect the presence of a gap between the fragments (Fig. 6.4), a poor fit of the wires against the bony contours (Fig. 6.5), a trochanterotomy that is too high or too low, or a split in the trochanter. One of these faults is present in two of three cases where there has been a problem (21 of 31 nonunions).

Moreover, in one of four nonunions, the trochanter had subluxated anteriorly without breaking all the wires, as if a fault in the tightening or the positioning of the wires had allowed it to slip forward (Fig. 6.5). In fact, the anterior fibers of the mm. glutei contract and pull the trochanter anteriorly during active flexion of the hip, as demonstrated by Charnley.

Finally, in 15% of these nonunions there had been difficulty in reducing the prosthesis because we tried to gain an increase in leg length at the same time. This can be associated with difficulties in reattachment of the trochanter, and in these cases special attention must be paid to its fixation. These technical points are of great importance. If two surfaces of good cancellous bone are not in contact there will be a delay in consolidation, with the risk that the wires will break. If all the wires are not under equal tension, the one under greatest stress will break first. After it has broken, it will be followed by the second, and so on.

Trochanterotomy makes it easier to implant the prosthesis in a perfect position. However, much care is needed when the trochanter is reattached.

Postoperative management is of great importance. We require partial weight bearing on crutches of all our patients for 30 days. In 13 of the 31 cases of nonunion this instruction was not followed and the patient had taken full weight during the first 15 days. Occasionally, the patient fails to cooperate, but he or she may also lack coordination and so be unable to carry out postoperative instructions.

The *underlying hip pathology* does not seem to have any influence on nonunion. The osteoporotic trochanters in rheumatoid arthritis unite as well as in other conditions. More problems result from trochanters that are very sclerotic or deformed by previous surgery, such as repeated trochanterotomy or intramedullary nailing.

6.2.2 *Clinical Significance of Nonunion*

Nonunion does not always have an effect on function. It was considered necessary to revise the trochanterotomy in only one-third of the patients, and function was satisfactory in the remainder.

Of the nine patients for whom revision was necessary, four had marked instability and two had recurrent dislocation. Revision was deferred in the two other patients, whose general condition was so poor that it was not felt justified to subject them to a second operation and a prolonged period of bed rest.

The Technique of Revision

Revision can be a difficult procedure. The trochanter is often very high, being pulled up by retraction of the

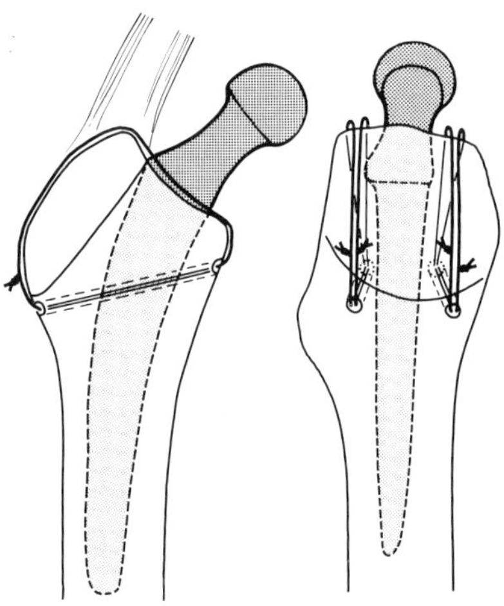

Fig. 6.6. Technique of revision of fixation of the greater trochanter with two wires passing on either side of the prosthesis (scheme)

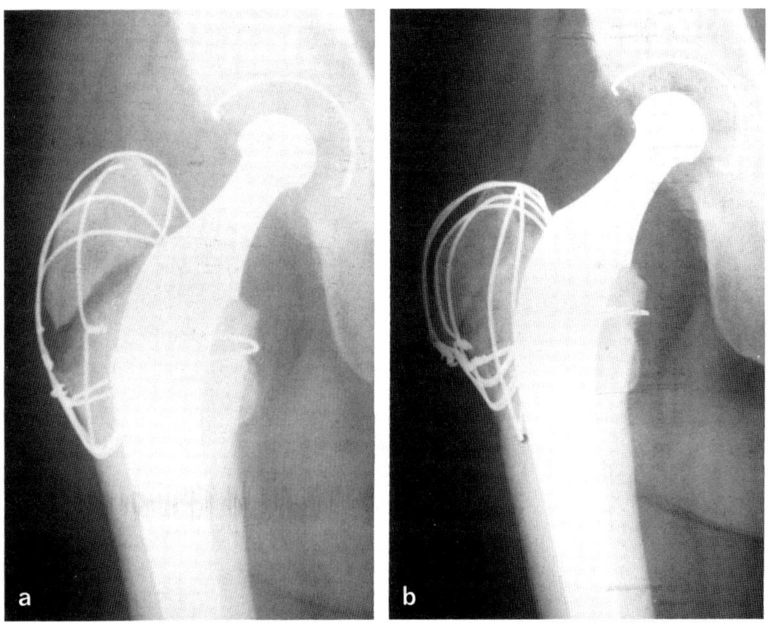

Fig. 6.7 a, b. Revision of trochanteric fixation using metal wires

mm. glutei, which cannot easily be restored to their normal length. A careful dissection of their anterior and posterior borders is necessary.
The surfaces of the osteotomy must be freshly prepared to ensure good bony apposition. We sometimes add a graft of cancellous bone to improve contact. The new wires cannot, of course, follow the same tracks, since the prosthesis is already in place. After a few attempts, we usually manage to pass two wires, one on each side of the prosthesis along drill holes, and one or two wires under the neck of the prosthesis that are tightened over the lateral surface of the trochanter (Figs. 6.6 and 6.7). This arrangement seems to provide firm fixation. Nevertheless, the patients remain in bed in traction for 2-3 weeks to reduce the stress on the trochanter and to allow consolidation to begin.

Results of the Revisions

Twenty-one revisions have been carried out in the department over 10 years.
Radiologically, the results are rather deceptive. Of the 21 revisions, 11 consolidated while ten were unsuccessful. The time at which the revision was carried out seems to be important. When revision was done within 3 months of the initial procedure, eight succeeded and three failed. When it was performed after 3 months there were 3 successes and 7 failures.
There is no doubt that the trochanter becomes retracted higher and the bony surfaces become more sclerotic the longer one delays. Therefore, we now revise the trochanterotomy as soon as nonunion has been diagnosed. For a long time we did not carry out early revisions because of the fear of introducing infection. However, there is only one case in which revision of the trochanterotomy could be implicated as a cause of sepsis.
Functionally, the results are better following revision. There was very good function in all cases where the trochanter consolidated. Of the ten failures of radiological union, four had a good functional result. Thus, there are finally six failures where patients have a poor functional result.

6.2.3 Conclusions

The unacceptably high failure rate stimulated us to look for another method of reattaching the trochanter. For all revisions over the past 2 years we have used a hook designed by Geneste and intended to prevent proximal migration of Küntscher nails. With slight modification, it hooks over the trochanter and holds it well. With the aid of a sagittal wire passing under the neck, this provides solid fixation that has resulted in consolidation in the six cases in which it has been used to date (Fig. 6.8). A modification of this design, in which the hook has been enlarged, is now in production.

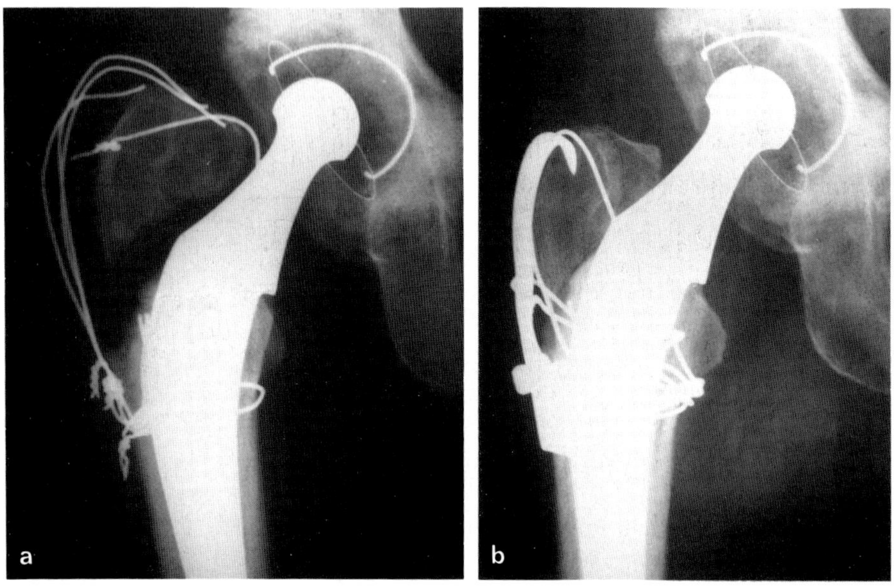

Fig. 6.8 a, b. Revision of trochanteric fixation by means of a lateral plate

6.3 Dislocation Following Total Hip Replacement

T. Arama and M. Postel

Dislocation following total hip replacement is a rare but always unfortunate complication, for which there is sometimes no satisfactory solution.

This study is based on two series. The first consists of 82 dislocations that occurred among the total hip replacements carried out in our department between 1970 and 1980. We shall consider only those protheses that dislocated and will see if they have any predisposing factors in common. The second is a series of 1300 prostheses made up of the different types described at the beginning of this book. By comparing those prostheses that dislocated with those that did not, we will see if there are any underlying etiological factors.

The incidence of dislocation is 1.7% among the hips operated upon over this period. This is greater than that in the series published by Charnley [1] in 1974 (0.7%), and less than that in the more recent publication by Picault et al. [2] in 1980 (4%).

6.3.1 Time of Occurrence and Types

Dislocation may occur at any time, but it most frequently presents before the 2nd month (50% of cases) or between 6 months and 1 year (one-third of cases). The first peak occurs early on, when there is little fibrosis around the hip and poor muscular control. The second peak incidence of dislocation is associated with a return to active life and no restriction on movement.

Two-thirds of dislocations are not recurrent and these are frequently those that occur early. One-third occur late and are occasionally preceded by signs of subluxation, noticed by the patient as a click. Dislocation may even occur very late - in one instance it presented after 8 years.

Nine of ten dislocations are posterior and the hip is then held in internal rotation. The few anterior dislocations presented in external rotation.

6.3.2 Predisposing Factors

The age and sex of the patients are not of significance, being the same in the group which dislocated as in the overall population. However, the following factors are more important.

There is no association with the underlying hip pathology, except when prostheses were implanted for a high congenital dislocation, and in fact, it is the difficult surgery involved in these cases, rather than the underlying condition, that is to blame.

The posterior approach of Moore may cause muscular imbalance to the advantage of internal rotators and will not forgive the slightest error in orientation.

Postoperative care and management played no role, except when there was failure of fixation of the trochanter.

Previously uncomplicated surgery did not predispose to dislocation. However, revision of total arthroplasty gave a slightly increased incidence of dislocation (3%).

Finally, trauma is occasionally blamed by the patients. This was seen in only one of ten cases and, with the exception of severe injury, it is seldom implicated.

6.3.3 The Mechanism of Dislocation

Three factors may be involved - poor orientation of the components, nonunion of the greater trochanter, and the "cam" effect.

Errors in Orientation. Orientation is not always easy to assess, although it is of great importance. The operation notes are often of little help. When an error in orientation has occurred the surgeon is unaware of it, and so, naturally, it has not been recorded. Throughout this series, the cup has only one metal marker that passes over its apex and which does not allow its position to be assessed on a simple AP radiograph. The more recent introduction of a circumferential marker has certainly helped in this respect, but this also requires other views which are not available in all cases. A technique for measuring the position of the components is described later.

It is difficult to define the ideal orientation exactly. However, we feel that the sum of the anteversion of both components should optimally be 20°, the cup and femoral component each contributing 10°.

Nonunion of the Greater Trochanter. This alone can lead to dislocation owing to the instability produced by muscle imbalance. Nonunion is found in 10% of dislocations (although it may also occur, of course, in the absence of dislocation). Six of the eight nonunions associated with dislocation have since undergone further surgery. In three cases consolidation was later achieved and no further dislocation occurred. The trochanter did not unite in three cases and dislocation recurred.

The "Cam" Effect. This is caused by an unyielding projection that extends in front of the anterior margin of the acetabulum. The neck of the femoral component impinges on this at the beginning of internal rotation and the head is thus levered posteriorly out of the cup.

These abnormal anterior projections may be bony or fibrous, such as an anterior osteophyte that has not been resected, a region of postoperative ossification, or very sclerotic scar tissue. Whatever their nature, it is usually impossible to demonstrate these ridges radiologically. We have seen them on three occasions when they were discovered during surgery and their removal effected a cure.

In practice, however, none of these underlying causes occurring in isolation can be implicated in three of four dislocations. Occasionally, the reasons for dislocation lie in the combination of several factors, each of which is present to a small degree. Thus, for example, on revising a Moore prosthesis implanted by the posterior approach, the external rotators are often of poor quality, and there is an imbalance between the external and internal rotators to the advantage of the latter. Each may not be serious by itself. If a total arthroplasty is then implanted with slightly inadequate anteversion of one or both components, this small error, which would have been tolerated in isolation, may combine with the above imbalance and result in dislocation. A similar though less obvious vulnerability may exist in obese patients with weak muscles, which become unbalanced as a result of the operative approach and are also poorly controlled. These patients would probably benefit from a course of intense physiotherapy to improve coordination.

6.3.4 *Treatment*

The treatment of a dislocated hip is always initially conservative, with reduction under general anesthesia. Strong traction on an orthopedic table is sometimes needed. This failed on three occasions, and open reduction was required. We treat an initial dislocation that occurs very early in the postoperative period by traction and hope that better scarring will develop posteriorly. The remainder are treated by skin traction for 24 h, which protects the stability of the hip until full muscle control is regained. We do not extend our treatment beyond this, as the majority of early dislocations do not recur.

In the case of a second dislocation, we measure the precise orientation of the components. The discovery of a significant abnormality provides a strong argument for surgery, which then has a high chance of success. Reoperation is more equivocal when no definite cause can be found, but if the frequency of redislocation is high, one may be pushed towards surgery in the hope of finding a treatable situation.

Obviously, the results of reoperation are to a large extent related to the causes of the dislocation and to whether any treatment has been possible. Of the 11 patients with malorientations that were diagnosed and revised, nine have had no recurrence while two suffered dislocation on the following day. The dislocations following detachment of the greater trochanter were always cured if consolidation was achieved. Excision of an anterior ridge that was producing a levering or cam effect always resulted in a cure.

The results were much poorer, on the other hand, when no underlying cause was found. Two cases of lowering of the greater trochanter and one involving reconstruction of the soft tissue posteriorly were not successful. In two instances the anteversion of the components was increased, even though their orientation was apparently correct, and no further dislocation occurred.

Fig. 6.10. Measurement of anteversion of a cup with a half-ring ▷ marker over the meridian

Roentgenograms required:
- Supine AP view of pelvis centered at the level of the joints
- Lateral view of the pelvis with the patient standing, the prosthesis being nearest to the plate

Radiographic measurements: On the *supine AP* view of the pelvis:
- The vertical is the line at 90° to the horizontal (taken to be a line joining two symmetrical points on the pelvis)
- The axis of the cup is the line joining the pole of the cup to the center of the prosthesis
- The pole of the cup is the tangential point on the meridian half-ring marker of a line that is parallel to the diameter of the cup

On the *lateral view* of the pelvis:
- The true vertical of the roentgenogram
- The axis of the cup, determined as above

Trigonometric result:
- The relationship of the angles made by the axis of the prosthesis to the vertical on the AP view (F), and to the vertical on the lateral vies (S) gives a geometric definition of the orientation of the cup
- The cup is anteverted if its axis faces down and forward and retroverted if it is directed down and backward on the lateral view

Comments: This technique allows cup anteversion to be measured to within 5°. If there are bilateral prostheses, the lateral standing view should be taken with the beam directed downward at an angle of 5°

Fig. 6.9. Measurement of anteversion of a cup with a ▷ marker ring around the equator

Roentgenograms required:
- AP view of pelvis, supine
- AP view of prosthesis, centered on hip

Radiographic measurements: Long axis *(D)* and short axis *(d)* of the equatorial marker ring

Results: Comparison of projected outline of the equatorial marker ring on roentgenograms of the pelvis and the hip enables degree of anteversion or retroversion of the cup to be determined
- Anteversion: (*d*) is shorter on AP view of the pelvis than on that centered on the hip
- Neutral: (*d*) is zero on AP view of the hip
- Retroversion: (*d*) is greater on AP view of the pelvis than on that centered on the hip

Tangent $\hat{A} = \frac{d}{D}$

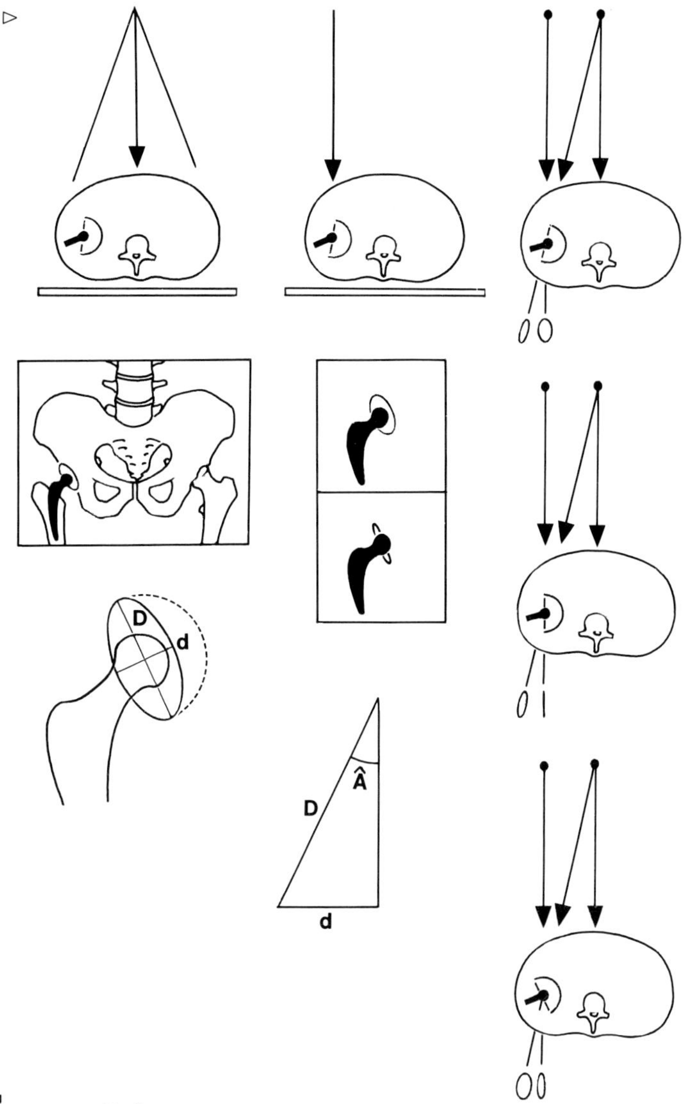

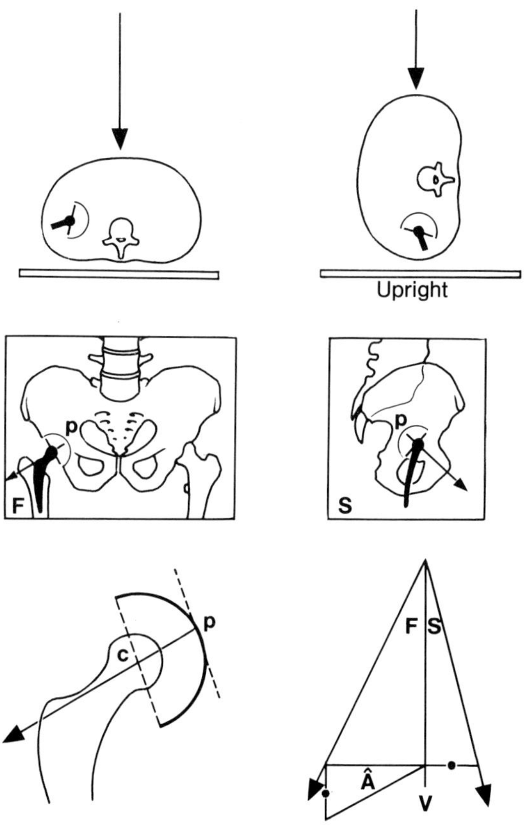

References

1. Charnley J (1979) Low-friction arthroplasty of the hip. Springer, Berlin Heidelberg New York
2. Picault C, Michel CR, Vidil R (1980) Prothèses totales de hanche de Charnley. Rev Chir Orthop 66: 57–67

6.4 Radiological Methods of Assessing the Orientation of the Components

A. Chevrot and G. Pallardy*

Measurement of the angles of the components of a total hip prosthesis have led to several interesting studies, especially concerning the Charnley-Müller

* Service de Radiologie "B" du Pr. G. Pallardy, Hôpital Cochin; 27, rue du Faubourg Saint-Jacques, F-75674 Paris Cedex 14

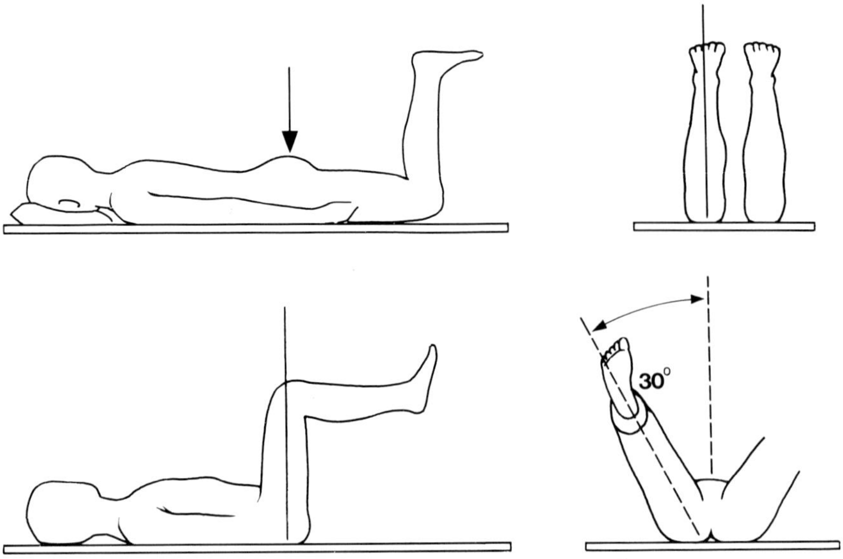

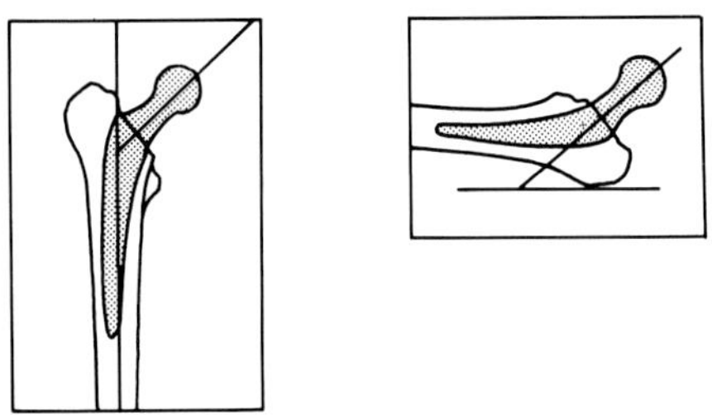

Fig. 6.11. Measurement of femoral anteversion by Dunlap-Ryder method

Roentgenograms required:
- PA view of the hip with the lower limb in zero rotation
- Lateral view of the hip in 30° of abduction using the Ducroquet view

Radiographic measurement: The cervicodiaphyseal angle and the angle of femoral anteversion can be measured directly from the roentgenograms

Results: Direct measurements are corrected using the Dunlap-Ryder table

prosthesis [11, 14]. A method using the radiopaque marker ring around or parallel to the equator of the cup has been published [9]. The Charnley prosthesis has a half-ring marker around the "meridian" and this makes the measurement of anteversion more difficult. There are also the more classical methods to determine the orientation of the femoral component.

6.4.1 *Assessment of a Cup with a Metal Ring Around or Parallel to the Equator*

An AP view of the pelvis in the supine position shows the ring as an elipse, with its long axis lying obliquely from above and facing outward (Fig. 6.9).
The tilt or degree of opening of the cup is shown by the angle that the long axis of this elipse makes with the horizontal. This usually approximates 45°. The degree of anteversion can be assessed by relating the long and the short axes of the elipse. However, one must make sure that the cup is anteverted and not retroverted. If the short axis of the elipse is longer on the AP view of the pelvis centered over the hip than on the AP view of the whole pelvis, then the cup is anteverted, and vice versa.
We do not use the method described by Gehlman [8] but prefer instead that of Goergen and Resnick [9] which makes use of how the radiograph has been centered. This can be applied to all cups with markers around or parallel to the equator.

6.4.2 *Assessment of a Cup with a Marker Around the Meridian*

The Charnley prosthesis has half a ring around the meridian whose ends are curved inward to define the diameter of the cup.
The pole P of the cup can be geometrically determined on the roentgenogram and is the tangential point on the meridian half ring of a line that is parallel to the diameter of the cup. The axis of the cup is the straight line that joins the pole to the mid-point of the diameter of the cup. On the AP view of the pelvis we

Angle of anteversion / Angle of inclination	5	10	15	20	25	30	35	40	45	50	55	60	65	70	75	80
100	1 101	9 100	15 100	20 100	25 100	30 98	35 99	40 98	45 97	50 96	55 95	60 94	65 94	70 93	75 92	80 91
105	5 106	9 105	15 104	20 101	25 103	31 103	35 103	41 100	45 100	51 99	56 98	60 97	65 96	70 95	75 94	80 92
110	5 110	10 110	16 109	21 108	27 108	32 106	30 100	42 105	47 104	52 103	56 102	61 99	66 98	71 97	76 95	80 93
115	5 115	10 115	10 114	21 118	27 118	32 111	37 110	43 109	48 107	52 105	57 104	62 102	67 101	71 99	76 96	81 94
120	6 120	11 119	16 118	22 117	28 116	33 115	38 114	44 112	49 110	53 108	58 106	62 104	68 103	72 101	77 98	81 95
125	6 126	11 124	17 123	23 121	28 120	34 119	39 118	44 110	50 114	54 112	58 109	63 107	68 105	72 103	77 100	81 96
130	6 130	12 129	18 127	24 126	29 125	35 124	40 123	46 120	51 117	55 116	60 112	64 109	69 107	73 104	78 101	82 96
135	7 135	13 133	19 132	25 131	31 130	36 129	42 126	47 124	52 120	56 118	61 114	65 112	70 109	74 105	78 102	83 98
140	7 139	13 138	20 137	27 133	32 131	38 132	44 130	49 127	53 124	58 120	63 117	67 114	71 111	75 107	79 103	83 100
145	8 144	14 142	21 141	28 139	34 138	40 136	45 134	50 131	55 128	59 124	64 120	68 117	72 114	76 110	79 104	83 98
150	8 149	15 146	23 146	29 141	35 143	42 141	47 138	52 130	56 134	61 129	65 124	69 120	73 116	76 112	80 105	84 100
155	9 164	17 152	24 151	32 140	38 148	44 145	50 142	54 130	58 137	63 132	67 128	71 124	74 119	77 115	81 108	84 102
160	10 169	18 153	27 157	34 155	44 153	46 151	52 147	67 144	61 141	65 134	69 132	73 128	76 122	79 116	82 111	86 103
165	13 164	23 164	33 161	40 159	47 158	53 156	57 153	62 148	67 141	68 140	73 135	76 130	78 122	81 119	83 113	86 106
170	15 169	27 167	37 166	40 164	53 163	58 159	63 157	67 154	70 150	73 145	76 142	78 134	80 130	83 122	85 118	87 113

can thus measure the angle F that the axis of the cup makes with the vertical (defined as the perpendicular to a line joining two symmetrical points on the pelvis, i.e., the ischial tuberosities).

This geometrical approach requires a projection of the prosthesis in a plane at right angles to the AP view of the pelvis, and for this we need a true lateral of the pelvis. The difficulty in defining the vertical plane (in both lateral and AP views at the same time) led us to suggest taking a strict lateral view of the pelvis while the patient is standing to enable use of the true vertical on the roentgenogram with reference to the AP view.

One can therefore determine the angle S (sagittal) that the axis of the cup makes with this vertical plane (Fig. 6.10). The degree of anteversion and tilt of the cup are given by comparing the angles F and S taken from the AP and lateral standing views of the pelvis. The amount of anteversion can be calculated either geometrically or trigonometrically or by reference to a table giving anteversion as a function of F and S (Table 6.3). We have devised a computer program from this trigonometric method.

6.4.3 Measurement of Anteversion of the Neck of the Femoral Prosthesis

Routine methods for measurement of anteversion of the neck of the femur are applicable to the femoral component. Where the hip can be flexed to 90°, we prefer the Dunlap-Ryder method (Fig. 6.11).

We use the Magilligan method (Fig. 6.12) when the hip has limited mobility. These two methods give us the angle between the neck and the diaphysis, which is not exactly the angle of the prosthesis because of the variable positioning of the prosthetic stem within the diaphysis.

Table 6.3. Table for calculating angle of anteversion of cup from angles F (taken from AP view of pelvis) and S (from lateral standing view). If axis PO is directed from above downward and from front to back on lateral standing view (i.e., if angle S is negative), then cup is retroverted

	0	10	20	30	40	50	60	70	80	90
0	0	0	0	0	0	0	0	0	0	0
10	90	45°	25°	15°	10°	8°	6°	4°	2°	0°
20	90	65°	45°	30°	20°	17°	12°	7°	4°	0°
30	90	70°	50°	45°	35°	25°	18°	12°	6°	0°
40	90	75°	60°	55°	45°	35°	25°	17°	8°	0°
50	90	80°	70°	65°	55°	45°	35°	25°	12°	0°
60	90	85°	75°	70°	65°	55°	45°	35°	17°	0°

Values have been rounded off to next highest

References

1. Bard M, Bernageau J, Djian A, Frot B, Massare C (1976) Examen radiologique d'une prothèse totale de hanche. J Radiol 57: 109-133
2. Beauvallet JP, Lord B, Marotte JH, Goutard LE, Elberg JF (1974) Contribution à l'étude radiologique des prothèses totales de hanche. Rev Chir Orthop 60: 4181-4232
3. Chanzy M, Brun M, Balmary G, Honnart F (1978) Les complications mécaniques des prothèses totales de hanche: Cah Reeduc Readapt Fonct 13: 175-182
4. Charnley J (1979) Low-friction arthroplasty of the hip. Springer, Berlin Heidelberg New York
5. Chevrot A, Najman G (1983) Les prothèses de type Charnley. Technique radiologique des mesures angulaires de la pièce cotyloïdienne. Rev. Chir Orthop 69: 483-485
6. Chevrot A, Najman G, Nicolas P, Bicharzon P (1983) Les aspects radiologiques normaux d'une prothèse totale de hanche scellée. J Radiol 64/11: 603-606
7. Dufour M, Abignoly AM, Chiousse E (1979) Radiographie des prothèses de hanche. Concours Med 101: 1947-1964
8. Duparc J, Frot B, Leroy P (1980) Méthode d'étude radiologique des prothèses totales scellées de hanche. In: Lequesne M, Massare C (eds) Maladie de la hanche. Vième Réunion Annuelle du GETROA. Laboratoires Ciba-Geigy, Wehr, pp 131-138

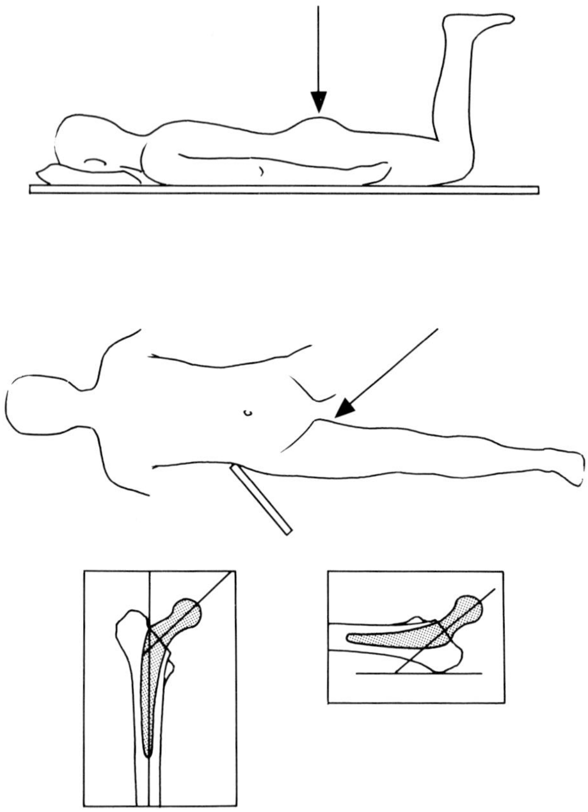

β↓	a→	80°	70°	60°	50°	45°	40°	30°	20°	10°
10°		10	11	12	13	14	15	19	27	46
15°		15	16	17	19	20	22	27	37	55
20°		20	21	23	25	27	29	36	47	64
25°		25	26	27	31	33	36	43	53	69
30°		30	31	34	37	39	42	49	60	73
35°		35	36	39	42	45	48	55	64	76
40°		41	42	44	48	50	52	59	68	78
45°		46	47	49	52	55	57	64	71	80
50°		51	52	54	57	59	62	67	74	82
55°		55	56	59	62	63	66	70	76	83
60°		60	61	64	66	68	69	73	78	84
70°		70	71	73	74	76	77	79	82	86
80°		80	81	82	83	83	83	84	86	88

◁

Fig. 6.12. Measurement of femoral anteversion by Magilligan method

Roentgenograms required:
- PA view with the upper femur in zero rotation
- Lateral of the hip using Arselin's view, with no femoral rotation

Radiographic measurements:
- The projected angle of anteversion
- The complement of the cervicodiaphyseal angle

Results: Calculated from Magilligan's table

Comments: Both the Dunlap-Ryder and the Magilligan method are suitable for assessment of anteversion of the neck of the femoral component of the prosthesis

9. Ghelman B (1979) Three methods of determining anteversion and retroversion of a total hip prothesis. AJR 133: 1127-1134
10. Ghelman B (1979) Radiographic localization of the acetabular component of a hip prosthesis. Radiology 130: 540-542
11. Goergen TG, Resnick D (1975) Evaluation of acetabular anteversion following total hip arthroplasty: Necessity of proper centring. Br J Radiol 48: 259-260
12. Green DL, Bahniuk E, Liebelt RA, Fender E, Mirkov P (1983) Biplane radiographic measurements of reversible displacement (including clinical loosening) and migration of total joint replacements. J Bone Joint Surg 65/8: 1134-1143
13. Langlais F, Postel M, Kerboull M (1979) Surveillance radioclinique des prothèses totales de hanches. E.M.C. 9: 14318 F10
14. Lewinner GE, Lewis JL, Tarr R, Compere CL, Zimmerman JR (1978) Dislocations after total hip-replacement arthroplasties. J Bone Joint Surg [Am] 60: 217-220
15. Postel M (1975) Les complications des prothèses totales de hanche. Encyclopédie médico-chirurgicale, Techniques Chirurgicales, Orthopédie, Paris, 4.3.05, 44668
16. Seidel H (1979) Diagramme de mesure et de position pour l'appréciation de la mise en place des prothèses totales de hanche. Chirurgie 50: 269-271
17. Seradge H, Nagle KR, Miller RJ (1982) Analysis of version in the acetabular cup. Clin Orthop 166: 152-157
18. Vacher H, Chevrot A, Menu Y, Baillet P, Andre C, Correas G, Pallardy G (1979) Etude radiologique de la cupule cotyloïdienne de la prothèse totale de hanche de type Charnley. J Radiol Electrol 60: 147

6.5 Aseptic Loosening Among Charnley-type Prostheses

J. Courpied and M. Postel

6.5.1 Definitions

Loosening is the failure of fixation of the prosthesis. This seemingly simple definition requires an appreciation of the fact that deterioration of the arthroplasty is not always associated with a similar change in function of the hip.

Table 6.4. Radiological abnormalities associated with Charnley-type prostheses

Acetabular signs	Femoral signs
1. No abnormality	1. No abnormality
2. Nonprogressive lucent zone	2. Localized, nonprogressive space between cement and prosthesis
3. Progressive lucent zone	3. Progressive space between cement and prosthesis
4. Change in position of cup	4. Change at bone-cement interface

What are the different features of the abnormalities seen on roentgenograms?

Abnormalities of acetabular fixation always arise at the cement-bone interface and never between prosthesis and cement in a prosthesis of this type. A clear space around the cup is the usual abnormality, and sclerosis or cysts are exceptional. This lucent zone reflects a poor bone-cement junction, which may be present from the outset and be of no significance or may appear secondarily and become progressive. It may also vary according to the angle of incidence of the roentgenogram. Therefore, it is the progression of the lucency, rather than its extent, thickness, or position that is considered significant. This assumes that roentgenograms taken at regular intervals are available. The radiological features of acetabular fixation can be classified into four groups (see Table 6.4), ranging from a perfect picture to one where a change in the position of the cup denotes obvious loosening, although this may not have been symptomatic initially. Nonprogressive lucent zones do not produce symptoms. They are usually localized and correspond to a similarly localized defect in the preparation of the acetabulum.

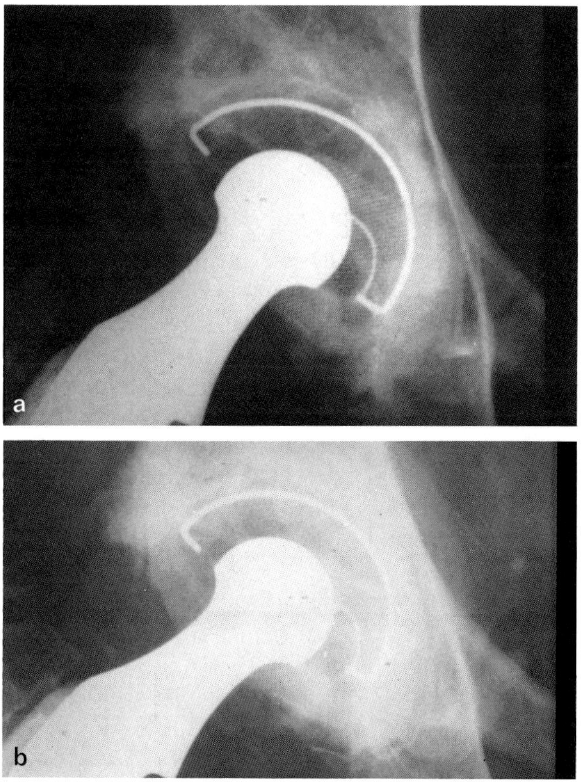

Fig. 6.13. a Operation in 1970, with good acetabular fixation. **b** Thirteen years later there is an extensive lucent area; this hip is not completely pain free and this lucent area is considered significant

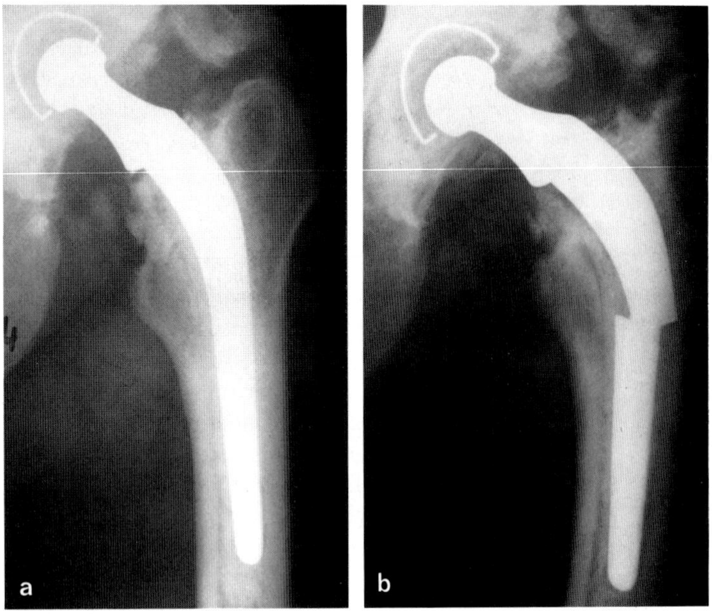

Fig. 6.14. Arthroplasty where the femoral component is aligned down the axis but is too small: **a** At 4 years there is a lucent zone between the cement and the prosthesis, with a slight tilt into varus. **b** At 6 years, it appears to be a rupture of the stem by flexion owing to the mobility of the upper part, while the lower part is firmly fixed in the cement

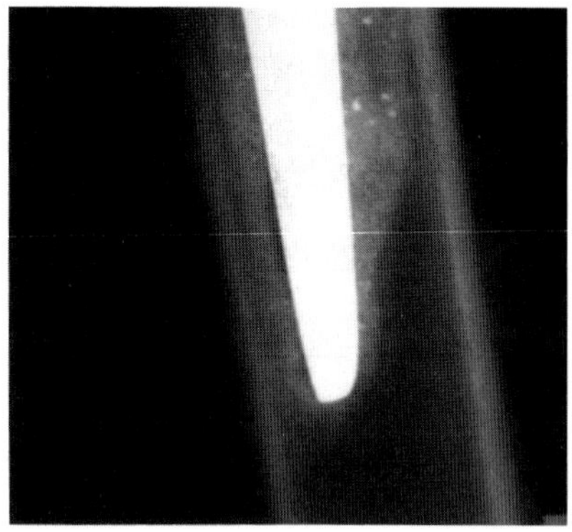

Fig. 6.15. The change at the bone-cement interface is a lucent area produced by medullary remodeling at the distal end of the cement

Lucent areas that progress are much more worrying, and if they are associated with a deterioration in function then loosening is certain, even if the position of the cup remains unchanged (Fig. 6.13).

The oblique obturator and iliac views which are so useful in the assessment of the resultant bony damage are, in practice, of little value in the diagnosis of loosening. This is because they are not taken routinely and therefore cannot show the progression of radiological abnormalities.

The study of femoral abnormalities is more complex, as these may arise in two situations: at the bone-cement interface or between the cement and the prosthesis. There are four types of femoral fixation (Table 6.4), ranging from a perfect picture, over a progressive or nonprogressive lucent zone between the cement and the prosthesis, to a lucent zone at the bone-cement interface.

Spaces between the cement sheath and the convexity of the femoral stem are associated with a slight tilt into varus and appear in the first 2 years, most frequently being localized and nonpregrossive. If they become worse, even though only gradually, true loosening will follow, with the occasional fracture of the stem of the prosthesis (Fig. 6.14).

True lucent zones at the bone-cement junction are very rare and are found only after revisions. These will be studied in a separate chapter.

False images can also be seen resulting from X-rays of variable penetration, or from medullary or cortical reactions to the prosthesis that are usually of no consequence. Medullary reactions usually present as an increase in density around the distal extremity of cement (Fig. 6.15). Cortical reaction is seen as a decrease in bony density and possible endosteal resorption, to be followed by a phase of ossification with a feathery appearance. This modification is very often associated with cortical thickening. Both these phenomena seem to be related to stresses exerted on the diaphysis (Fig. 6.16).

We have not found arthrograms to be of great help. Those that we have made have given us little additional information. In the end, it is clinical examination and repeated standard AP roentgenograms of the hip which provide the best overall interpretation of these features.

All these signs signify loosening. They may be of purely mechanical or septic origin, and it is of importance to differentiate between the two. The radiological features and their progression, together with clinical examination and laboratory investigations, will enable the distinction to be made.

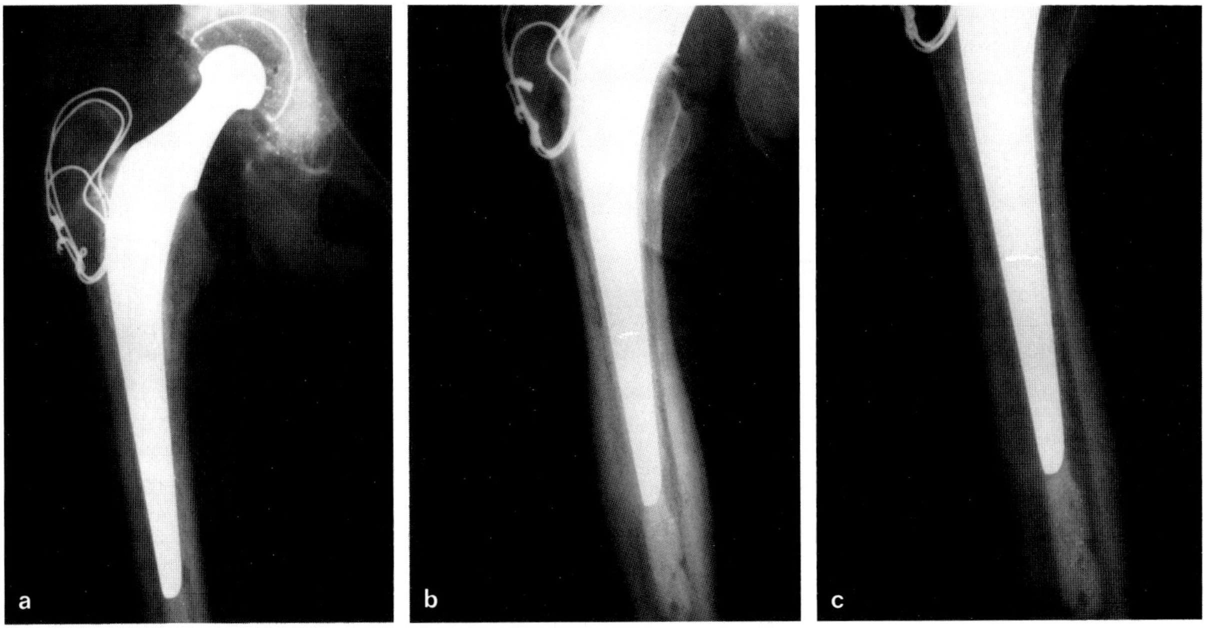

Fig. 6.16. **a** Total arthroplasty in 1976 with a well-fitting stem; thickening of the medial and lateral cortices begins after 1 year. **b** At 3 years the thickening has progressed and in addition there are endosteal changes that remain unchanged in 1982 (**c**). This does not represent an empty space, as a network of bone can be seen, but is undoubtedly a bony reaction to the prosthesis

6.5.2 Radiological Abnormalities Occurring in Our Series

Following the definitions that we have described above, we have studied problems of fixation among 1031 Charnley or modified Charnley prostheses implanted between 1970 and 1980. Among these, 806 are known to be aseptic (325 Charnley and 481 Charnley-Kerboul), 182 having been followed up for 10 years or more. The other patients either had a shorter follow-up or have died.

There were six loose cups; this represents 0.7% of those cases with a known outcome. Three of these have been revised, while the others are still being relatively well tolerated.

In our study of the femoral component we shall consider the Charnley and the Charnley-Kerboul prostheses separately. Among the former there were 18 loosenings (5.5%), while there was no instance of femoral loosening among the Charnley-Kerboul prostheses, which is quite remarkable.

Problems Related to the Cup

There were six loosenings, and in 11 cases we found progressive localized lucency at the bone-cement junction. All the abnormalities occurred early, presenting during the first 4 years postoperatively. Clinical symptoms were few. The average pain score among those that were loose was 4, two patients being asymptomatic. Among those with a lucent area at the cement-bone interface eight were completely asymptomatic, while the three others in whom the lucency was more marked had a pain score of 5. Thus, if we consider those three cases with some pain as probable loosenings over the long term, we have a total of nine failures of cup fixation (1.1%).

We have looked for factors that might explain these problems with the cup. The characteristics of the cup itself are probably not to blame, given the very low rate of cup loosening. The lucent zones are more common in arthroplasties carried out for juvenile or infantile arthritis, as mentioned earlier. The age and weight of the patient and the range of movement of the prosthetic hip do not have a significant influence. Wear of the cup, to be covered in another chapter, does not seem to be a factor in producing acetabular loosening over the period of follow-up available to us. On the other hand, there are two technical points that are most important - the preparation of the acetabulum and the exact position in which the cup is cemented. We have already described how the acetabulum should be prepared. When we try to cement a cup into hard, sclerotic, unreactive bone, where the cement penetrates poorly or where there are no effective keying areas, the immediate postoperative roentgenogram will often show an extensive lucent zone, and this is a poor prognostic sign. We have 35 cases of this typs, and among them are four of the six loosenings in our series.

The position in which the cup is finally cemented also seems to play an important role. If it is too high and too lateral, the risk of loosening is considerably increased. There was only one loosening among the 600 cups in a good position, while among the 200 that were badly placed, five became loose. This may be due to an alteration in the forces acting on the hip during walking, or it may simply result from bad fixation within a bony cavity that is too small and the use of too much cement, together with grossly inadequate keying points.

In conclusion, the reasons for the loosening of the six cups are divided between poor preparation of the bony cavity and poor positioning of the cup – two of the six cases having both these faults. On the other hand, those arthroplasties in which there were no technical errors on the acetabular side did not develop any abnormalities of fixation of the cup throughout their follow-up (500 of the 800 arthroplasties).

Study of Femoral Fixation

For the *Charnley prostheses,* excluding all revisions, there were 325 aseptic arthroplasties with known follow-up among the 500 prostheses carried out in 1970–1971. Three hundred have been followed up for more than 5 years and 175 for more than 10 years.

Spaces between the cement and prosthesis appeared early in 25% of cases and remained nonprogressive in 16% of cases. In 12 they progressed slowly (3.7%) and were therefore a cause for concern. They resulted in loosening in 17 cases (5.2%), requiring ten further operations, six of which were for fracture of the femoral stem.

Table 6.5. Radiological abnormalities associated with femoral components of Charnley-type prostheses

Type of arthroplasty (primary)	Nonprogressive lucency at cement-prosthesis interface	Progressive lucency at cement-prosthesis interface	Loosening (within cement)	Abnormality at bone-cement junction
Charnley (325)	54 (16%)	12 (3.7%)	17 (5.2%)	3 (0.9%)
Charnley-Kerboul (481)	5 (1%)	0	0	9 (1.8%)
Well-fitting femoral component (350)	0	0	0	9 (2.5%)

Finally, and very rarely, abnormalities appeared at the cement-bone interface (0.9%; Table 6.5).

In our study of the underlying causes of these femoral loosenings the following factors did not seem to be significant: the type of arthropathy and the underlying pathology, the relation of the lever arms in Pauwel's equilibrium after arthroplasty, whether the prosthesis was supported against the calcar or not, the length of femoral neck left after resection, or even the amount of residual neck that was subsequently resorbed (this is a factor that we shall cover together with wear of the cup in another chapter).

The positioning and fit of the femoral stem in relation to the diaphysis is a factor of cardinal importance. Loosening is much more frequent if the stem is in varus (nine of 127 cases), although a femoral component positioned in valgus or along the axis of the diaphysis will not be immune from loosening within the cement (eight of 198 cases).

When the femoral component was introduced into the diaphysis as a tight fit, its size being close to that of the medullary canal, there was neither any loosening nor any space between the cement and the prosthesis. We have 25 cases of this type among this series of Charnley prostheses.

The femoral problems of the *Charnley-Kerboul prosthesis* are studied in connection with our group of 700 prosthesis. There are 481 primary arthroplasties with no sepsis, 250 of which have been followed up for more than 5 years.

There has been no femoral loosening. Overall, the femoral component fits the diaphysis much more closely than with the Charnley prosthesis. However, in a few cases the fit is not perfect, and among these there are several localized nonprogressive lucent zones between the cement and the prosthesis. These represent 1% of the whole series.

In 1.8% of cases we noted changes at the cement-bone interface, while this occurred in only 0.9% of the Charnley prosthesis. This tendency was even more marked when we considered only those femoral components where the stem was a good fit within the diaphysis among both Charnley and Charnley-Kerboul prostheses. In 350 such cases there was no loosening, and no problems were seen at the interface between the cement and prosthesis, but in nine cases there were changes at the bone-cement junction (2.5% of cases) which have remained completely asymptomatic up to the present (Table 6.6).

As previously mentioned when we defined the radio-

Table 6.6. Diaphyseal changes in Charnley-type prosthesis

Fit of femoral stem	Changes at bone-cement junction	Cortical thickening
Stem too narrow (456 THR)	0.9%	12%
Well-fitting stem (350 THR)	2.5%	25%

THR, Total hip replacement

logical features, these changes can be understood as lucent areas related to cortical remodeling. They may correspond to a restructuring of the endosteum and may be related to a change in the stresses acting on the diaphysis produced by the presence of a rigid prosthetic stem of large caliber. Cortical thickening seems to be related to the same causes (Table 6.6).

In conclusion, among the prosthesis reviewed to date we have found only a few femoral lucent areas of no significance and an incidence of less than 1% of cup loosening. These mechanical problems can be overcome if the arthroplasty is carried out using the strict technique that we have described and using a prosthesis that fits the new hip perfectly. The few diaphyseal changes that we have noticed do not seem to jeopardize femoral fixation.

7 Revision Surgery for Aseptic Loosening of Total Hip Replacement - Acetabular Reconstruction

7.1 Introduction

M. Kerboul

To consider further surgery upon a total hip arthroplasty implies that the first procedure has ended in failure. This failure is due to movement of the components relative to the bone to which they may or may not have been cemented. In the absence of infection, failure occurs for two main reasons: poor operative technique or an unsatisfactory prosthesis which has high built-in friction or whose components are poorly adapted to the bone. Failure is also often blamed on the cement or on poor bony ingrowth into the irregularities on the surface of the prosthesis. These factors are often necessarily related: they lead to functional failure as a result of movement of the components and this causes bony damage to a varying degree. To reoperate implies that one has the intention and ability to do better than on the first occasion, that one has understood the reason for the failure, and that one has the means to improve on it. If this is not so, the second procedure will be no more effective than the first because in surgery, as elsewhere, similar causes inevitably produce the same effects. One must therefore have a better prosthesis, be confident of mastering the technical problems, and have the means of correcting any bony damage, be it acetabular or femoral.
We shall now discuss the solutions that we have found to these problems and the thoughts that they have stimulated. No doubt, there are other methods of solving these problems; the solutions that we shall describe have the advantage of having been tried and shown to be effective.

7.2 Problems Related to the Acetabulum

M. Kerboul

7.2.1 The Lesions

Acetabular damage always occurs with certain prostheses, and we ourselves contributed to this, as we initially used a large number of metal-on-metal prostheses. Once the original and then the modified Charnley prostheses had become the only type of arthroplasty used at Cochin, loose cups became rarities and never resulted in severe bony destruction. Since then, such cases have come to us only from outside sources. This had enabled us to approach the problem with a lighter heart, although it has not, of course simplified the procedure.
The *surgical approach* is the first problem presented by such a multi-operated hip. This is tedious and must be by sharp dissection through dense, sclerotic tissue, with areas of ossification where the vessels and sciatic nerve may be at risk.
Removal of the Components. The extraction of a metal cup that has migrated deeply carries the risk of inflicting damage on the walls of an acetabulum that are already thin and perforated, especially if the instruments are not handled gently. However, if one is too gentle and hesitant, no progress will have been made 2 h later. Force can be used safely only when the operator is experienced and there is good exposure (one must be able to see well in front, behind, above, and below).
On the other hand, the extraction of plastic cups is always easy. They usually come away from the cement by simple traction; occasionally one may even find that a cup has migrated and is lying free in the buttock with no trace of cement on its convexity. A cup that is firmly attached to its cement can always be separated by means of a gouge. Breaking up the cement will then enable it to be removed piecemeal without exacerbating any underlying bony damage.
Extraction of uncemented cups is always a straightforward procedure. They usually come away from their

bed by gentle traction once the outer rim has been freed. They rarely resist for long. There may be a washer that has to be unscrewed and the necessary instruments must be available.

It is not uncommon to find that a cup has migrated medially and is close to, or sometimes in direct contact with the iliac vessels, which can be compromised or become ulcerated. Removal of the cup may then precipitate a dramatic hemorrhage; this possibility must be anticipated prior to surgery and one must be prepared to deal with it.

Once the prosthesis has been removed and the acetabulum has been cleared of cement and fibrous tissue, an *assessment of the damage* can be made. This damage is the result of resorption and is caused by movement of the prosthesis against the bone. In some prostheses there may also be chemical osteolysis. This is most frequently caused by particles of cement, rarely by polyethylene, occasionally by metal. Metal produces black staining of the tissues, even some distance from the joint, and can result in necrosis of the periarticular muscles.

Whatever the etiology of the acetabular damage, the medial wall is frequently perforated and all or part of the roof and the anterior and posterior walls are missing. At worst, there may be a transverse fracture through the remanants of the old acetabular cavity, which is then divided into two separate parts.

If one likes to make "classifications", these lesions can be assessed according to their size and position and arranged in different types, degrees, or stages. This is of theoretical interest only, because in the end all defects must always be repaired. All attempts to cement a cup back into a destroyed acetabulum that has not previously been reconstructed will sooner or later inevitably end in failure.

Reconstruction requires a supply of bone and the equipment with which to perform osteosynthesis. Bone can be taken as an autograft from the ipsi- or the contralateral iliac crest (so avoiding extensive detachment of the mm. glutei), or as a homograft from arthritic femoral heads that have been removed during previous total arthroplasties and that have been stored in a freezer.

In the acetabulum, a cruciate plate is used for the osteosynthesis. This provides solid fixation where there is nonunion following a transverse acetabular fracture. In other instances it can provide a metallic support for an acetabulum that has been reconstructed by bone graft. It has the added advantage of automatically recentering the hip when it is used correctly (Fig. 7.1).

7.2.2 *Technique and Indications for Acetabular Reconstruction*

In the early days we were bewildered and almost at a loss when faced with massive acetabular damage, especially where there was a transverse fracture of the acetabulum.

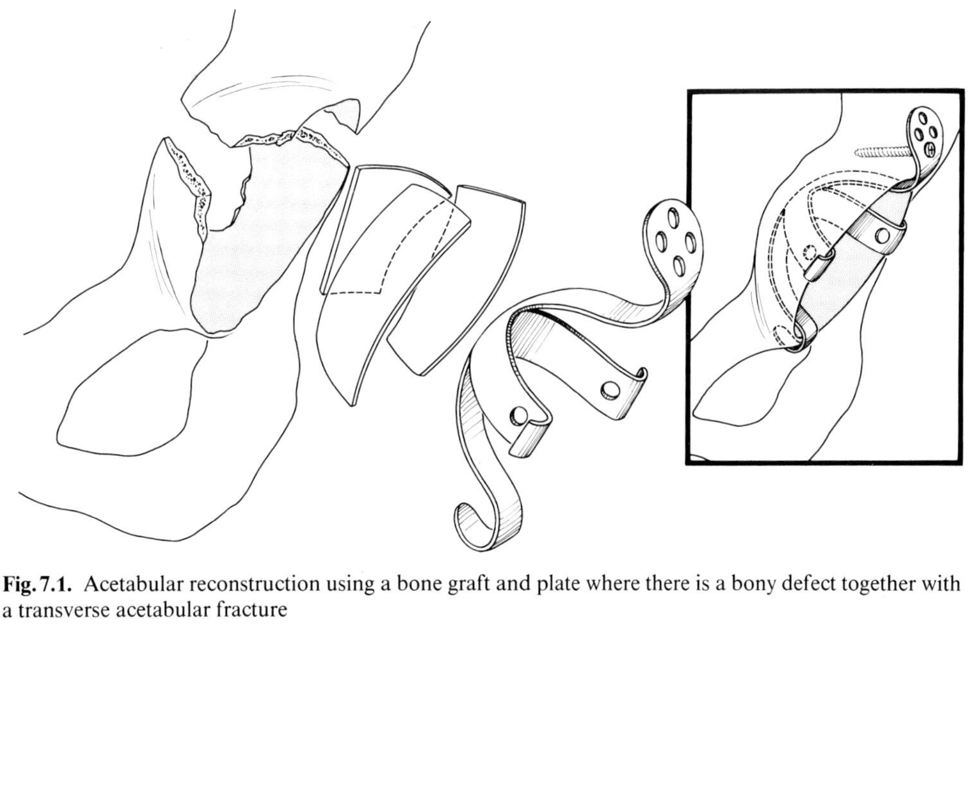

Fig. 7.1. Acetabular reconstruction using a bone graft and plate where there is a bony defect together with a transverse acetabular fracture

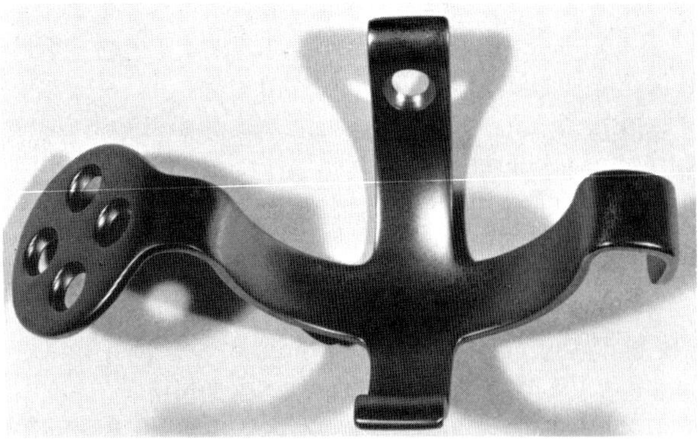

Fig. 7.2. The acetabular plate

Our first attempts, using a metal mesh to repair the defect or a screw to hold the transverse acetabular fracture, ended in complete and early failure. It took us some time to appreciate that there was only one solution to this problem: to fix the transverse acetabular fracture with a special plate and to fill the defect with bone graft. It was not until 1975 that we were able to produce a suitable plate. This had four arms and a concavity that matched the acetabulum. It was held to the inferior margin by a hook and to the iliac bone by four screws (Fig. 7.2).

This plate was first used for massive acetabular damage with a transverse fracture and an extensive bony defect caused by a sliding band prosthesis with a loose cup. We felt in advisable to carry out the acetabular reconstruction in two stages, in view of the extent of the damage. In the first stage, the old prosthesis and cement were removed and the acetabulum was reconstructed with an autogenous bone graft and a plate. Six months later, we were able to implant a new arthroplasty in an excellent anatomical environment. The reconstructed acetabulum had become perfectly solid and sound. Seven years later, the functional and radiological result remains perfect.

The use of autogenous bone brings additional complications to the operation. To take a graft from the iliac crest of the same side means that the mm. glutei have to be extensively detached, and this compromises the final stability of the hip. If the graft is taken from the opposite iliac crest the patient has to be toweled up twice, and this prolongs the procedure considerably. We had been tempted to omit the graft and to use only a plate together with a large wire mesh to prevent medial migration of the cement across the defect. In spite

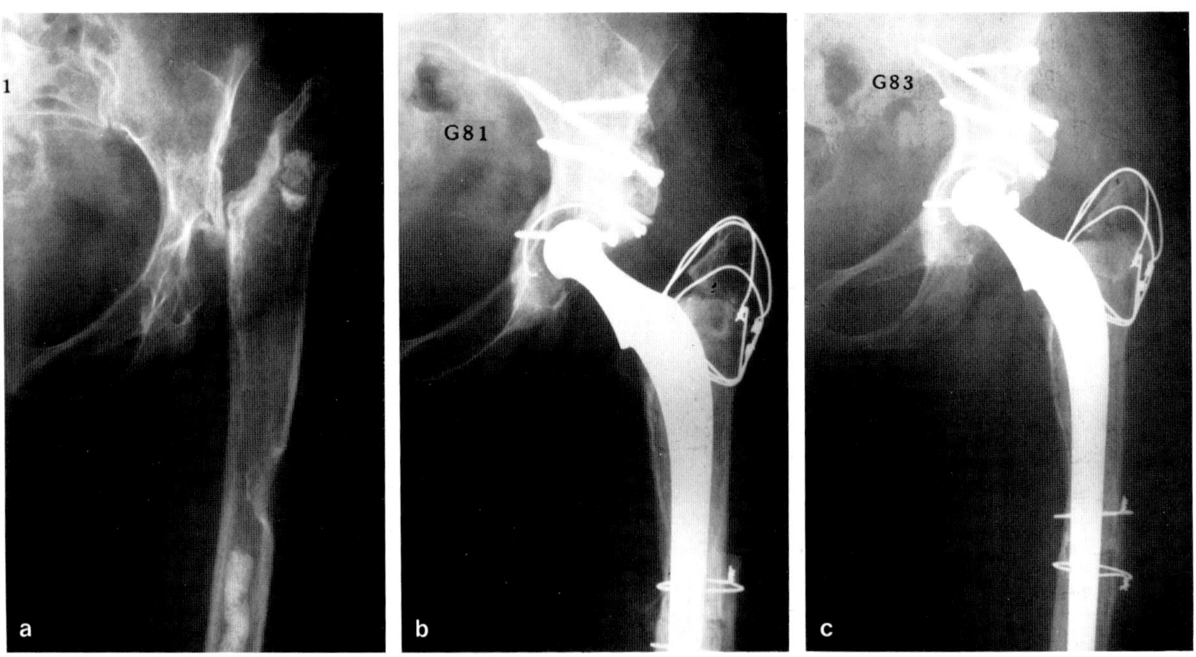

Fig. 7.3. **a** Severe acetabular damage following the repeated failure of a prosthesis in a patient with Recklinghausen's disease whose femur is 5 cm too long. **b** The result 6 months following acetabular reconstruction by homo- and autograft, together with shortening of the femur, and the implantation of a new prosthesis. **c** The grafts have been well incorporated and the femoral osteotomy has consolidated 2.5 years postoperatively

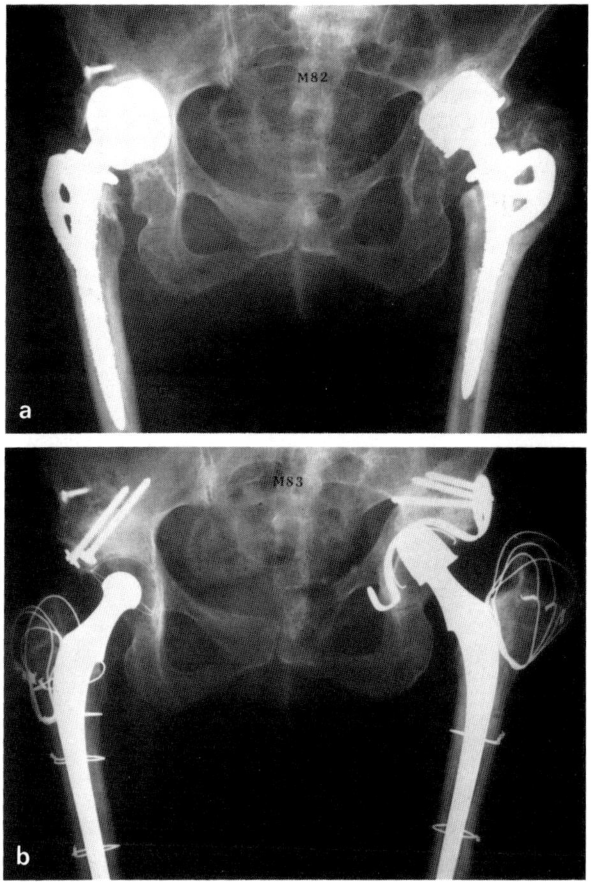

Fig. 7.4. **a** Bilateral failure of uncemented prostheses. Both cups are loose and the femoral component on the left has fractured. **b** The acetabulum has been reconstructed in the selected position by filling the superior defect with homograft. Fixation was achieved by screws on the right and by a plate on the left. Removal of the femoral components was possible only by making a large window in the cortex. The grafts have consolidated perfectly 1 year after both operations

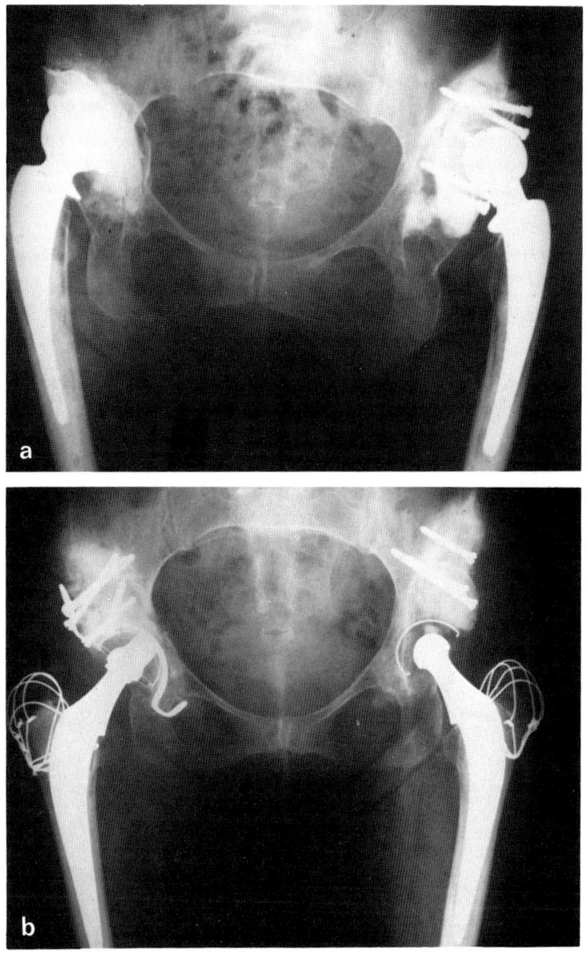

Fig. 7.5. **a** Severe bilateral acetabular destruction following failure of several prostheses. **b** Acetabular reconstruction, with a plate on the right but no plate on the left and using large amounts of homograft

of the initial impression of relatively solid cup fixation, this progressively deteriorated and resulted in failure with a fracture of the inferior arm of the plate.

Bony reconstruction is therefore absolutely essential. However, the amount of graft that it is possible to take from the iliac crest of an elderly patient will obviously be insufficient to fill a defect that is of any significant size. If the patient is young and the defect small, then bone from the iliac crest may possibly suffice.

During 1975, we began to use frozen femoral heads, most often alone, but occasionally together with fragments of autogenous bone. The femoral heads were cut into slices or shaped into larger fragments by a saw, bone cutters, or circular reamers. They could then fill defects in the walls or the roof of the acetabulum. The graft was orientated with its cancellous surface against the bone and was held in place either by screws or by the plate (Fig. 7.3).

The plate is not always necessary, especially when there is only a defect in the roof with a remaining horizontal buttress of solid bone higher up (Fig. 7.4). A large molded fragment of femoral head can be wedged under a solid rim of iliac bone and screwed into place. This may provide support that is solid enough to allow one to dispense with the metal plate.

However, the plate does give the reconstruction immediate and long-lasting rigidity by enabling the bone graft to be wedged beneath it, and by its firm fixation to the ilium by the hook located under the inferior margin of the acetabulum and the screws superiorly (Fig. 7.5).

The plate is indispensible when the defect involves the medial anterior and posterior walls and of course where there is a transverse acetabular fracture or non-union (Fig. 7.6).

When the defect is very extensive and a large quantity of graft is required, a mixture of auto- and homograft may be used.

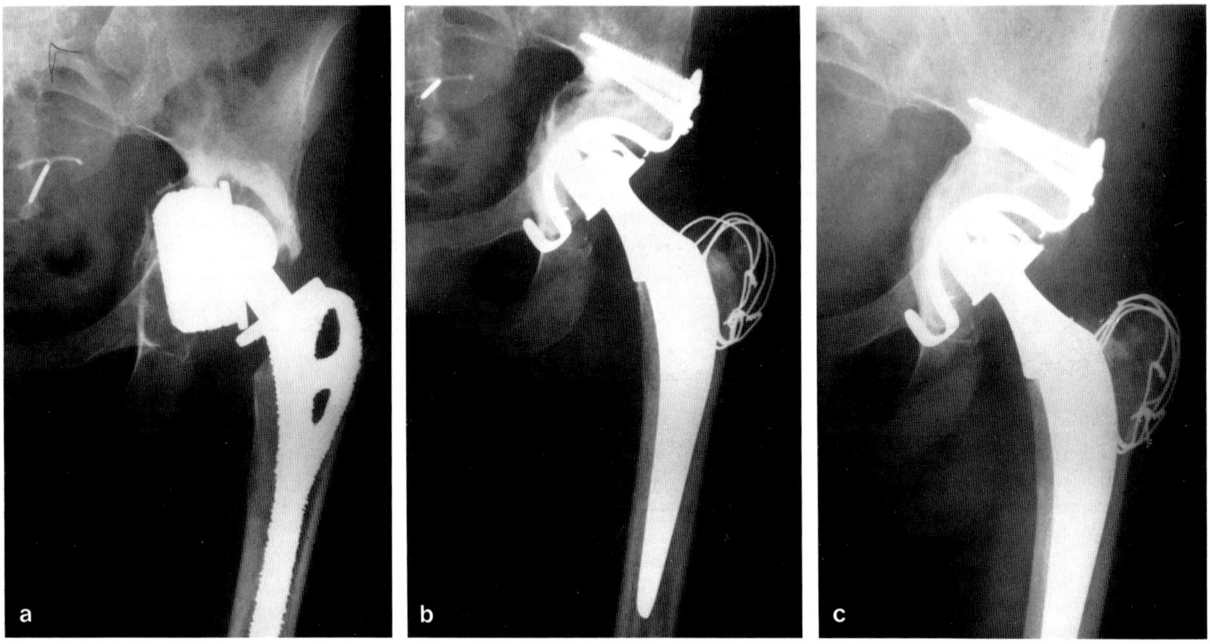

Fig. 7.6. a Failure of an uncemented prosthesis with an ununited transverse acetabular fracture and a widespread bony defect. **b** Acetabular reconstruction with homograft and plate. **c** Perfect incorporation of the grafts 3 years after surgery

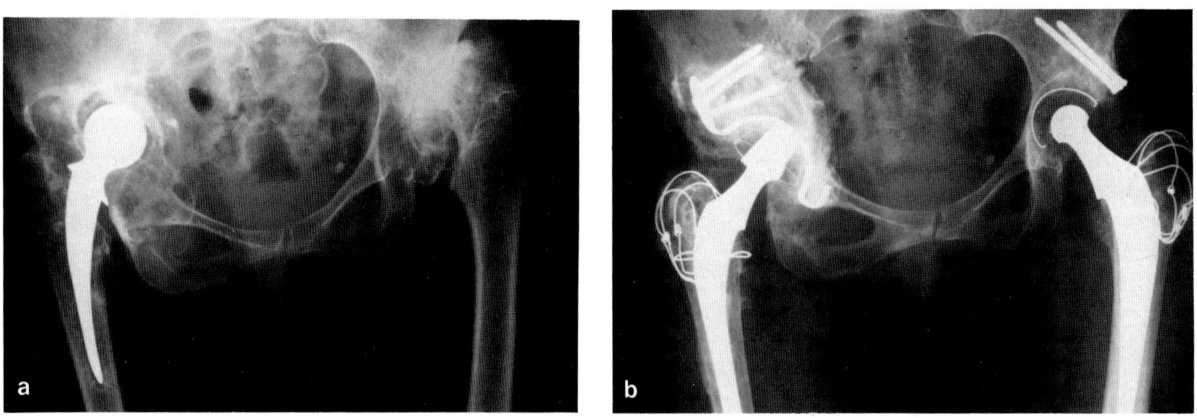

Fig. 7.7. a Massive bony defect of the right acetabulum following failure of a total arthroplasty. **b** Acetabular reconstruction using a mixture of autograft (the femoral head of the opposite side) and homograft

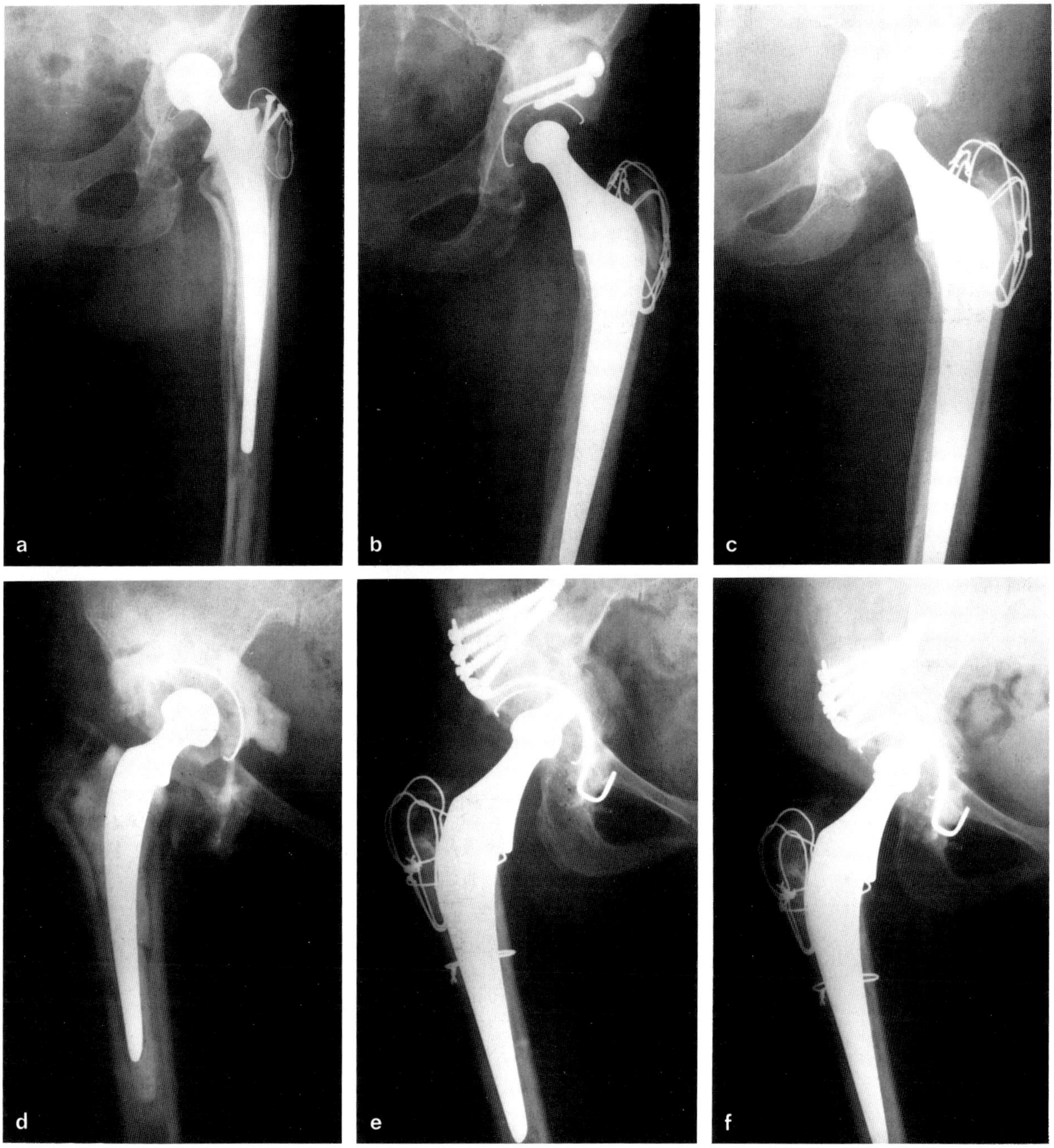

Fig. 7.8. **a** Septic loosening with serious osteolysis of the femur and extensive acetabular destruction. **b** Acetabular reconstruction using homograft and a new total arthroplasty. **c** The roentgenogram 5 years after surgery. **d** A further example of septic loosening with more extensive acetabular damage. **e** Reconstruction of the new joint, and **f** the radiological result at 2 years

In some instances autograft can be provided by an arthritic femoral head taken from the opposite side. Fragments of a femoral head that has been removed during a previous arthroplasty and stored in a deep freeze can be mixed with those of the autograft to enable extensive lesions to be repaired. Rarely, the obturator ring may be disrupted by destruction of the inferior margin of the acetabulum, and the hook then has no grip inferiorly. In this case a graft can be cut to size and wedged in between the pubis and ischium to form a support for the hook (Fig. 7.7).

The acetabulum may be grossly enlarged and weakened but have no significant perforations or gaps. It is then better to strengthen and thicken the walls with grafts and to reinforce the roof with a metal plate, rather than to implant a large cup. We were encouraged by the excellent viability of these homografts, which seemed to be rapidly incorporated into the underlying bone. We therefore extended their use to cases with possible infection where there was also gross acetabular damage, and this was equally successful. In these cases we also occasionally used a plate (Fig. 7.8). After 10 years of experience, we are still pleasantly surprised by the excellent appearance of these grafts, which seem solid and unaltered. They seem to become incorporated into weight-bearing areas, where they contribute to the integrity of the structure, although they soon become partially resorbed in other situations where an excessive amount of graft has been used unnecessarily (Fig. 7.9).

The plate does not seem to disturb the dynamics of the ilium. It is open, although rigid enough to provide an immediate firm osteosynthesis, and it remains sufficiently deformable so as not to alter the elasticity of the ilium. It is therefore perfectly suited to these acetabular reconstructions, as is shown by the quality and durability of the results. Whatever satisfaction the surgeon and patient may derive from the reconstructions, it is preferable for both to avoid these problems by reoperating on loosenings before widespread destruction can occur, and to prevent mechanical failure of the arthroplasty by using the correct technique and a prosthesis whose reliability has withstood the test of time.

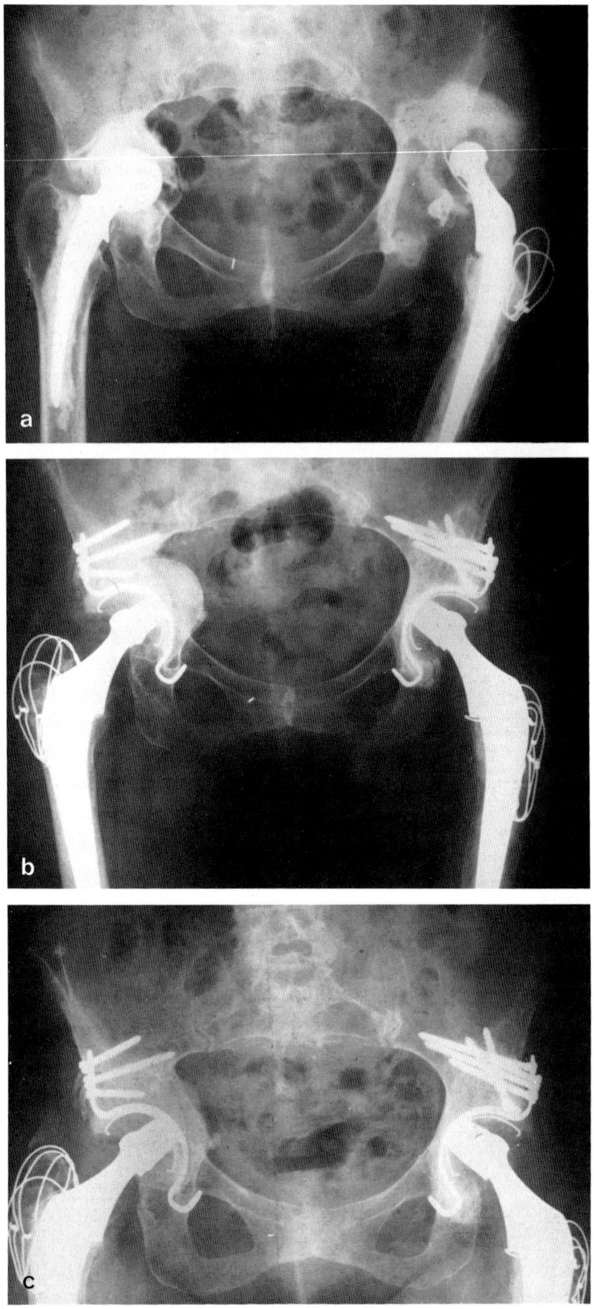

Fig. 7.9. **a** Bilateral loosening that is aseptic on the right and septic on the left. **b** Bilateral acetabular reconstruction using a homograft and plate. **c** Perfect consolidation of the grafts after 4 years; the graft on the right was unnecessarily large, and has been partially resorbed

7.3 The Femoral Stage of Total Hip Revision

M. Postel

In all revisions we have tried to be as sparing and conservative as possible regarding the femur and so to produce a reconstructed hip that resembles a routine prosthesis.

7.3.1 Revision of Cemented Prostheses – Removal of Cement

The *removal of the femoral component* after the hip has been dislocated presents no problem. The prosthesis comes out of its sheath of cement after a few sharp blows with a punch. However, if the femur is very fragile, one must take care that all force is accurately transmitted along the axis of the femur.

Removal of the Cement. When the prosthesis is definitely not infected it may be sufficient to remove only cement that is loose or that will obstuct the introduction of the new prosthesis. If there is the slightest doubt that infection may be present, all the old cement must be removed.

Above all, one must be sure of the position of the stem of the old prosthesis within the medullary canal. Many stems do not lie exactly along the axis, usually because they have not been perfectly centered but sometimes because of the sagittal curve of the femur. Whatever instrument is used, it is most important that it be orientated in such a way as to give the least risk of creating a false passage. Lateral and AP roentgenograms of the whole length of the prosthesis are required.

Powered instruments are dangerous in spite of all precautions that might be taken and carry a high risk of producing large false passages. They may be used as a convenient method of enlarging the cavity within the cement sheath. However, they cut a cylindrical hole within a square or rectangular cross-section and take a long time before they can enlarge the diameter sufficiently.

If the femoral stem has been perfectly centered in the diaphysis, then drills may be useful to attack the far end of the sheath that is difficult to remove using chisels, but they are otherwise of use only over a short range (Fig. 7.10).

We have tried many of the large number of guides and centering devices that are available but have given them all up for the moment. Although effective over the first 4 cm, where they are not required, they become less efficient the further that one goes down the femur, which is exactly where they are most needed. In fact, we work mainly with a selection of chisels and a hammer (Fig. 7.11).

In the upper femur, where the cortex is thin and where the cement lies next to cancellous trochanteric or subtrochanteric bone, one must take great care not to pass immediately between the bone and the cement. This would soon result in serious bony damage. It is wiser to attack the cement with a thin chisel of the Muller type and to direct it along the radius of the cross-section of the femur. This will split the cement sheath into several segments that can then be easily detached from the bone. We continue as far distally as possible using this method, although this is not usually more than 5–6 cm. As we progress further down, we use a long chisel of the Letournel type and direct it alternately along the radius and at the outer border of the

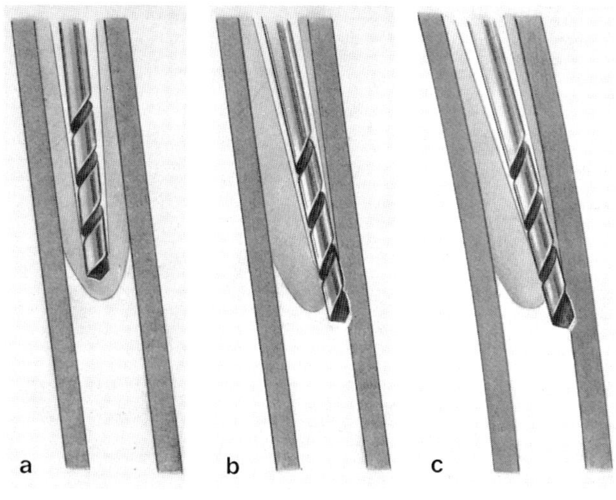

Fig. 7.10. **a** When the stem of the prosthesis has been perfectly centered down the medullary canal a drill is not dangerous. When the stem has not been centered (**b**), or more seriously, if there is significant curvature of the femur (**c**), then any rotating instrument is dangerous

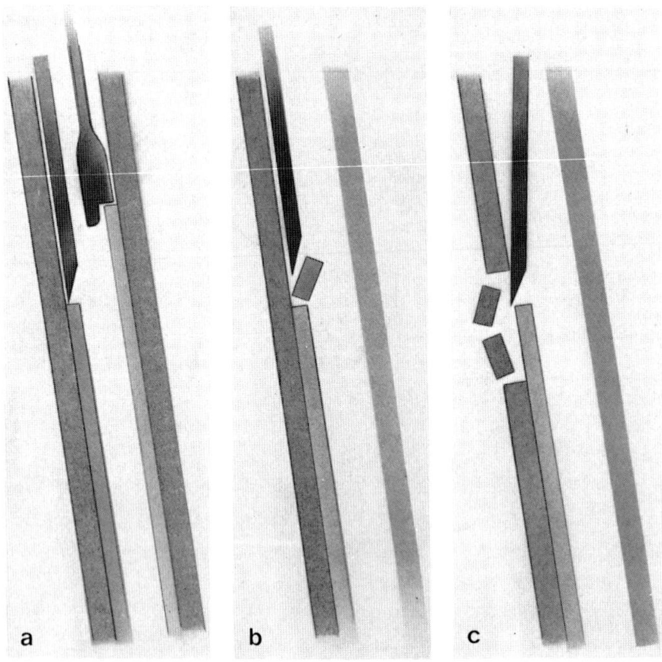

Fig. 7.11. **a** The cement is broken up with a chisel directed radially. **b** It can then be attacked using a chisel whose bevel is turned toward the canal and that is held firmly against the cortex. **c** If the chisel lies obliquely against the cortex there is a risk of penetration and of forming a false passage

cement. However, the thickness of the bevel and the distance at which one has to work make it impossible to use the optimal angle of attack, and so the bevel has to be directed toward the medullary canal. This tends to make the chisel run outward and to create a false passage. One must advance only in small steps, a millimeter at a time. In this way the cement is detached in small pieces. These are picked up with a fine, long forceps. The canal is irrigated with saline of Dakin's solution and an aspirator is used to remove blood and debris.

A well-directed, portable operating light will enable one to see a long way down, and fiberoptic light is often useful. When the end of the sheath is reached, the last 2 cm of cement often become free and can sometimes be lifted out with a forceps or retrieved with a hook. In an uninfected case this can just be tapped further down.

The canal is then cleared of any false membrane and debris by means of a curet or with long rasps. This procedure is completed with a burr on a power drill.

7.3.2 Diaphyseal Windows

We got to great lengths to avoid making windows in the diaphysis. However, a window may be necessary if there is an obstruction proximally, or in a septic case where all foreign material must be removed.

The window is cut with an oscillating saw, after we have carefully checked the correct level. The lid is finally replaced and held by cerclage wires before the prosthesis is cemented into position.

7.3.3 False Passages

False passages may occur whatever method is used. It is essential to recognize them and not to increase the damage, as they must be taken into account in carrying out the reconstruction. They are usually suspected when the note of the chisel changes or because the chisel suddenly no longer meets any resistance. They can easily be located with a fine, long, curved instrument, or with a roentgenogram if necessary. Failure to recognize a false passage risks leaving an area of residual weakness that may result in a fracture (Fig. 7.12).

7.3.4 Uncemented Prostheses

Sometimes uncemented prostheses are not well fixed and can be removed easily using a punch. Then only the false membrane that has formed around them remains to be cleared out by means of a curet, rasp, or reamer. When they cannot be moved, a long window

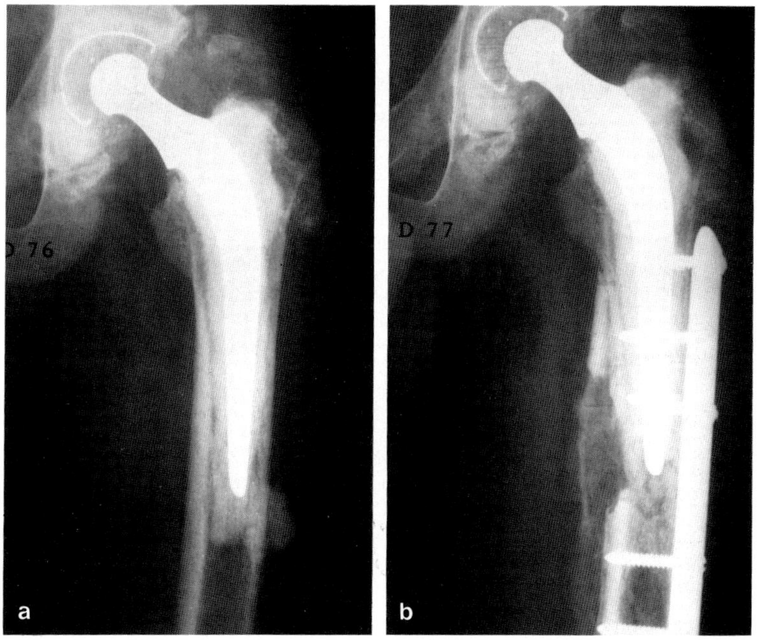

Fig. 7.12. **a** A false passage that is small but in a bad position. **b** Fracture of the femur 1 year later

must be made, extending the whole length of the stem and continuing 2 cm distal to the tip, which will allow the prosthesis to be knocked upward from below. Such a window is cut on the lateral surface of the femur and has not as yet given rise to any problems, although it is biomechanically undesirable.

The window is made with an oscillating saw; it must be wide enough to allow a blade to be passed between the prosthesis and the bone, so dividing any structure that joins the two. Removal of the window is not usually difficult, although bony ingrowth can occasionally cause problems. The separation of the prosthesis from the medial cortex is a delicate procedure if the stem is well fixed. This can be done only with a chisel that may also be used as a lever. However, the femur is very weak at this stage and great care is needed. The lid is then carefully replaced and held by cerclage wires.

*7.3.5 **Broken Prostheses***

Frequently, the distal fragment can not be removed using a forceps alone. If made of steel, the fragment can be drilled down the middle; the hole is then tapped, and a thread is inserted enabling the fragment to be extracted. However, this is not possible if the prosthesis is made to stellite.

We have occasionally made use of a trephine that is large enough to encircle the fragment of metal. It is then drilled into the cement deep enough to enable the fragment to be grasped and removed with a forceps. A window in the diaphysis usually has to be made in addition (Fig. 7.13).

*7.3.6 **The New Prosthesis***

The same principles used for a primary prosthesis apply, and we select a prosthesis of normal length that fills the medullary canal to the maximum. The cortices of a femur in which a prosthesis has come loose are often thin, sclerotic, and fragile. It is then inadvisable to use rasps in making a bed for the definitive prosthesis. It is better to use a small burr on a power attachment to enlarge the size of the medullary canal and to smooth down any ridges that may obstruct the insertion of the prosthesis. The stem must extend 2–3 cm distal to any false passage to prevent the risk of secondary fracture. This may require a stem that is 200–250 mm in length. It can be difficult to implant a long rectangular stem into a femur that has a marked sagittal curve, and a stem of considerably smaller size may be required. When it is not possible to use a stem of sufficient length to bridge the false passage, it may be wise to reinforce the femur with a plate or a graft held by cerclage wires.

The diaphysis may be incomplete or weakened over a

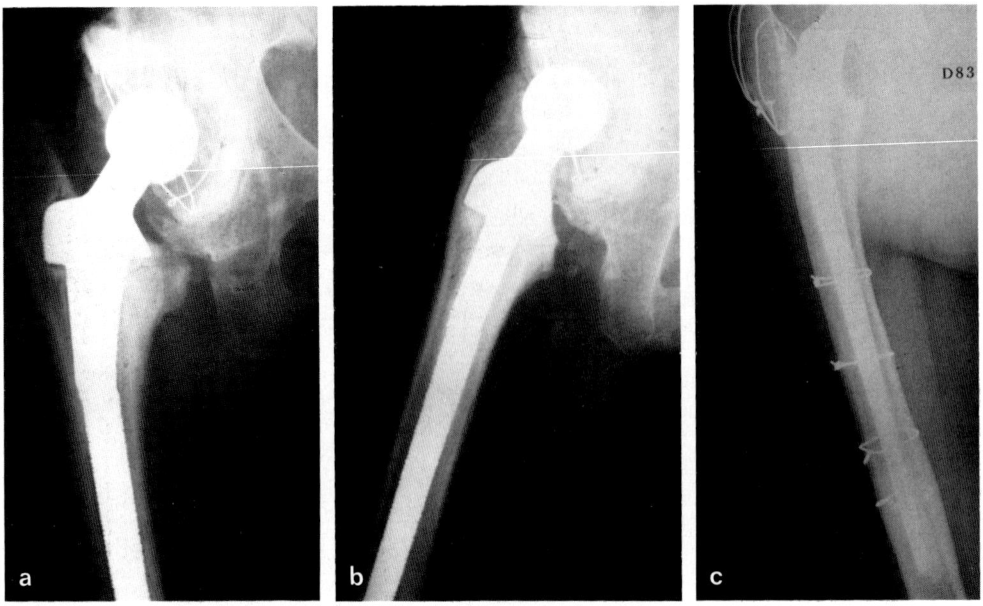

Fig. 7.13. a, b Fracture of an uncemented prosthesis; the stem could be removed only by making a lateral window. **c** The curve of the femur forced us to use a new prosthesis of a relatively small diameter

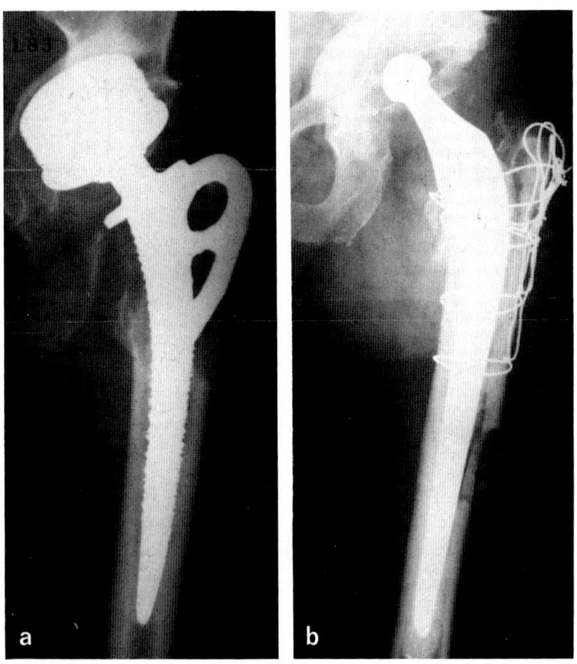

Fig. 7.14. a The superolateral cortex has been completely destroyed by a metallic granuloma. **b** A distally placed window was needed to remove the prosthesis. A strip of bone was freed and slid proximally to reconstruct the upper cortex and provide an area of support for the trochanter

large area as a result of an extensive lesion or following a surgical mishap. It can be reinforced by an autograft taken from the iliac crest or, more commonly, by a homograft held by cerclage wires.

Occasionally, the area around the trochanter is weakened or has disappeared. It can then be helpful to move a longitudinal segment of the lateral femoral shaft up proximally, thus giving a good site for reattachment of the trochanter. The remaining distal defect is filled with homograft (Fig. 7.14).

The patients are kept in bed slightly longer than usual (15 days) following these complex reconstructions of the femoral cortex, and full weight bearing is delayed by a few weeks.

There may be such widespread damage that it is impossible to carry out the repair in one stage. The femur may then be reconstructed around a Küntsher nail without the prosthesis, which is subsequently implanted as a second procedure.

There are also femora whose shape and length have been so altered by earlier surgery that it is impossible to introduce a prosthesis of sufficient width and of adequate length down the medullary canal. We have corrected the deformity in several such cases by carrying out a transverse osteotomy during the revision. Together, the prosthesis and the cement have provided adequate fixation. We took care to prevent any interposition of cement between the two fragments, and consolidation occurred without any problem (Figs. 7.15–7.17).

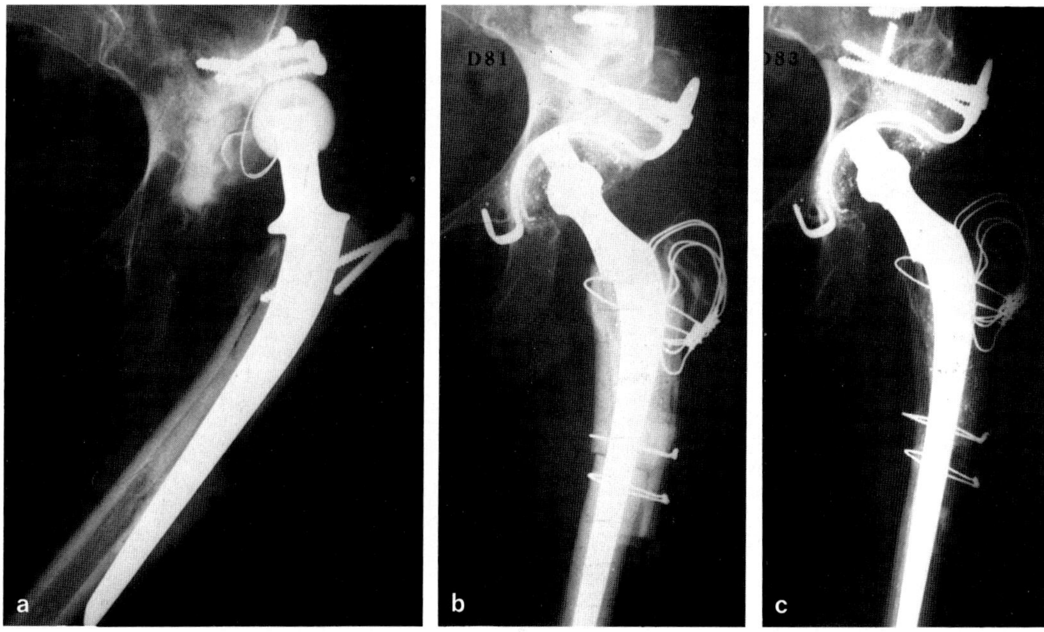

Fig. 7.15. **a** A false passage and a defect laterally with a very long prosthesis. **b, c** The femur was too long (after shortening of the opposite side), and a long stem was used with a shortening asteotomy that was reinforced using a fragment from the diaphyseal resection

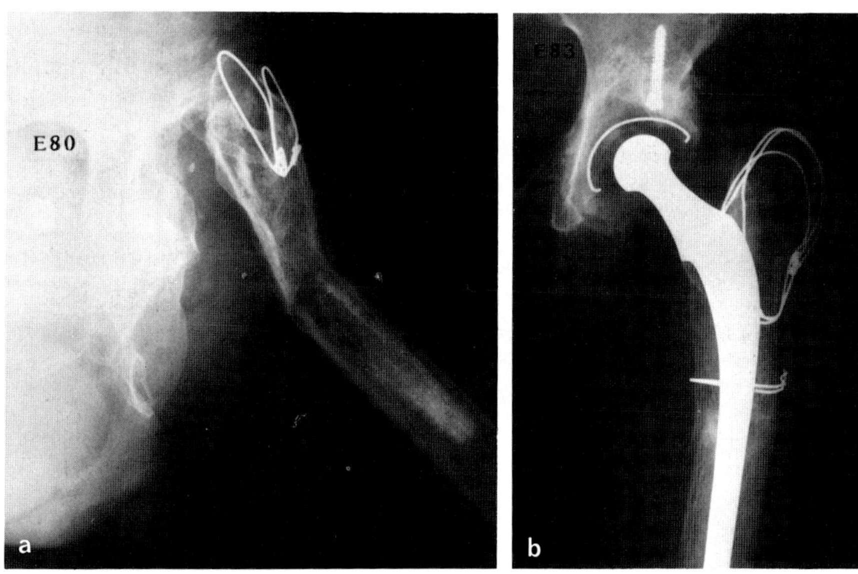

Fig. 7.16. **a** A femoral osteotomy was needed to allow insertion of the prosthesis. **b** Consolidation occurred uneventfully

Finally, all the hips that we have undertaken to correct have been reconstructed without recourse to the use of massive prostheses. Autografts and homografts give us great flexibility. They are the best investment for the future and are therefore to be preferred.

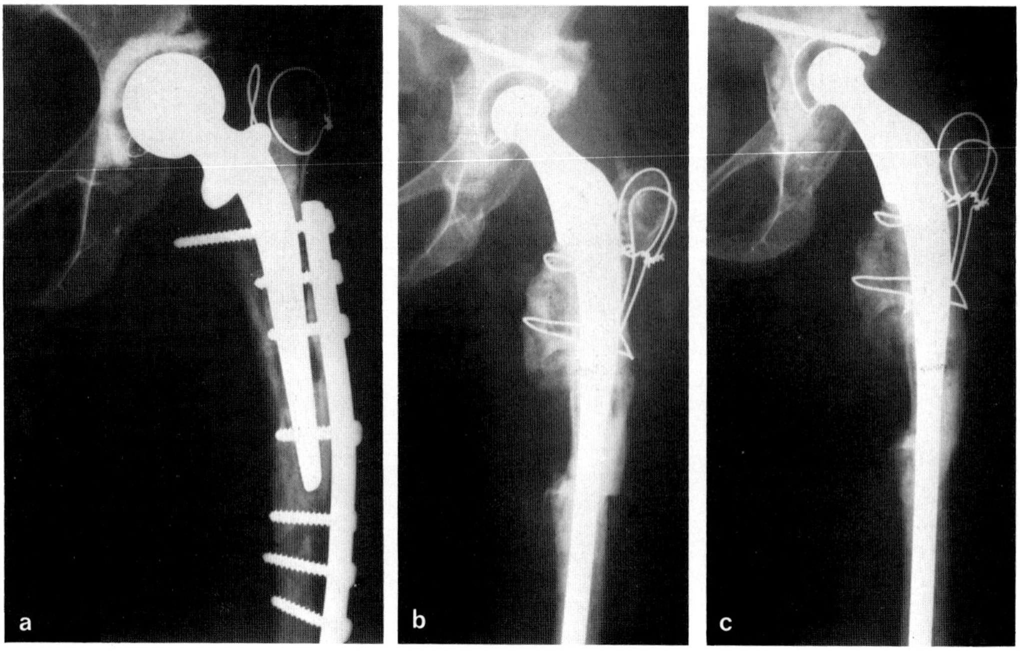

Fig. 7.17. **a** A loose prosthesis with considerable damage to the medial cortex. An old femoral fracture, held by a plate that has bent. **b** A low osteotomy was needed to allow insertion of the femoral component. The subtrochanteric region has been completely resorbed and has been reconstituted by a homograft held by cerclage wires. **c** The result 2 years later

7.4 Acetabular Reconstruction by Homograft as a Part of Total Hip Revision

C. Hedde and M. Postel

The destruction of the bony acetabulum that frequently accompanies a failed total hip replacement is one of the major problems of revision surgery. It is essential to restore the bone stock that is required to fix the new cup in a good position. Since 1973, we have achieved this by the use of homografts made from stored femoral heads. The increase in their use since 1979 (Fig. 7.18) reflects not only the increase in the number of revisions carried out in our department but also a greater confidence in the method. At present they are used in one-third of revisions. We have studied the reliability of this technique in the first 65 cases which have been followed up for at least 1 year.

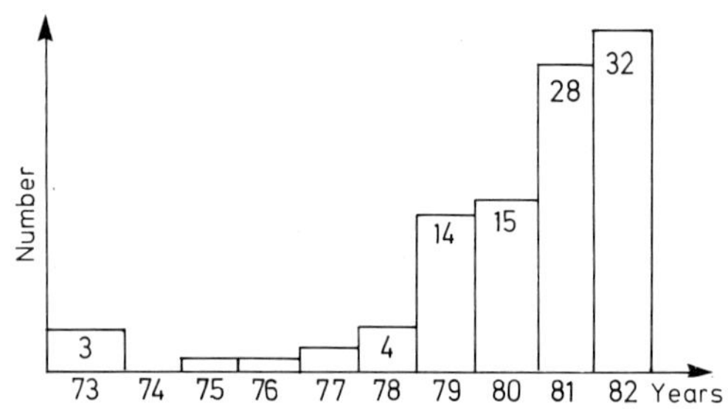

Fig. 7.18. The increase in the use of homografts for acetabular reconstruction in our department

7.4.1 The Homograft

Experimental studies on the biology of bone grafts show that they progress in the following manner. The postoperative hematoma becomes organized and is accompanied by a local inflammatory reaction. There is then a proliferation of vascular granulation tissue that progressively invades the graft.

Mesenchymal cells of endothelial origin differentiate into osteogenic cells. Incorporation of the graft, in the true sense, comprises the resorption of the grafted bone by osteoclasts together with the formation of new bone by osteoblasts.

There are several special features associated with homografts. The initial inflammatory reaction is pro-

▷

Fig. 7.19. **a** February 1977: large bony defect in the medial wall of the acetabulum. **b** June 1977: reconstruction using a large homograft that protrudes into the pelvis. **c** March 1978: outline of the graft undergoing remodeling. **d** February 1984: Fusion seems to be complete and remodeling continues

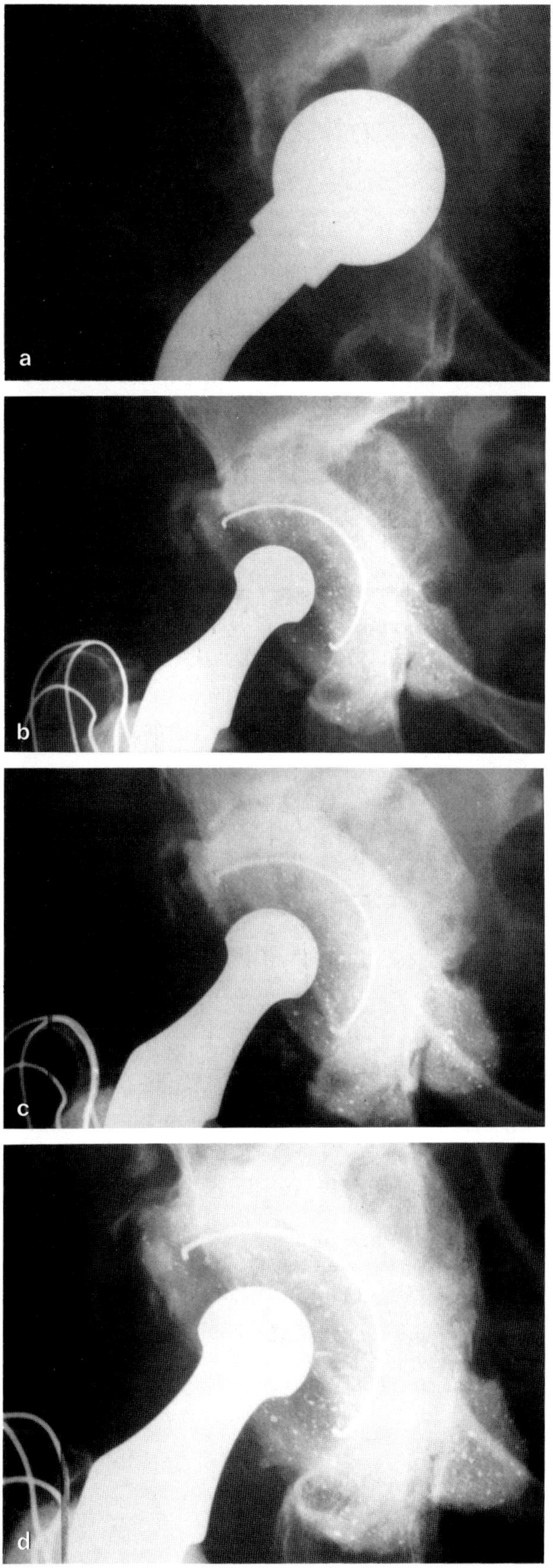

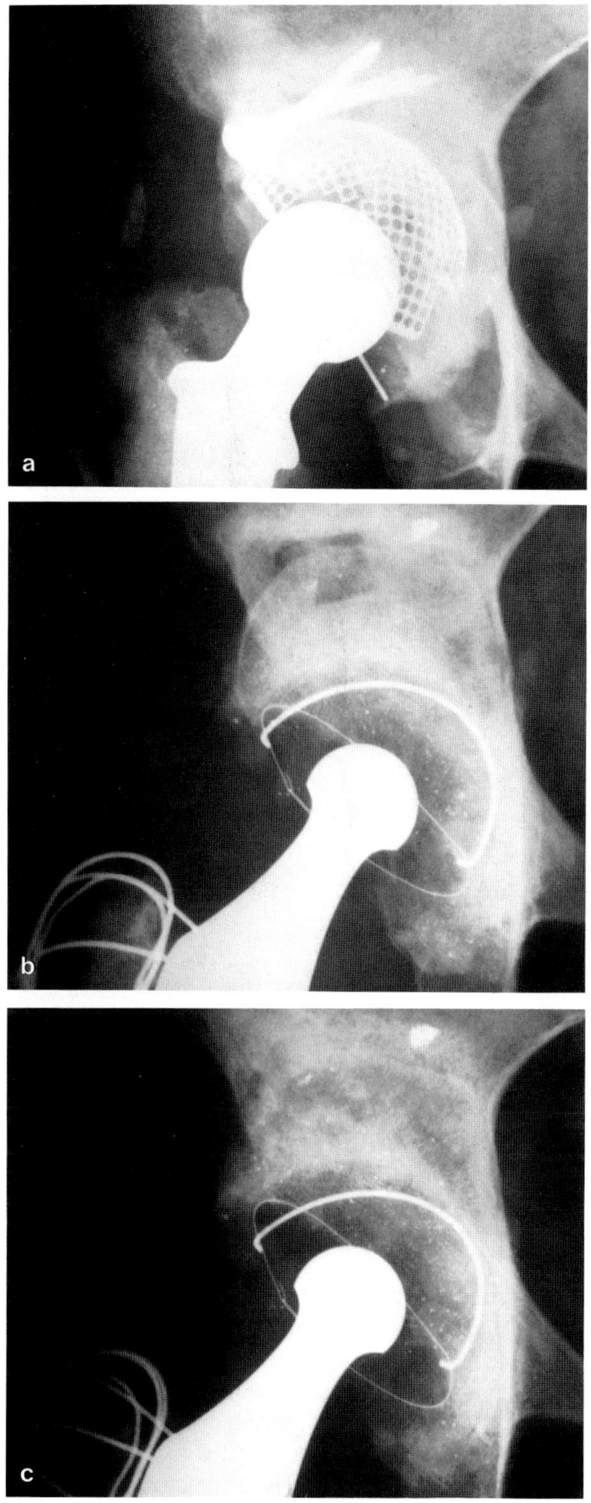

Fig. 7.20. **a** September 1982: large defects of the roof. **b** October 1982: repair using a large portion of a femoral head; outline is clearly visible. **c** October 1983: the homograft has become fused and the roof seems to be solid. There is no longer any gap between the iliac bone and the homograft

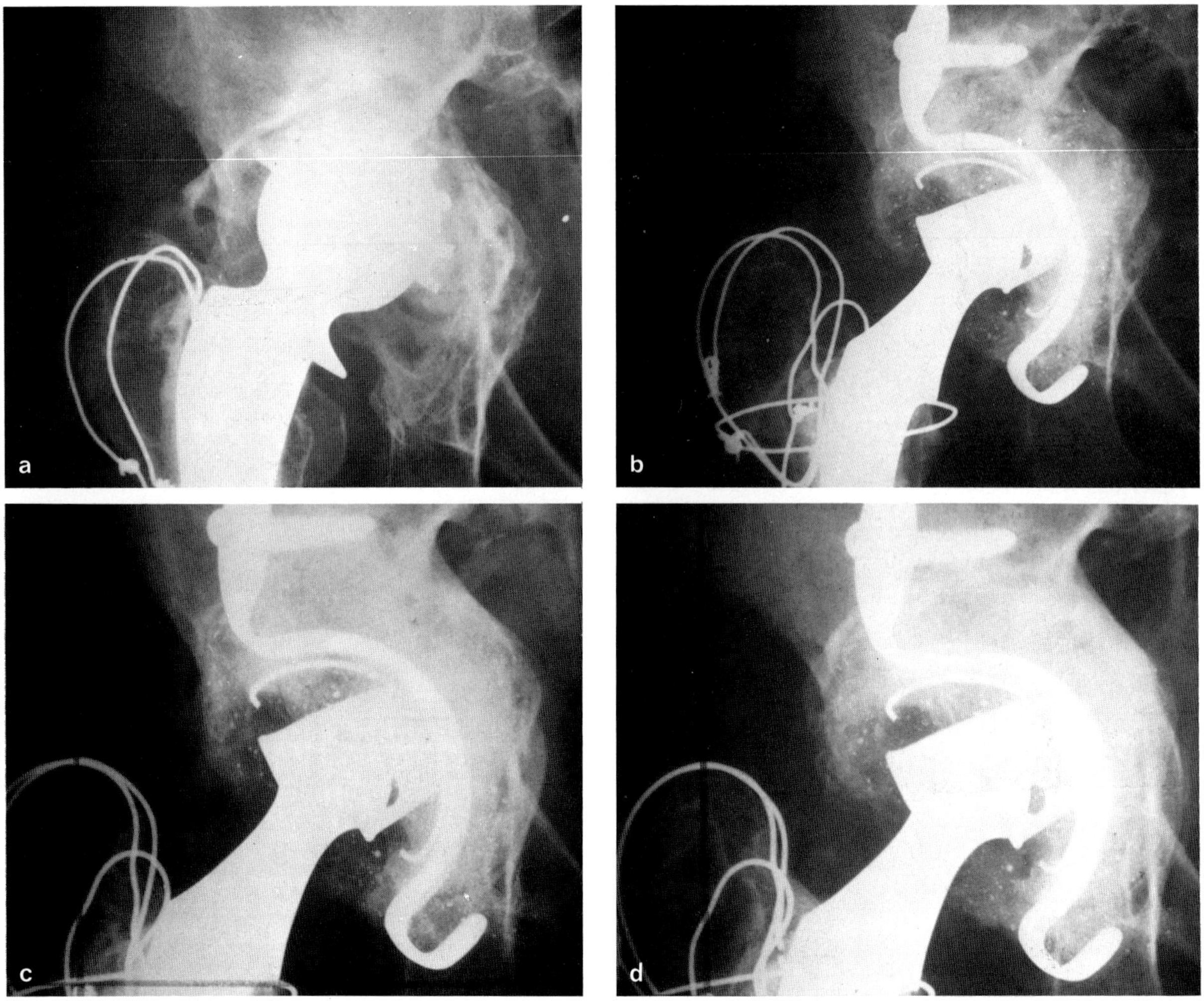

Fig. 7.21. a April 1980: the acetabulum has been greatly enlarged as a result of "metallosis". **b** June 1980: reconstruction using a homograft held in place by a plate. **c** October 1980: acetabular remodeling is beginning. **d** March 1984: remodeling of the homograft medially is now apparent. Consolidation seems to have occurred

longed (4-6 weeks), and reconstitution is twice as long as for an autograft. A rejection reaction may be suspected when there is partial resorption of the graft, but a generalized immunological reaction has never been described. The main theoretical risk is the introduction of infection by a contaminated graft.

Rigid aseptic precautions are therefore taken in the handling of grafts. The head is removed in ideal conditions such as are found during a total arthroplasty for osteoarthritis in a young patient free of infection or malignancy. Bacteriological swabs are cultured both aerobically and anaerobically over the next few weeks. If these prove to be positive, the head is obviously rejected. The head is stored inside three receptacles. It is first placed in a sterile glass jar that is hermetically sealed. This jar is then placed inside two sterile cellophane envelopes, the outer one of which is also heat sealed. The package is immediately placed in a freezer at $-36\,°C$ for 24 h, after which it is stored at $-20\,°C$. We have never used material that has been stored for more than 12 months, although this period could no doubt be exceeded.

When the head is to be used, the two envelopes and the jar are opened and the head is given to the scrub nurse. A new swab is taken from the head for culture. The head is cleaned of any remnants of synovium, freshened, and cut into the required shape or broken up into fragments to fill the bony defects and to reconstruct the acetabulum.

7.4.2 Radiological Progression

The radiological progression of the grafts is variable. This depends partly on the conditions under which they are used. These vary greatly, from blocking a simple perforation of the acetabulum (16%) or filling a large perforation of the medial wall or a sizeable cavity in the roof (59%) to replacing a vast bony defect (25%). In some cases (15/65), the grafts cannot be seen on a roentgenogram as they either are obscured by the cement or are too small. In other instances, they show no evidence of remodeling although they can be seen on a roentgenogram (8/65). The remainder (42/65) are seen to undergo changes. Partial resorption may occur between 6 and 12 months, and the grafts then become stable by the end of 2-3 years. This resorption is usually that of an unnecessarily large ridge of graft that protrudes into the pelvis or is situated around the acetabular rim. Except in one case where the graft seems to have disappeared, remodeling tends toward the restoration of normal anatomy (Fig. 7.19).
In the majority of cases, the zone of separation between the iliac bone and the graft disappears after 2-3 years as if fusion had occurred. There is sometimes even the impression of callus formation (Figs. 7.20 and 7.21). Over this period it is common to see a change in the density and structure of the graft. This overall progression suggests that a process of consolidation and reconstitution is occurring.
There were four cases of recurrent loosening. However, it does not seem likely that this was related to the homografts. In two cases the revision prosthesis was of the metal-on-metal design, and in three instances the acetabular reconstruction was grossly inadequate. Responsibility for these failures seems to lie more with poor technique than with the graft itself. Further surgery was required in only one of these cases and the homograft was found to be fused to the acetabulum.
There are two hips that are possibly infected at present. None of the seven cases which had previously been infected or which were still infected at the time of revision are giving rise to any anxiety at 12 months following surgery. Thus, it seems that the postoperative course is not affected by the use of homografts in this respect. The functional results fall within the average obtained among all of our revisions.
The usefulness of these grafts and the virtual absence of any unwanted secondary reactions has resulted in their being employed with increasing frequency.

7.5 Results of Revision of Aseptic Total Arthroplasty

J. P. Courpied

Between 1973 and 1980, 149 total hip revisions for aseptic loosening were performed in our department using the Charnley-Kerboul prosthesis. The number of revisions carried out is increasing, with more than 120 hips revised between 1981 and 1983.
The majority of the 149 revisions were carried out for failure of the metal-on-metal type of prosthesis, which had problems with the cup. The main problem with the Charnley prosthesis was loosening of the femoral component. The other types of metal-on-plastic prostheses presented with loose cups, although there were frequently problems with the femoral component as well. In 15 cases the prosthesis had already been previously revised. The average time between the previous arthroplasty and the revision was 5 years, and the average age of the patients was 63 years.

7.5.1 The Operation

The operative difficulties encountered are dependent on the state of the hip, and in nearly half of the cases there were severe acetabular lesions, often with a loss of bony continuity. Serious destruction of the diaphysis was less common (Table 7.1). Reconstruction was often necessary; 32 major acetabular and five femoral reconstructions were carried out, one of which was performed in two stages.
The number of occasions on which the femur was damaged during surgery gives a good indication of the technical problems encountered. Damage to the femur has very serious repercussions on the outcome of the arthroplasty. There were 22 perforations of the femoral shaft that sometimes passed unnoticed during the operation and seven diaphyseal fractures, six of which required a long femoral stem.
Revision is always a major procedure that lasts an average of 2 h, 30 min, but on ten occasions it reached or

Table 7.1. Lesions associated with loosening

Acetabulum	- 60 damaged acetabula with 44 large perforations and 5 transverse fractures - 10 small perforations
7 periarticular ossifications (type III)	
Femur	- 8 major diaphyseal lesions - 3 fractures of the diaphysis - 10 fractures of the prosthetic stem

exceeded 3 h. In half of the patients, blood loss during surgery and over the first 24 h was in excess of 4 l. Following the revision, the lower limb was approximately 2 cm too long or too short in ten cases, while leg length was corrected satisfactorily in the remaining cases.

A long femoral stem was used on 20 occasions and gave consistently good results. The indications were as follows: three fractures of the shaft associated with loosening as the original indication for revision, six peroperative fractures caused by false passages produced during removal of the cement, nine localized cortical fissures, and support of an extremely thin femoral cortex on two occasions. At no time did we use a massive prosthesis.

Table 7.2. Functional results of the revised arthroplasties

			Results at latest examination
Very good (PMS: 18)	96		96
Good (PMS: 16–17)	34	2 ⟶	36
Average (PMS: 15) (1 loose cup)	9	4 ⟶	13
Poor (PMS 12–14) (3 probable infections + 1 femoral loosening)	4		4
Bad (PMS < 12) 4 infections + 1 loose femoral component + 1 femoral stem fracture	6 ⟶	Revision	0

PMS, Sum of scores for pain, mobility, and stability

7.5.2 *Functional Results*

More than half of the patients had a follow-up of over 5 years, 14 were lost to follow-up between 2 and 7 years, and seven died between 2 and 5 years after surgery (Fig. 7.22).

We had no deaths or early infections in this series. Two cases of phlebitis and four of pulmonary embolism resolved uneventfully. There were four late infections that presented between 1 and 4 years postoperatively and required four further procedures. Three patients with suspected infection have not yet undergone surgery. The addition of antibiotic to the cement seems to have been effective, as there has been only one definite and one suspected case of sepsis among the 94 cases in which it has been used. Among the 55 cases in which there was no antibiotic in the cement, there were three definite and two suspected cases of sepsis.

Among the aseptic complications were six dislocations, occurring between 2 months and 1 year postoperatively. There was only one case in which the dislocation recurred. This involved a previous nonunion of the greater trochanter in association with the loose prosthesis and was successfully treated by surgery. There were six nununions of the greater trochanter in addition to that in the patient just referred to. Five have been successfully reoperated upon and the sixth does not require revision.

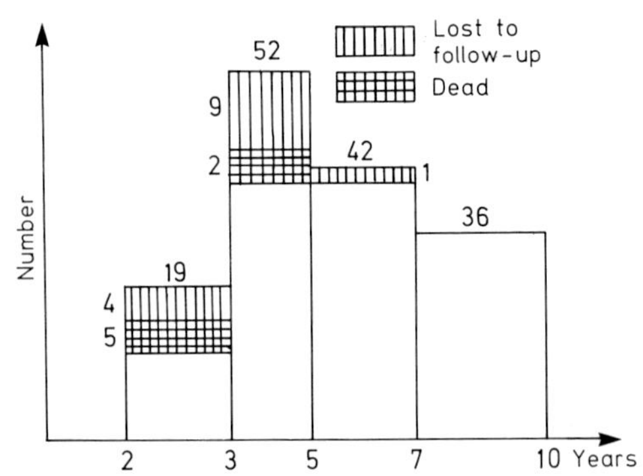

Fig. 7.22. Follow-up of 149 revision arthroplasties

Five diaphyseal fractures occurred between 3 months and 4 years after surgery. Although these were not immediate complications of the arthroplasty, they were definitely caused by weakening of the femur. Fixation by a plate was needed in three cases.

The functional results in this series are good or very good in the majority of cases: 88% of hips are pain free, 86% score 6 for movement, and 78% are completely stable. The good or average results are due to imperfect stability caused by repeated damage to the musculature, and also to episodes of pain of uncertain origin. These may be related to small cracks in the cortex, or to holes following previous plating that have allowed some cement to extrude outside the femur. In two instances movement was reduced by large areas of periarticular ossification. The poor results are with the three hips with probable infection and the one case of femoral loosening that has not yet been revised. Finally, there were six bad results, all of which required reoperation: four infections, one aseptic femoral loosening, and one fracture of a femoral stem. After further surgery, the four infected hips had results classified as average and the other two had good results (Table 7.2).

At present, therefore, we have 132 good or very good functional results and 13 average results. The hips with poor function will certainly have to be revised, and we hope that they will then move up into a higher category.

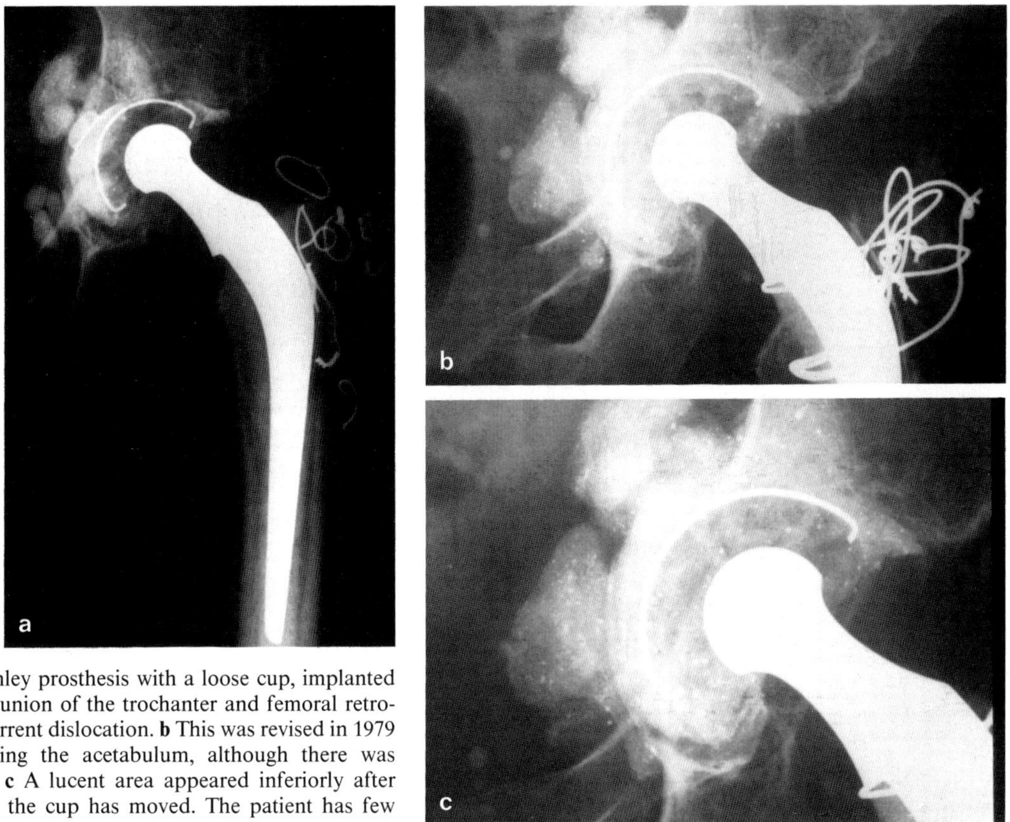

Fig. 7.23. **a** A Charnley prosthesis with a loose cup, implanted elsewhere, with nonunion of the trochanter and femoral retroversion causing recurrent dislocation. **b** This was revised in 1979 without reconstructing the acetabulum, although there was some loss of bone. **c** A lucent area appeared inferiorly after 2 years and in 1983 the cup has moved. The patient has few symptoms and has therefore not undergone further surgery although the cup is definitely loose

7.5.3 Radiological Results

There is a correlation between the radiological results and clinical findings. On studying the progress of the uninfected hips we note that the absence of any radiological abnormality corresponds with the best results. One loose cup gave an average result, one loose femoral component gave a poor result, and the bad results were caused by a second loose femoral component and a fracture of a femoral stem (Table 7.2).

The Cup

Of 127 cups that have been revised, 118 have been followed up for over 4 years. These can be divided into three groups according to the degree of previous bony damage: those where there had been very little previous acetabular damage (60 cases), those where the acetabulum had been poorly reconstructed in the presence of considerable previous damage (28 cases), and those with a good reconstruction (30 cases). In the first group the only abnormal radiological feature was one localized lucent area that was progressing slowly. The second group produced one loosening that has not yet been revised (Fig. 7.23) and two cups with lucent zones. In the third group there have been no loosenings or radiological abnormalities.

The Femoral Component

There were 142 revisions of the femoral component, 128 of which have been followed up for over 4 years. This is more than the number of cups revised, as there were 15 isolated femoral revisions for loose Charnley prostheses. Five femoral reconstructions were carried out and all of these had a good result. Among the femoral components that we have revised there are now two loosenings, one femoral stem fracture, and eight cases with radiological abnormalities that are at present asymptomatic. These problems can be related to several factors (Table 7.3).

A poor fit of the femoral component within the diaphysis resulted in a nonprogressive gap between cement and prosthesis in two cases and in one case of loosening that was revised after 2 years.

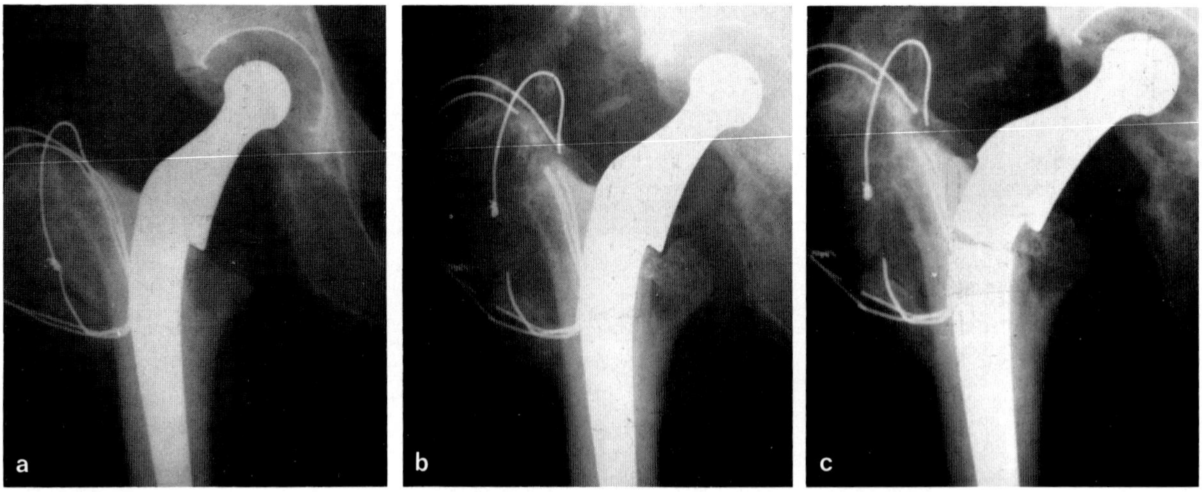

Fig. 7.24. **a** Revision of a metal-on-metal prosthesis implanted in 1973 in an obese patient. **b** Seven years later, no lucent zone at the cement-bone junction and no sinking of the femoral component. **c** In 1982 the stem fractured, although the prosthesis is not loose

Table 7.3. Probable causes of femoral complications among the revised arthroplasties

Cause	Radiological signs
Bad fit of the stem within the diaphysis	1 loosening 1 femoral stem fracture 2 spaces between prosthesis and cement
Alterations to the femur cortex	
- Cracks in the cortex	3 diaphyseal fractures 1 lucent area between prosthesis and cement
- Thin cortex, sclerosis	2 diaphyseal fractures 1 loosening 5 lucent areas at the cement-bone interface

The femoral stem fracture was not associated with loosening but seemed to be caused either by a prosthesis that was not strong enough for that particular patient or by metal failure (Fig. 7.24).

Alterations to the bone itself seem to have been a factor. There were cracks in the cortex which caused the three secondary diaphyseal fractures and resulted in one poor femoral fixation. It may be that the poor condition of a femoral cortex that has been modified by previous surgery is to blame. Good preparation of the bone is difficult to achieve in such cases, and perhaps this explains the second loosening of the series, the two diaphyseal fractures, and the five abnormalities that were seen at the bone-cement junction (Fig. 7.25).

Table 7.4. Incidence of diaphyseal changes among femoral components with a good fit within medullary canal

Original prosthesis	- Cortical thickening	25%
	- Lucent area at the cement-bone interface	2.5%
Revision prosthesis	- Cortical thickening	8%
	- Abnormality at the cement-bone junction	4.5%

Abnormalities at the bone-cement interface seem to be partly dependent on the quality of the bone and on the amount of preparation that is therefore possible. It is interesting to compare the radiological features of the well-fitting femoral stems from among the original prosthesis with those found among the revisions (Table 7.4). In the first instance, where the cortical bone has not been subjected to previous surgery, the response to the stresses imparted is seen mainly as cortical thickening and, to a lesser extent, as lucent areas related to cortical remodeling. Among the revisions, where the cortex has already been assaulted, there is less cortical thickening, while worrying changes at the bone-cement junction occur more frequently, although at the moment they have caused no problems. True lucent zones are seen more often in revised prostheses, while in the original prostheses there is more likely to be just a modification of the endosteum. Of course, one can make only hypotheses from these figures, but it is logical that a cortex damaged by revision surgery will react less favorably to changes in

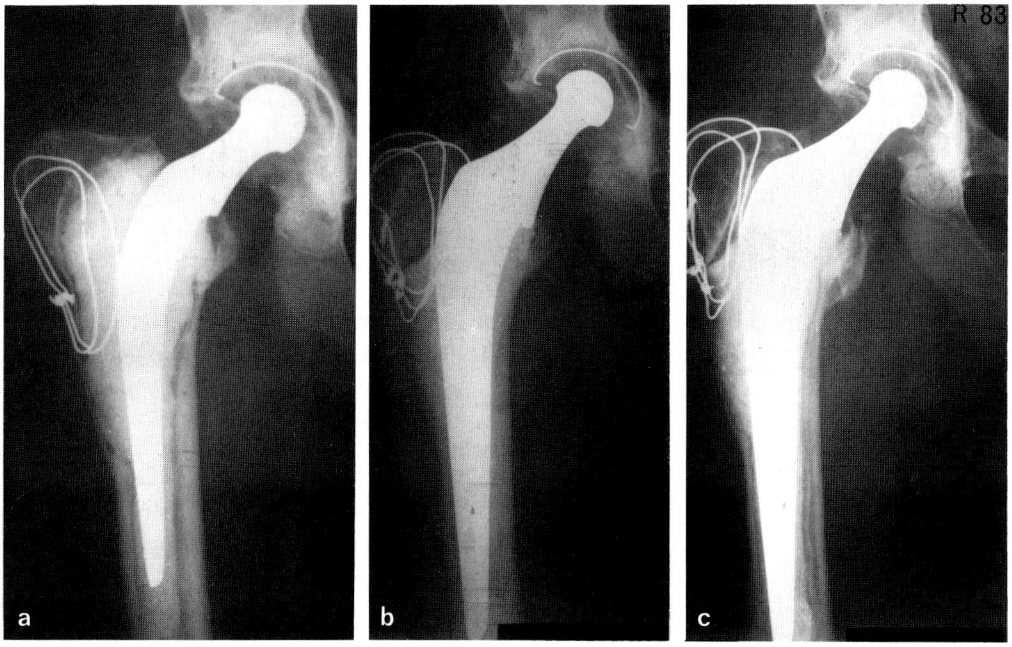

Fig. 7.25. **a** Loosening of a Charnely prosthesis that had already been revised. Loosening occurred first within the cement and then between the cement and bone. **b** A new revision was carried out in 1979. **c** A lucent area appeared at the cement-bone interface 4 months later, followed by loosening in 1983. This has not yet undergone further revision

the stresses to which it is subjected. This could lead to resorption, with unfortunate results.

In conclusion, there were only four serious aseptic complications among this series of revision arthroplasties, and there was good function in the majority of cases. We have 113 good or very good results among the 128 patients who have been under regular follow-up. The quality of the result is completely dependent on the quality of the reconstruction. It must be emphasized, however, that complications are slightly more frequent and the results slightly poorer than following a first total arthroplasty.

7.6 Conclusions

M. Postel

In concluding this study of total hip revision a few points deserve special emphasis.

7.6.1 Indications

Some indications are obvious. A painful prosthesis with radiological signs of loosening requires urgent revision, the condition of the patient permitting. Other indications are not so well defined. Should one, for example, revise all infected prostheses? This question is not relevant if there is pain and when the damage is progressing, but antibiotics may reduce the symptoms to a tolerable level, and although this simple treatment will not cure the problem deep within the hip, it may enable an old, tired patient to retain his or her prosthesis and maintain a reasonable level of function.

The problem is even more difficult when the patient is doing well clinically but there is definite radiological evidence of loosening and a gradual progession of the bony lesions. There is then little doubt that delaying surgery will make the reconstruction more difficult. To reoperate on a patient who is asymptomatic but whose roentgenograms are giving increasing cause for concern is a difficult decision for the surgeon and one that the patient finds difficult to accept. Caution is perhaps the best policy. Regular checks of all total prostheses is a rule that must be strictly followed.

The overall results of revisions are slightly poorer than those of primary prostheses: the incidence of loosening is slightly higher, a number of hips are still painful, and stability is seldom perfect. A proportion of roentgenograms arouse concern over the outcome in the long term. Not all these factors can be taken into account in deciding on the indications for revision. The decision can be made only after a careful study of the file and a long discussion with the individual patient.

These facts have great relevance to the present indications for total hip replacement. The problem of arthroplasty in the young is an increasing one. As the life expectancy of a prosthesis is limited, the possibility of a later revision often arises during the discussion of the indications for surgery, assuming that the proposed prosthesis will be worn out after 15 or 20 years. It would be easy to say that a revision is possible and that the patient would be able to embark on a long period of excellent function once more. But it would be dishonest to pretend that revisions are simple "routine exchanges" and to ignore the fact that the second prosthesis is unlikely to be as good as the original prosthesis.

7.6.2 Technical Problems

We are being presented with an increasing number of failed arthroplasties that require a difficult revision. Occasionally, these lesions are simply the result of too long a delay, and regular follow-up would have enabled an earlier operation, for instance before an acetabulum could have fractured. This demonstrates how vital it is that all patients be followed up, and this point must be understood by the patients themselves.

However, problems often arise from the prosthesis. Stems that are too long can cause widespread damage to the femur. Many of the commonly used prostheses have stems that are unneccessarily long, with no mechanical justification. In others there is an excess of cement that is difficult to remove. This is a reason for using a plug to block the femoral canal, ideally made of bone. Some prostheses require the removal of unjustifiable quantities of bone and are unnecessarily destructive. We believe that in designing or choosing a prosthesis, one must bear in mind that it is highly likely that a revision will be necessary. Without prejudicing the quality of the primary prosthesis, one must look to the future so that any revision procedure will be as simple as possible.

On the technical side, we are convinced that the best revisions result from accurate reconstruction of the hip. The new hip will then bear the closest possible resemblance to the original arthroplasty. The aim is therefore to reconstruct a skeleton that approximates the normal as closely as possible. We find that homografts usually enable us to use prostheses of normal dimensions and obviate large amounts of cement, large components, or superfluous materials - metal or otherwise - that can never be a substitute for bone.

8 Infective Complications of Total Hip Replacement

8.1 Introduction

J. Evrard

Although infective complications of total hip replacement have already been mentioned, they are worthy of a chapter in their own right because of the problems that they present in both diagnosis and treatment. Before studying infected arthroplasties in detail we shall consider their incidence, significance, and cost.

The incidence of infection is difficult to assess. Eftekhar [1] produced figures from several American hospitals that varied from 0% to 11%. However, they were drawn from a wide spectrum of operative conditions; some used the Charnley tent and some gave prophylactic antibiotics, while others used both or none at all. This explains the wide differences in the percentage of infection reported.

We can provide two statistics from our own department that seem to be of more value:

- Among the first 500 Charnley prostheses implanted at Cochin, there were 17 infections (3.3%). To this must be added 15 doubtful cases of infection, giving a rate of more than 6%.
- The survey from the Group Studying the Prophylactic Treatment of Infection in Joint Replacement (GETPIA) included 415 patients from our department, 11 of whom were infected (2.6%). This was a randomized study and can be divided into two groups. The group given prophylactic antibiotics included one infection (0.4%), while there were ten infected cases in the placebo group (4.8%).

The gravity of these infections is clear. They require admission to hospital and involve repeated surgery. In our series, the mortality directly attributable to infection was 3%. The cost to society is high. The figure of $ 25000 per year in the U.S.A. quoted by Nelson [2] seems to be reasonable.

A classification is necessary in order to study the clinical types of infection. The classification most commonly used at present, especially in the English literature, does not appeal to us, as we do not think that superficial infections should be in a separate group. If the infection is really superficial then it is of no significance; conversely, a serious infection is not superficial. Similarly, infected hematomas should not be put into a separate category, as they fall into the group of deep infections.

We therefore distinguish between:

- Early infections, which may be acute or subacute
- True late infections, similarly acute or subacute
- Secondary infections, which are the most common. They progress chronically and may appear months or years after surgery, in a variety of presentations, and may eventually produce an acute purulent discharge.

References

1. Eftekhar NS (1973) The surgeon and clean aid in the operating room. Clin Orthop 96: 188–194
2. Nelson JP (1980) Musculoskeletal infections. Surgical infections. Surg Clin North Am 60: 1

8.2 The Patients

C. Gaudillat

We have studied 264 patients with infected hip replacements treated at Cochin between 1968 and 1980. In 186 patients the primary arthroplasty had been performed at Cochin, while the 78 other cases were referred to us for treatment, the prosthesis having been implanted elsewhere.

A study of the septic complications in our department, according to the year in which the prosthesis was implanted (Fig. 8.1), shows that there was a progressive increase until 1974 (20–30 septic cases a year), after which there was a rapid fall to less than 20, and even as few as ten cases a year. The introduction of routine prophylactic antibiotic therapy from 1975 onward is undoubtedly the reason for this dramatic fall. The failure to recognize possible chronic infections is not likely to have been a factor over such a long period, as these whould have had time to manifest themselves

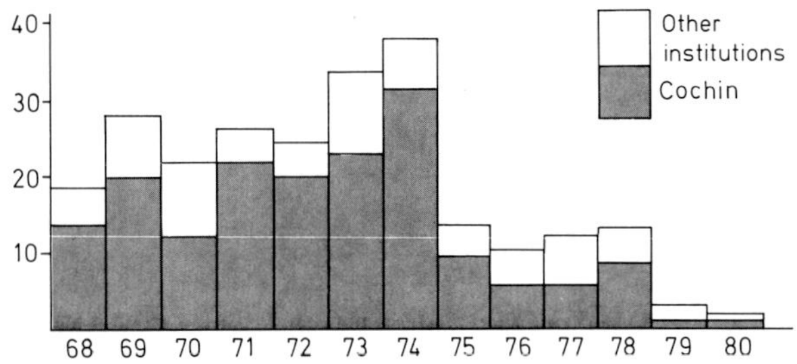

Fig. 8.1. Cases of sepsis treated annually at Cochin (including referrals from other institutions)

between 1975 and 1978. On the other hand, this could possibly have played a part in the years from 1979 to 1980.

At the time of diagnosis of the infection, 187 patients had only one prosthesis; 72 patients had two arthroplasties, and in only two of these cases was the infection bilateral.

In 14 patients, a prosthesis was implanted into the other side after treatment of infection in the first hip, and in 13 cases no problems have arisen. Only one patient gave cause for concern 3 years later, although no definite diagnosis of infection was made.

We have looked for any factors that may predispose to infection. If we compare the 186 infected arthroplasties from Cochin with the series of uninfected arthroplasties reviewed earlier, we find no significant difference among the two groups concerning age, obesity, underlying pathology, blood loss, or duration of the operation. Paradoxically, there was a slightly lower incidence of infection in long and difficult procedures, but these were usually performed by more experienced surgeons.

The only predisposing factor was diabetes: 5% of the patients with infected arthroplasties were diabetic as compared with 2% in the uninfected group.

Among all the patients whom we have followed up, 30 are known to have died. (This figure is no doubt much higher among the more aged. Among those over 75 years of age, half have been lost to follow-up over the 3-year period, especially those who came from the provinces, have retired, or lived in nursing homes.) Fifteen of these patients died after the infection had been cured, and in 15 patients the infection was still present at the time of death, which was directly due to infection in eight of the 15 (3% of all infected patients). It was caused by septic shock, acute adrenal insufficiency, or other medical complications; one patient died immediately postoperatively. The cause of death in the other seven patients was malignancy in six cases, hepatitis in one.

Is there any evidence that an impaired state of immunity predisposes to the persistence of infection? This was definitely so for a woman with a severe infection who died from aplastic anemia; she was also receiving chemotherapy. No definite conclusions can be reached in other cases.

Finally, it should be noted that among the 1313 total arthroplasties carried out at Cochin that have been studied in detail, 720 of the patients were given systemic prophylactic antibiotics, and of those, 1.8% required revision because of infection; 593 did not receive prophylactic antibiotics, and 3.4% of this group required revision for sepsis, twice the above figure.

8.3 Early Infection

J. Evrard

Early infection is an uncommon occurrence, following gross contamination of the wound during surgery, and it is usually iatrogenic. We shall study the 28 such cases that have been seen at Cochin from 1968 to 1980.

Infection can appear very early, during the first 4 days postoperatively, or slightly later, at the end of the 1st month. Less commonly, it may be delayed, presenting between the 30th and 90th days (Table 8.1).

In the most typical case, the clinical picture rapidly develops into the acute condition. There is acute pain and high, fluctuating pyrexia, and there may also be systemic signs. On examination, there are the local signs of a thigh that is red, hot, swollen, and painful. There may al ready be a discharge from the suture line, and a swab may be taken for culture and sensitivity. One or a series of blood cultures should also be taken.

Early subacute infection is less common; five of the 28 cases presented later, at 10 or more days postoperatively. The signs of infection are less marked; the fever is only 38°-38.5 °C, and local signs are minimal or even absent.

In difficult cases where it is not clear whether the hip is really the cause of the pyrexia, the joint should be aspirated without delay.

Table 8.1. Date of onset of early infection

23 in the first month	18 immediate
	5 between the 12th and 26th days
5 between the 1st and 3rd months	

Table 8.2. Bacteriology of early infection

Staphylococcus aureus	16
Staphylococcus epidermidis	4
Streptococcus	3
Pseudomonas aeruginosa	1
Escherichia coli	2
Anaerobes	4 (2 *Clostridium perfringens*)
Other gram-negative organisms	3

Whatever the clinical presentation, radiological examination is of no help at this stage, because the infection is limited to the soft tissues. Signs of bony involvement will appear only later on, if the infection is allowed to progress.

Bacteriological investigation enabled the organism to be identified in all cases studied (Table 8.2), and in six patients two organisms were found. The causal organisms were most frequently gram-positive, and *Staphylococcus aureus* predominated. A few *Staphylococcus epidermidis* and *Streptococcus* were isolated, as were a few anaerobes (two *Clostridium perfringens*). When gram-negative infections occurred they were usually associated with one of the above organisms.

All patients underwent further surgery after a variable interval, and the wound was cleaned and the prosthesis conserved. Before surgery, the majority of patients were treated with a short period of strict bed rest, together with traction if the pain was severe. Large doses of the antibiotic to which the organism was sensitive were given intravenously, if possible, and the wound was treated with alcohol dressings. Following this treatment, it was usually possible to operate a few days later under optimal conditions.

This operation to debride the wound was carried out early, and experience showed that the chances of success rapidly decreased when the period between the onset of signs of infection and surgery exceeded 35 days (Table 8.3). Early operation enabled the prosthesis to be saved in nearly 50% of the cases. When surgery was delayed for over 35 days this fell to less than 25%.

However, early intervention is not the only factor that affects the quality of the result. The way in which the procedure is carried out plays a major part. We shall describe the operation in detail later on, but it should be stated here that one must employ painstaking care to clean and excise all infected tissue, layer by layer, from the skin right down to the prosthesis. There must be a perfect view of the prosthesis itself.

The femoral component must be dislocated to give good exposure of the cup. The junctions between bone and cement and cement and prosthesis must also be meticulously cleaned.

Finally, the wound is closed over a continuous irrigation system (saline and antibiotic) that provides mechanical lavage and a therapeutic level of antibiotic locally.

The majority of those procedures that were successful had been carried out in this way. Conversely, incomplete cleaning without exposure of the prosthesis, that was not followed by continuous irrigation or that was carried out too late, usually led to a recurrence of the infection that sooner or later necessitated the removal or an exchange of the prosthesis.

Following revision, antibiotic therapy is continued for several months (at least 2–3), depending on the sedimentation rate. It is possibly as a result of the effectiveness of this antibiotic therapy that gram-positive infections *(Staphylococcus* and *Streptococcus)* have been cured more frequently than gram-negative infections. This differs from our experience with débridement of chronically infected prostheses and is possibly peculiar to this series.

The overall results are shown in Table 8.4. Of the 28 patients, 13 retained their prosthesis (44.8%); the majority of these seem to have been completely cured (Fig. 8.2) after a follow-up of 2–7 years.

It is important to emphasize that the incidence of early infection has decreased steadily since 1968 (Table 8.5). This remarkable improvement in the reduction of early complications has been due to (a) technical progress enabling the operating time to be reduced, and (b) perfection of aseptic precautions

Table 8.3. Treatment of early infection

28 Revisions (6 repeated)
21 before 15th day: 10 prosthesis retained (47.6%)
7 between 35th and 90th days: 2 prostheses retained (28.5%)

Table 8.4. Early infections: results

12 prostheses retained (4 still doubtful)	= 12
2 prostheses exchanged (1 failure)	= 1
14 prostheses removed	
Patients "cured" with a prosthesis in place	13 (44.8%)

Table 8.5. Decrease in incidence of early infection

Period	No. of cases
1968–1972	16
1973–1976	9
1977–1980	3

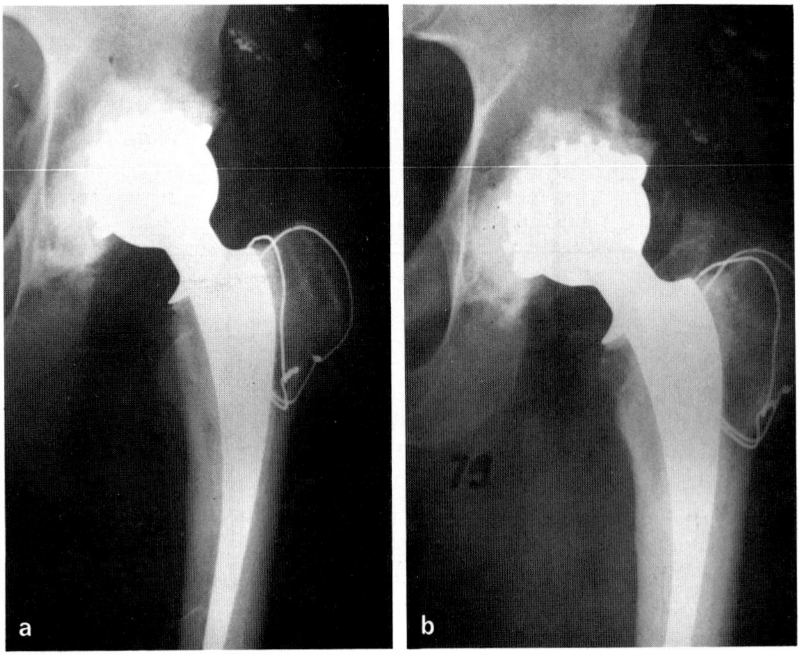

Fig. 8.2. a One month after a débridement carried out on the 15th day postoperatively for signs of acute early infection (pain, pyrexia of 39 °C, ESR 120, WBC 10000). *Staphylococcus aureus* was cultured from swabs taken during the débridement. **b** Six and a half years later the patient remains cured, both clinically and radiologically

during surgery. Finally, the use of prophylactic antibiotics has been particularly effective in the fight against operative infection. Thanks to this, early infection should practically disappear.

8.4 Acute Infection of Late Onset

J. Evrard

This is another rare type of infection that occurs quite unpredictably. These *true* late infections are completely unrelated to any contamination that may have occurred during surgery. They are spread hematogenously by septicemia or simple bacteremia and affect any massive foreign body, which in this case is the prosthesis. We found 13 definite cases of late acute infection which were characterized by the sudden onset of localized infection in an arthroplasty that had been functioning perfectly until then. An asymptomatic interval between the implantation of the arthroplasty and the appearance of infection is absolutely fundamental to the diagnosis.

In all cases, pain was notably absent or minimal (scoring 6 or 5 according to the Merle d'Aubigné system) during the years preceding the onset of the infection. This is clear evidence of late infection, and the time to onset, following the original arthroplasty, was 2–7 years in our series (Fig. 8.3), the average time interval being 4 years.

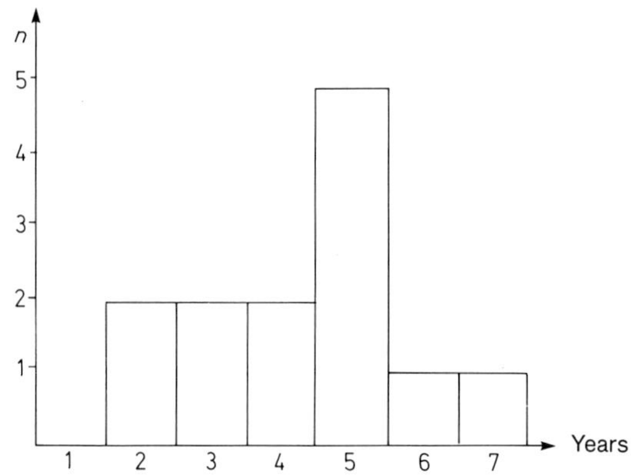

Fig. 8.3. Time of onset of acute late infections (average interval, 4 years)

The portal of entry was usually identified (seven of 13 cases), and the hip was clearly the site of a true metastatic infection, spread from a distant focus. Blood culture was positive in one of two cases. In a typical case the organism was detected in the original lesion, in the blood, and then at the site of the prosthesis (Table 8.6).

In other cases it is the mode of onset that enables the diagnosis to be made. The typical clinical picture is the sudden presentation of an acute arthritis, occurring several years after surgery, in a prosthetic hip which had previously functioned perfectly. Extreme pain prevents or severely restricts any movement of the hip; there is a high, fluctuating pyrexia and the

Table 8.6. Late acute infections: portal of entry and bacteriology

	From site of infection	Blood culture	From prosthesis
Postoperative infection			
Insertion of a pacemaker	*Staph. auereus*	+	*Staph. aureus*
Prostatectomy	*Pseudomonas aeruginosa*		*Pseudomonas aeruginosa*
Acute arthritis			
Opposite hip	*Streptococcus*	+	*Streptococcus*
Knee	*Streptococcus*		*Streptococcus*
Postabortion infection	*Streptococcus*	+	*Streptococcus*
Acute cholecystitis	?	+	*Klebsiella*
Infective gastroenteritis	?		*Staph. aureus*

Table 8.7. Late acute infections: bacteriology

Staphylococcus aureus	3
Staphylococcus epidermidis	2
Streptococcus	4
Pseudomonas aeruginosa	1
Escherichia coli	1
Klebsiella	1
Unidentified	1

sedimentation rate is in excess of 40 mm in the first hour.

Unfortunately, none of the patients but one were seen during this acute phase; they presented several weeks or months later. By this stage, radiological changes were often already present and were similar to those seen in chronic infection, as will be described later.

A bacteriological diagnosis was reached in all cases except one. Three patients had fistulas at the time of admission, in which the causative organism was found. The hips of the other ten patients were aspirated, and eight positive results were obtained. The same organism was usually found when the hip was explored, and organisms were found in one of two patients from whom the previous aspirate had been negative. Table 8.7 lists the organisms that were isolated; they are quite different from those found in early acute infection.

A variety of different treatments were used (Table 8.8), for reasons that will become clear later. In all cases, specific antibiotic treatment was instituted and continued over a long period. On only three occasions was bacteriology negative, the specimens taken peroperatively having remained sterile.

Table 8.8. Late acute infections: treatment and results

Débridement 3 → 1 Success
Débridement 3 → 2 Failures → 1 Removel of prosthesis (died)
2 Failures → 1 Change of prosthesis
Exchange of prosthesis 4 → 4 Successes
Removal of prosthesis 6 → 5 Successes
Removal of prosthesis 6 → 1 Failure (died before revision)

Table 8.9. Late acute infections: results

11 Cures → 6 with the original prosthesis
11 Cures → 5 following removal of the prosthesis
} 9 with satisfactory function
2 Failures → 2 deaths (1 caused by infection)

The joint was cleaned and debrided in three cases, producing a definitive cure in one instance. The success of this procedure depends on how soon it is carried out after the onset of infection (up to 30 days), on how thoroughly it is performed (including dislocation of the prosthesis to allow the whole wound to be cleaned), and on the sensitivity of the causative organism *(Streptococcus)* (Fig. 8.4a–c). The two other cases ended in failure and required further surgery. The reasons underlying these failures are that the surgery was incomplete and too late, and that the organisms were among the most virulent – a *Staphylococcus aureus* and a *Klebsiella*.

These two failures have been revised. The prosthesis was removed in one case, but the patient died postoperatively as a result of septic shock. A new prosthesis was implanted in the second patient, but this had to be changed a second time following a recurrence of the infection.

The prosthesis was changed in four cases, and all of these are successful at present.

Finally, the prosthesis was removed straight away in six cases. Five of these patients have been cured of their infection, and three of them have a satisfactory functional result. One patient returned with a residual infection which would have justified further surgery, had he not died following a myocardial infarction.

Overall, 11 patients have been cured, six of whom have retained their prostheses, and nine have a functional result that is good or acceptable. Two patients died, one because of a complication related to the infection (Table 8.9).

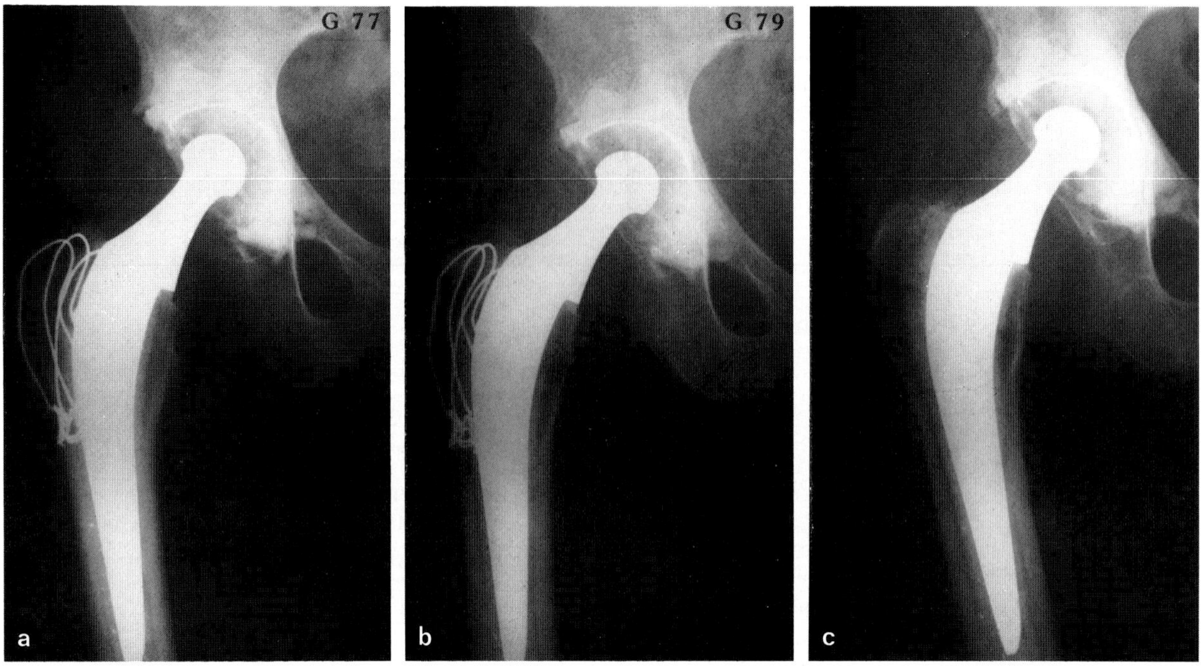

Fig. 8.4. **a** Postoperative radiograph. No complications. **b** Two years later, following knee infection, acute infection of the hip. Drainage shows streptococcus. Reoperation 15 days later. **c** Five years later: clinically and radiologically good results

Table 8.10. Late acute Infections: relation of the causative organism to the final result

	Prosthesis removed	Prosthesis conserved
Staph. aureus	2	1
Staph. epidermidis	0	2
Streptococcus	2	2
Pseudomonas aeruginosa	1	0
Escherichia coli	0	1
Klebsiella	1	0
Unidentified	1	0

Some conclusions can be drawn from this series, although it is not large. It is most important to realize that true acute infection of late onset is an emergency. Thorough surgical débridement must be carried out as soon as possible; it is this that will give the prosthesis its best chance of being saved. If the patient is seen more than 30 days after the onset of infection, there is no chance that simple débridement will be successful; it is useless even to attempt it. The choice is then between removing the prosthesis and exchanging it for a new one. The problem is identical with that presented by chronic sepsis, as in both instances the infection has progressed to the chronic stage.

Without pre-empting the chapter on treatment, we can say that the choice of treatment was determined partly by the type of organism involved (Table 8.10), but more so by the time at which the patient presented (Table 8.11). The earliest cases - until 1976 - were treated by removal of the prosthesis, but after this we exchanged the prosthesis when ever possible. The prosthesis was then removed only where the insertion of a new arthroplasty was contraindicated, usually because of the generally poor condition of the patient.

Table 8.11. Late acute infections: changing pattern of treatment

	1973-1976	1977-1980
Prostheses conserved	0	6
Prostheses removed	4	3

8.5 Diagnosis of Chronic Infection

C. Gaudillat and P. Deplus

This study includes 220 prosthesis where infection progressed and the diagnosis was made only a relatively long time after surgery (a minimum of 3 months).

A review of the operative procedure reveals no particular features, apart from the frequent absence of prophylactic antibiotic cover. One hundred and seventy patients received no pre- or postoperative cover, 20 were given antibiotics only postoperatively, and no record was made in the remaining 30 cases.

The immediate postoperative course was usually uneventful, and 75% of the patients were apyrexial by the 10th day. Only 25% had a temperature that gave slight cause for concern. However, 17 hematomas required evacuation, 18 wounds discharged before they healed spontaneously or resolved following antibiotic therapy, and there was one case of septicemia arising from the urinary tract. (The same colibacillus was found in the hip 3 years later.)

It is instructive to look at the time interval between the appearance of the first signs of infection and the point at which the diagnosis was made (Fig. 8.5). A definite diagnosis was arrived at in the 3rd year in 88% of patients and in the 2nd year in 68%. The decision to explore the hip was made an little later. In 64% of patients this was made in the 2nd year and in 88% in the 3rd year. On the other hand, the first worrying symptoms occurred much earlier; 88% of patients had abnormal signs from the 1st year onward; but at this stage they did not attract attention.

In 70% of patients the postoperative course was slightly abnormal from early on. The patient may have been slow in discarding the second cane, or there may have been a persistent pain that gradually increased. Pain was not acute or disabling and produced only minimal symptoms among patients who had been much more handicapped during the long years prior to the arthroplasty. The important point is that either a perfect result was not achieved, or else the hip began to deteriorate after the first few months.

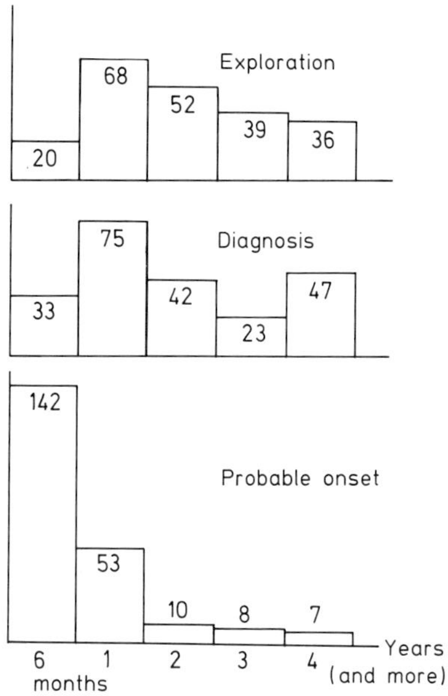

Fig. 8.5. Time interval between onset and exploration

The radiological signs were equally nonspecific (40%), and it was necessary to look for them carefully, knowing what importance should be attached to them and their progression: a small lucent area around the cup, blurring of the calcar, a minimal periosteal reaction.

One or more febrile episodes for which there is no other explanation may rarely attract attention (18%).

What are the different factors that point to the diagno-

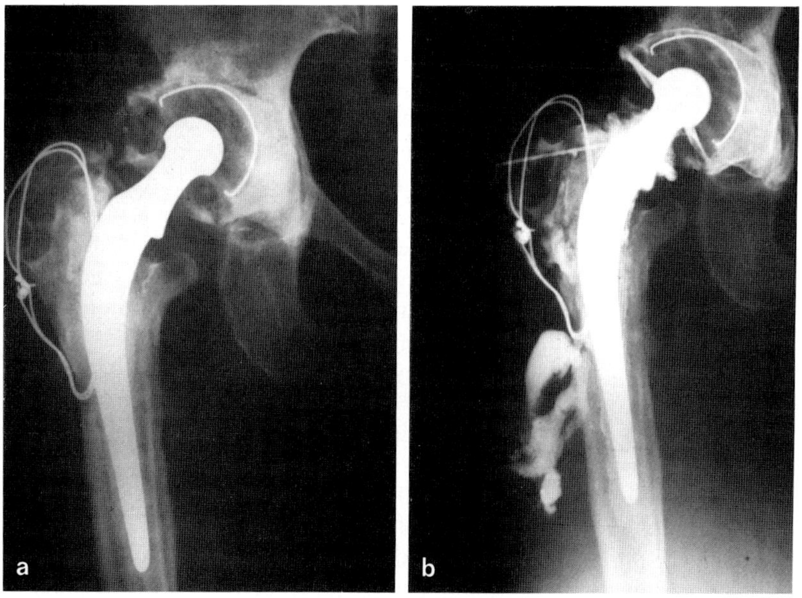

Fig. 8.6 a, b. Arthrography. **a** Clear radiological signs of infection – resorption of the calcar and periosteal reaction. **b** Arthrography shows precise details. Both components are loose, the exit holes of the trochanteric wires have become enlarged, and there is an abscess cavity over the lateral aspect of the diaphysis

sis? *The presence of a fistula* is sufficient to confirm sepsis. This is most commonly associated with pain in the hip, with or without radiological changes. The organism was isolated in three out of four such cases, although often only after a number of swabs had been taken. Eighty-two patients in our series had a fistula (40%). This figure is misleadingly high, because 60 patients operated upon elsewhere were referred to our department precisely because they had developed such a fistula following arthroplasty.

In the absence of a fistula, it is most frequently pain that leads to the diagnosis of infection (133 hips among the 138 that had no fistula). In 52 cases, pain occurred together with a high sedimentation rate and radiological signs that were highly suggestive of infection. In 25 cases, the pain was associated only with radiological signs suggestive of infection. Six cases manifested the local or general features of infection.

In these cases the strongly suspected diagnosis of infection was confirmed before surgery by aspiration of the hip on one out of three occasions. In the remainder, the diagnosis was confirmed by the macroscopical findings, with or without a positive culture. We shall return to this later.

For the remaining 55 patients (50 of whom had pain), the roentgenograms were abnormal but did not allow a definite diagnosis to be made. In 51 cases the diagnosis was reached either by aspiration of the hip to produce a turbid fluid, by positive bacterial cultures, or by arthrography (Fig. 8.6).

8.5.1 Radiological Signs

No hip was radiologically normal. The majority of radiological signs were nonspecific if taken in isolation, but significant when they occurred together and were progressive. They often appeared early (6 months–1 year) and progressively became worse, but their infective nature was frequently not appreciated until 1 or 2 years later.

The incidence of radiological signs seen at the time of exploration can be classified as follows: an extensive lucent zone around the cup (78%), resorption of the calcar (56%), periosteal reaction (50%), an extensive femoral lucent zone (44%), femoral cysts (25%), ossification (25%).

Acetabular abnormalities were by far the most common, in the form of an extensive and progressive lucent zone at the bone-cement junction (78%). In 14 cases this was the only radiological sign, and there was then the problem of whether this was in fact an aseptic loosening (especially in metal-on-metal prostheses, where the clinical picture is of little help). There were occasionally lesions that were slightly more suspicious, such as cysts around the acetabulum (16%).

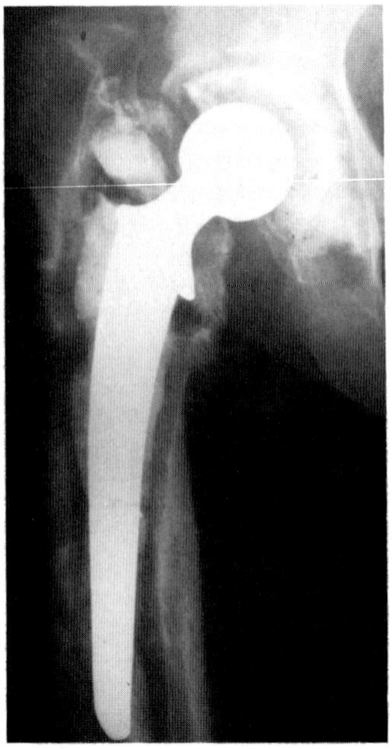

Fig. 8.7. Major loosening of both components

A cetabular lesions often occurred together with femoral abnormalities (65%), such as involvement of the calcar (62%), periosteal changes (58%), or a femoral lucent area, which then signified loosening of both components (Fig. 8.7).

Femoral signs were the only radiological abnormalities seen in 30 cases. Resorption of the calcar (124 cases) (Fig. 8.8), at worst resulting in the progressive destruction of the whole cortex, was nearly always associated with lesions of the acetabulum (80%) or of the periosteum (63%). It occurred in isolation on only two occasions.

Periosteal reaction (116 cases) (Fig. 8.9) is even more significant when it occurs on both the medial and the lateral side of the femur, and far from the regions of stress (such as the tip of the prosthesis) or directly in relation to a cyst. These periosteal reactions are most often associated with other femoral abnormalities such as involvement of the calcar or resorption around the wires reattaching the trochanter (one out of four cases). They rarely occur in isolation.

The following femoral abnormalities are never seen in isolation:

- An extensive femoral lucent zone between bone and cement was present in 97 cases, and in one out

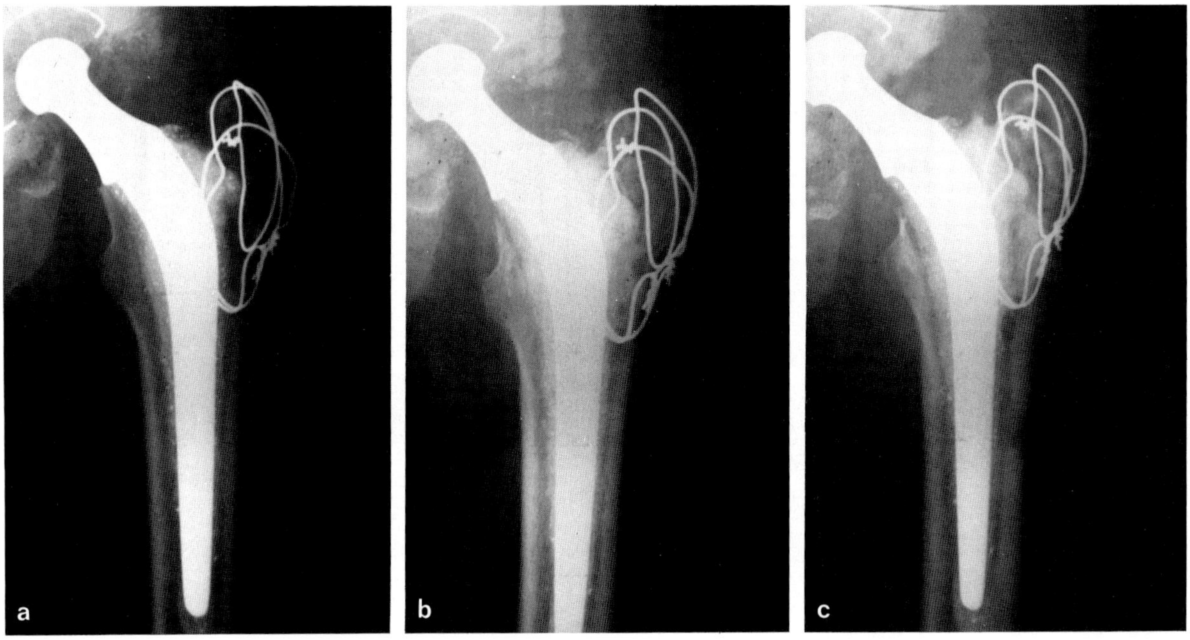

Fig. 8.8 a–c. Resorption of the femoral neck. **a** Postoperative roentgenogram. **b** At 3 months the calcar is being eroded. **c** At 15 months there is now marked resorption, with the full radiological picture of sepsis

of two such cases there was also resorption of the calcar and periosteal reaction.
- Endosteal cysts (Fig. 8.10) are rare but are perhaps the only truly specific sign of osteoclastic activity directed against a pyogenic infection. They are usually seen in association with other extensive femoral lesions.

Ossification was seen in 25% of cases. It was type II or III in only 16% of cases, which is nevertheless clearly more common than in the study as a whole.
Early diagnosis is made by recognizing these signs and their progression from the outset. However, abnormalities seen on radiological examination do not allow the diagnosis to be confirmed beyond all doubt. The diagnosis remains dependent on bacteriology and histology.

8.5.2 Bacteriology

Table 8.12 shows the spectrum of organisms that were isolated. The following points are of interest:

- The low incidence of *Staphylococcus aureus,* compared with that in the acute infections
- The wide range of organisms and, in particular, the presence of some that have until recently been considered nonpathogenic (*Staphylococcus albus, Cory-*

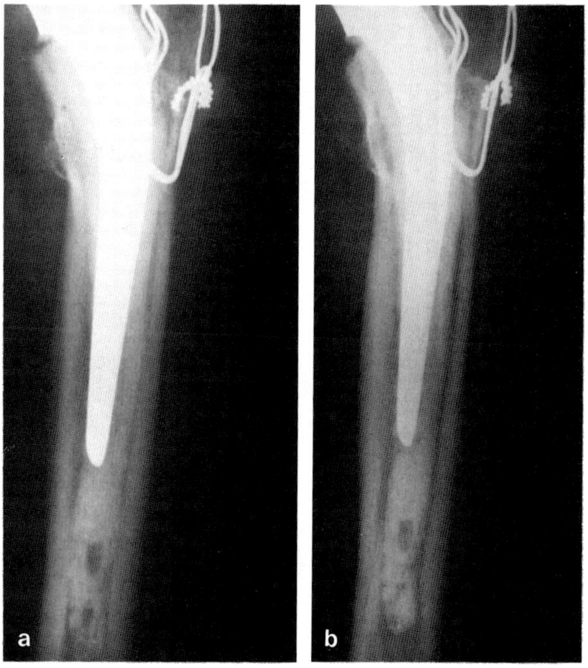

Fig. 8.9 a, b. Periosteal reaction. **a** At 4 months postoperatively there is a localized reaction on the medial surface of the diaphysis. **b** Six months later, this has become obvious

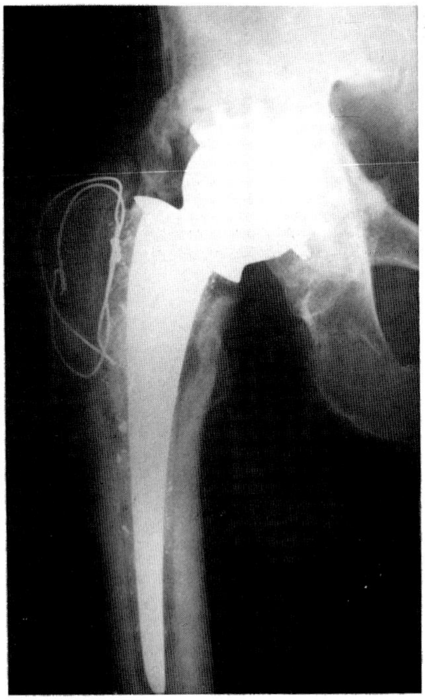

Fig. 8.10. Femoral cysts. There are two endosteal cysts, one medially, near the lesser trochanter, and the other laterally, near the tip of the prosthesis

Table 8.12. Preoperative bacteriology from fistula, blood culture or aspiration

Organism	Percent of cases (n=220)
Staph. epidermidis	28
Staph. aureus	12
Streptococcus	12
Pseudomonas aeruginosa	5
Escherichia coli	5
Corynebacteria	5
Others	5
Negative or unknown	24 (51 cases)

nebacteria). Their isolation means that the prosthesis must be considered infected until there is evidence to the contrary, even if contamination of the specimen is suspected. Sensitivities must be obtained as soon as possible and specific long-term antibiotic therapy may be indicated while surgery is under consideration. It is a good prognostic sign if cultures from peroperative specimens are negative.

- The incidence of swabs that were negative or not taken because the diagnosis was not suspected (one in eight)

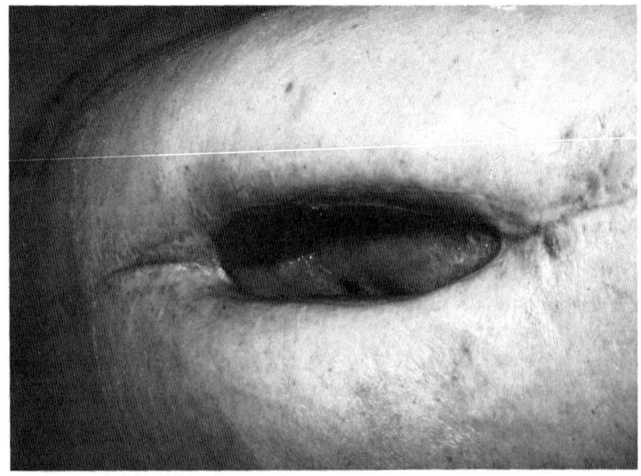

Fig. 8.11. Tuberculous superinfection following total hip replacement. After removal of the prosthesis and attempted coaptation, the wound was left open. There is suppuration with *Pseudomonas aeruginosa*

As might be expected, the distribution of bacteria in the group of specimens taken preoperatively is identical with that in the specimens taken during surgery.

As mentioned earlier, some patients who had already been treated with antibiotics had negative cultures preoperatively, although peroperative specimens were later positive (18 of 51 cases).

Several hips with fistulas that had been treated as having pyogenic infections were later diagnosed as having tuberculous infections. Had the specimens been cultured in the appropriate medium, treatment could have been instituted a few weeks earlier (Figs. 8.11 and 8.12).

During surgery, the surgeon can assess how securely the components are fixed and can identify any pus, turbid fluid, suspicious granulation tissue, or false membranes. Some surgeons systematically take specimens for histology, while others do so only if there is some doubt as to the diagnosis. As a result, histological examination was carried out in only one out of two cases. This showed granulation tissue that was inflammatory in 44% of cases and suppurative in the remaining 46%. Histology was negative on 12 occasions.

Taking our 220 cases overall, the diagnosis in 206 patients was reached from a combination of many factors. On the other hand, histology was the only positive finding indicating infection in two cases, and peroperative bacteriology was the only positive finding in 12 cases (against a clinical and radiological background of loosening of the cup in a metal-on-metal prosthesis).

Chronic infection is a rare occurrence (0.5%) that raises questions concerning peroperative contamina-

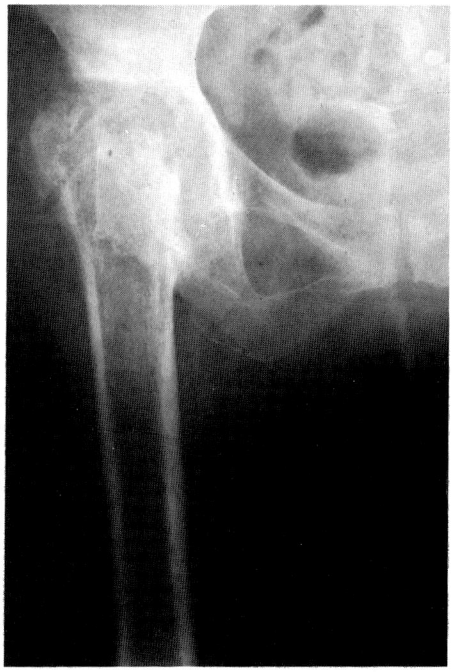

Fig. 8.12. Roentgenogram of case in Fig. 8.11. Two years later, after four explorations, the diagnosis of tuberculosis was reached by histology. This was confirmed as the condition progressed; the wound healed completely after 1 year of the appropriate treatment

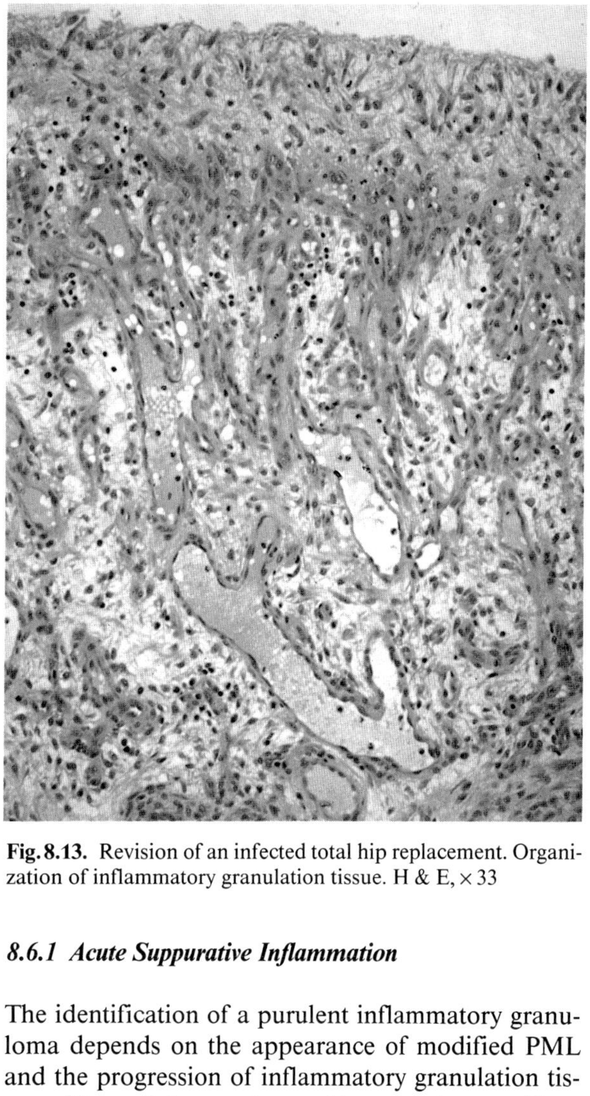

Fig. 8.13. Revision of an infected total hip replacement. Organization of inflammatory granulation tissue. H & E, × 33

tion. The incidence of such contamination has been shown by samples taken during the GEPTIA survey. The isolation of bacteria during a routine arthroplasty was not usually associated with subsequent infection. In summary, early radiological signs are most important, and if there is the slightest suspicion of infection, the hip should be aspirated and arthrography carried out. During exploration of the hip, the diagnosis can be confirmed by taking several specimens for bacteriological culture and histology.

8.6 Histopathology and the Diagnosis of Infection

M. Forest

This involves the analysis of the newly formed joint capsule and the membrane surrounding the cup and the femoral component. The specimens taken reflect the stage of progression of the infection. There are several diagnostic pitfalls of which one must be aware, and in any case, histology can never be a substitute for bacteriological analysis.

8.6.1 Acute Suppurative Inflammation

The identification of a purulent inflammatory granuloma depends on the appearance of modified PML and the progression of inflammatory granulation tissue with a cellular exudate and invasion by a capillary network (Fig. 8.13). This granuloma developing within the new capsule has the following features:

- It is usually distinct from neighboring histiocytic reactions.
- It often includes a marked superficial exudate forming a fibrinous layer (Fig. 8.14).
- It is often associated with localized tissue destruction and with cytolysis that releases lipid bodies and cholesterol crystals, leading to the formation of a secondary fat granuloma (Fig. 8.15).
- It is often localized and is sometimes very superficial. The purulent inflammatory reaction may form microabscesses within the fibrous tissue or be localized outside the capsule within the peripheral fat.

It may extend into the surrouding bone as a purulent osteitis. This can frequently be extensive, involving all

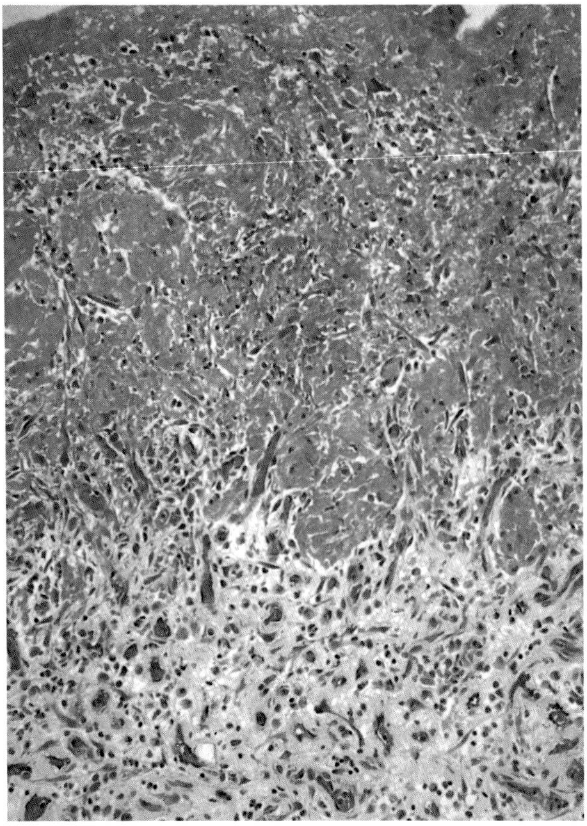

Fig. 8.14. A fibrinous superficial exudate over a cellular inflammatory reaction. H & E, × 33

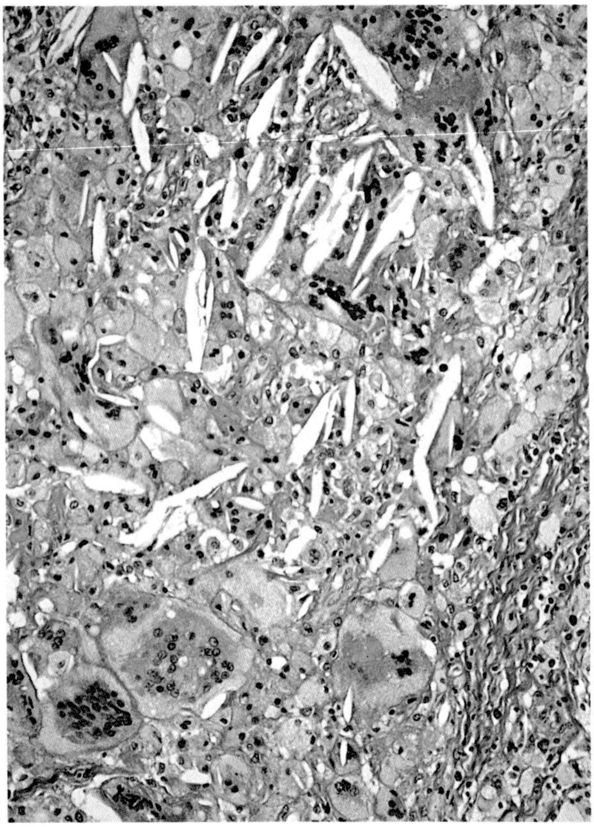

Fig. 8.15. A lipophagic granulome related to a purulent infection; many cholesterol crystals. H & E, × 66

of the lacunae. Zones of resorption by osteoclasts lie predominantly along the surfaces of the lamellae and are not solely at the bone-cement interface or at the junction between bone and the interposed tissue membrane.

8.6.2 Chronic Inflammation

This may be either diffuse or localized. There is cellular infiltration of lymphocytes or plasma cells (Fig. 8.16), and the latter is frequently accompanied by diffuse edema, separating the layers of collagen, and by capillary network invasion.

To support the diagnosis of infection, these lesions must be analyzed not only cytologically but also according to their structure and topography.

It is not sufficient to identify an invasion of lymphocytes or a new capillary network in isolation. The major diagnostic pitfalls are as follows:

- Isolated islands of reactive lymphoid tissue are occasionally found in residual synovial structures.
- Layers or islands of lymphoid tissue that are found around the margin of the joint capsule are usually a sign of involution of the surrounding muscle.
- Satellite infiltrates of lymphocytes are often related to the histiocytic granulomas seen in "metallosis" (Fig. 8.17).
- Multiple capillary outgrowths are a part of tissue repair that are seen in the normal response to surgery.

Whether the inflammation is acute or chronic, it may be masked by a histiocytic granuloma or covered with an extensive layer of fibrous tissue following organization of the fluid exudate. Acute inflammatory lesions that are superimposed on chronic inflammation are easily recognized by an invasion of leukocytes that are associated with localized exudates.

8.6.3 Rapid Diagnosis of Infection

Some departments routinely use methods enabling frozen section diagnosis of infection [4, 5]. The relia-

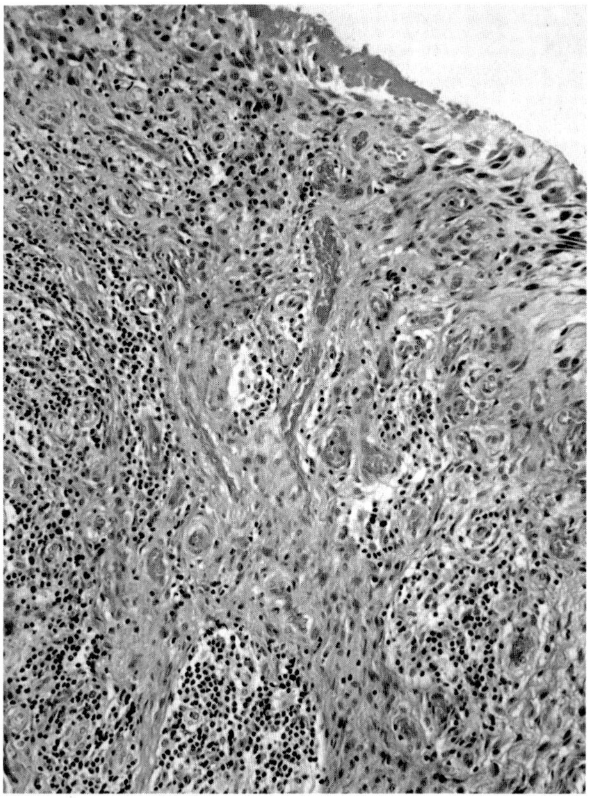

Fig. 8.16. Chronic inflammatory changes. Superficial layers of plasma cells. H & E, × 33

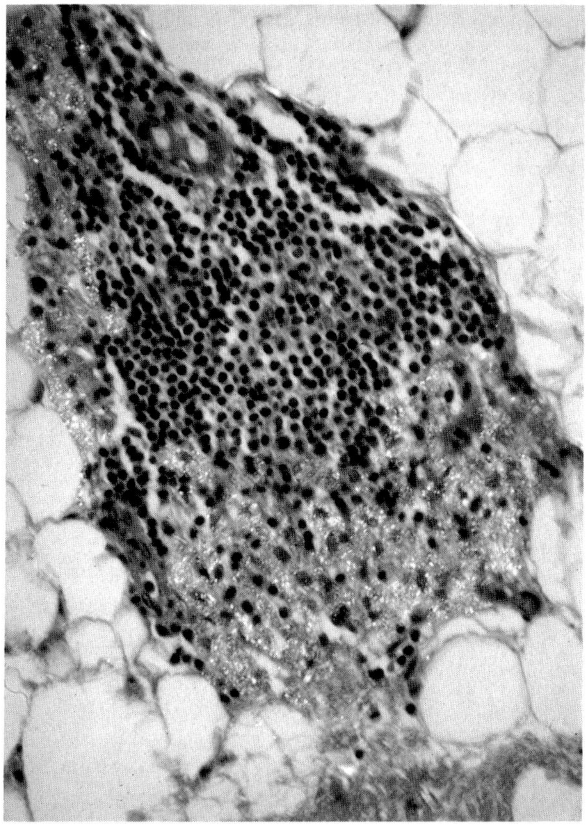

Fig. 8.17. An island of lymphoid tissue seen as part of a histiocytic response to metal. H & E, × 66

bility of the results that can be obtained from such methods depends on several factors:

- The area that can be studied on frozen sections is limited and occasionally is not representative.
- It is often technically difficult: there is encrustation with fragments of cement or polyethylene; there is an excess of lipids in the new capsule, with large areas of necrosis.

Since 1971, we have employed a method using tissue imprints [1-3]. This involves the fresh specimen being pressed against a series of microscope slides to leave a film of cells. The best-quality imprints are then taken after removal of foreign material and any metaplastic ossification. After fixation and staining by routine cytological methods, this technique allows the rapid identification of:

- An invasion of modified PML.
- An invasion by histiocytes that may also be present.

The Gram stain is used occasionally, but it is difficult to interpret and carries a risk of false positives because the preparations are often contaminated by debris from the lysis of the surrounding cells.

Two pitfalls should be avoided: the appearance of an infection deeply embedded in fibrous tissue that is therefore inaccessible to cytology, and the incidence of false positives in a specimen of synovium from active rheumatoid arthritis.

The identification of chronic inflammation in frozen section histological examination has too many diagnostic pitfalls, and the diagnosis should be made only by the proper histological assessment of several representative sections.

References

1. Bloustein PA, Silverberg SG (1977) Rapid cytologic examination of surgical specimens. Pathol Annu 2: 251-278
2. Forest M, Postel M, Tomeno B (1975) Interêt de la cytologie sur empreintes en pathologie osseuse. Rev Chir Orthop [Suppl 2] 61: 262-268
3. Ghandur-Mnaymneh L (1983) Tissue imprints in surgical pathology with a modified fixation procedure. Hum Pathol 14: 929-930

4. Mirra J, Amstutz HC, Matos M, Gold R (1976) The pathology of the joint tissues and its clinical relevance in prosthesis failure. Clin Orthop 117: 221–240
5. Pizzoferrato A, Sozarino L, Lambertini V (1980/81) Histopathological grading suggestion for the evaluation of the intolerance in hip joint endo- and arthroprostheses. Chir Organi Mov 76: 147–171

8.7 Methods of Treatment

J. Evrard

A number of methods of treatment are available to manage these different forms of infective complications. They can be divided into two groups, according to whether the aim is to conserve the prosthesis or not.

8.7.1 Conservation of the Prosthesis

The simplest method of treatment is obviously nonsurgical and consists of the administration of antibodies. This line of treatment may be used in two very different situations, and the expected outcomes are equally opposite.

In the case of early infection (or true late infection) with no evidence of pus or signs of osteitis, i.e., a subacute infection seen early on and at a purely inflammatory stage, well-managed antibiotic treatment can theoretically render the infection completely quiescent. In practice, this form of management is inadvisable other than in combination with surgery, and we always prefer to carry out an exploration and débridement of the wound in addition.

In the case of a subacute infection that has become chronic, whether there is a discharge or not, one can sometimes produce symptomatic relief with antibiotic therapy. This is only a palliative form of treatment, and it must be understood that it will not lead to a cure. However, it may enable the patient to regain an acceptable level of function and to avoid further surgery. A variety of reasons (usually the patient's general condition) may oblige us to follow this purely symptomatic line of treatment.

Exploration of the hip, on the other hand, is an active surgical approach. By this we mean a planned surgical procedure with the aim of carrying out complete débridement and toilet of the prosthetic joint and the whole operative field.

Exploration is applicable mainly in infections that are seen early, before there is any bone involvement. It must be done as soon as possible after a period of preliminary preparation, involving immobilization in traction and large doses of antibiotics of the appropriate sensitivity. This will enable the procedure to be performed under the optimal conditions. Surgery must be carried out early, usually within 30 days, and must include comprehensive débridement and cleaning, layer by layer, down to the prosthesis, with excision of all tissue that is suspicious, necrotic, or infected. The prosthesis is dislocated so that the area near the cement can also be cleaned completely, avoiding if possible division of the mm. glutei or revision of the trochanterotomy.

This procedure is carried out in acute or subacute infection, regardless of the time of presentation. At this stage only soft tissue is affected, and we do not feel that it is necessary to remove the prosthesis and cement or to change the prosthesis.

In addition to this definitive operation, which gives a good result in one out of two cases, there are other, less reliable procedures which one may have recourse to in special cases.

Late Exploration. This is the same operation described above (with the additional removal of the wires holding the trochanter), but it is carried out some time after the onset of the infection and when there is a low-grade infection with only minimal bony involvement.

This operation is completely illogical and has a very slender chance of success. It may nevertheless be indicated when one wishes to conserve an infected prosthesis that is functioning well by carrying out a less traumatic procedure.

Simple Débridement. This is in contrast to the systematic and complete exploration that extends right down the hip, and is a lesser procedure that is aimed at cleaning out lesions that are supposedly localized. It is appropriate only where there is a truly superficial infection, whose existence as a real entity has already been discussed, and more especially in cases of residual infection following removal of the prosthesis.

The most radical operation is obviously revision, or exchange of the prosthesis. This does not differ in principle from revision for aseptic loosening that has already been described, but it involves several additional specific points. First of all, it entails the extremely rigorous débridement of the soft tissues (excision of the fistula track, all abscess cavities together with their fibrous walls and diverticula, and as much of the new capsule as possible). Having removed the prosthesis and its cup, we proceed to remove the cement in its entirety. Removal of the cement from the acetabulum is usually straightforward, although cement within a perforating key hole may occasionally create problems. Removal of cement from the femur is usually a long and difficult task. It is not always possible to remove all of the cement from above, and rather than risk making a false passage, it is preferable to make an anterolateral window that will enable the distal fragment to be lifted out. The lid of the bone is then replaced and held with two or three cerclage wires. This obviously weakens the diaphysis, and it may then be necessary to use a long-stemmed prosthesis that will extend below the level of the window.

The new prosthesis is implanted using cement to which an antibiotic has been added (gentamicin, cephaloridine). The débridement and preparation of the bony surfaces usually makes necessary a new prosthesis of a larger size than the one that has been removed.

We routinely close the wound over a continuous irrigation system that enables any hematoma to be drained and maintains the concentration of the antibiotic locally.

Finally, long-term systemic antibiotic therapy must be continued until the sedimentation rate returns to normal. This must be for a least 6 months and is often for 1 year or longer.

We will not discuss the time of reimplantation of the prosthesis here. We usually carry out the procedure in one stage, following the débridement, as we do not think that a few months' delay significantly reduces the likelihood of rekindling any infection. Reconstructions of the femur or acetabulum, where there are extensive bony lesions, may provide an indication for the prosthesis to be implanted as a second procedure.

8.7.2 Removal of the Prosthesis

The most common procedure is *simple removal* of the prosthesis. In doing this, we prefer to divide the mm. glutei rather than to carry out a trochanterotomy. Débridement of both the soft tissues and the bone is then done as described above. If there is any periarticular ossification it is preserved, as it may help to stabilize the hip and can sometimes result in complete ankylosis.

After the mm. glutei are opposed with absorbable sutures, the wound is closed over a continuous irrigation system and the patient is kept in traction for 30–45 days.

The hip must be quite stable if a satisfactory functional result is to be achieved. Unfortunately, this is very difficult to predict. If there is significant telescoping at the end of the procedure, it is likely that there will be

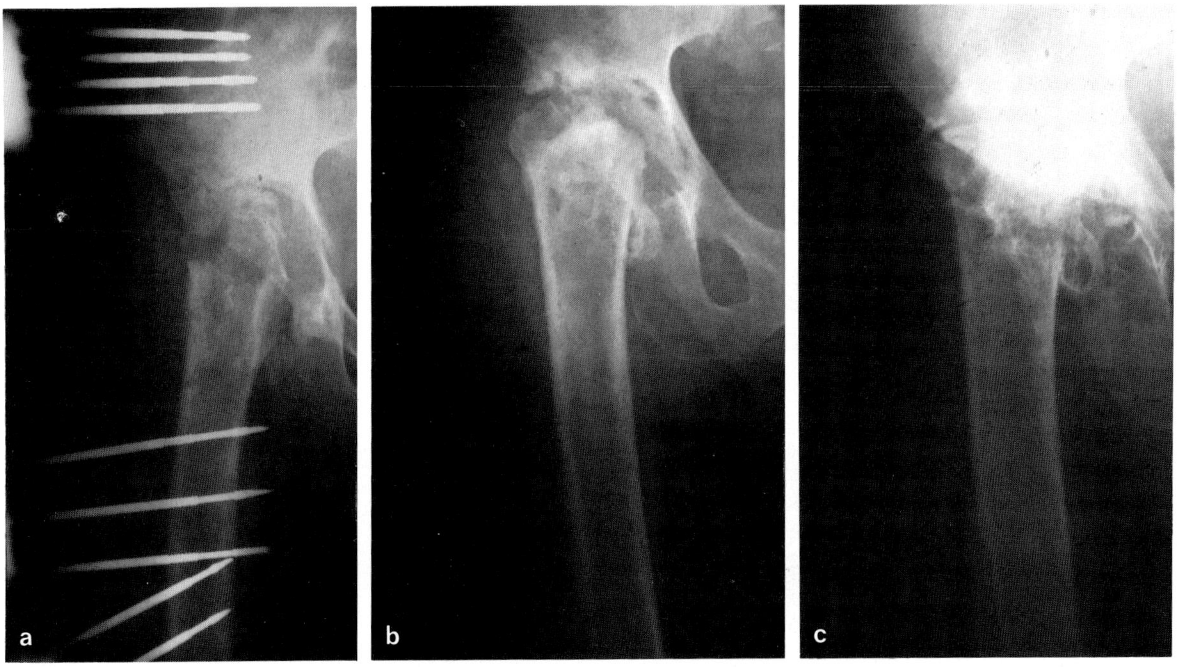

Fig. 8.18 a–c. Trochantero-iliac coaptation. **a** Postoperative roentgenogram: the coaptation is held in place by a Hoffmann external fixator. **b** After 5 months, the femur remains in position and there is surrounding fibrosis. **c** Radiograph 10 years later: a new joint has developed. In spite of this, the functional result is poor. The hip is slightly painful; the patient walks using one crutch and has never been able to return to work

instability. One must therefore try to create as much fibrosis as possible to unite the femur with the iliac bone beneath the acetabulum.

Trochantero-iliac coaptation was devised Letournel and Brunet [1] to compensate for instability in a hip from which a prosthesis has been removed. We have used the technique described by Marotte and Lord [2]. The operation is long, arduous, and hemorrhagic. The upper end of the femur must be brought up into the acetabulum without excessive abduction, and must be held in place to prevent later displacement.

To achieve this, the medial surface of the femur must be prepared medially, the lesser trochanter divided, and the acetabulum hollowed out by shaping the roof obliquely upward and medially. The upper aspect of the greater trochanter is then freshened, and rigid fixation is achieved by a Hoffmann fixator with a triangular configuration and kept in place for 6 weeks (Fig. 8.18).

This operation can be carried out at the same time as the removal of the prosthesis. It is a particularly difficult procedure and carries a definite risk. There were five deaths among the 99 cases presented by Letournel and Brunet [1].

We prefer to carry out coaptation as a secondary procedure if removal of the prosthesis has given an unsatisfactory result because of poor function or infection. The indications are then clearer, and the operation is easier to perform and less extensive. In fact, we hardly ever use this technique now, as the results are frequently disappointing.

8.7.3 Residual Infections

Finally, there are residual infections that recur following earlier treatment of an infected prosthesis. If the infection recurs following the exchange of a prosthesis, one has the choice of either removing the prosthesis or changing it once more. The choice is frequently dependent on the general condition of the patient and also on his or her own wishes - to have a good hip, or not to undergo further surgery.

This is why "second-generation infection" is especially regrettable when it occurs after an operation that one hoped had been sufficiently radical. There are several possible presentations. The most common is the reappearance of a fistula. A roentgenogram of the fistula must be made to determine the cause of the recurrence; it usually arises from fragments of cement that have been left behind after incomplete débridement (Fig. 8.19).

Occasionally there is an extensive area of ulceration, which is the price to be paid for deliberately leaving a wound open in the hope that it will drain better. The wound will not heal spontaneously and secondary suture is required.

More rarely, we have found areas of residual osteitis

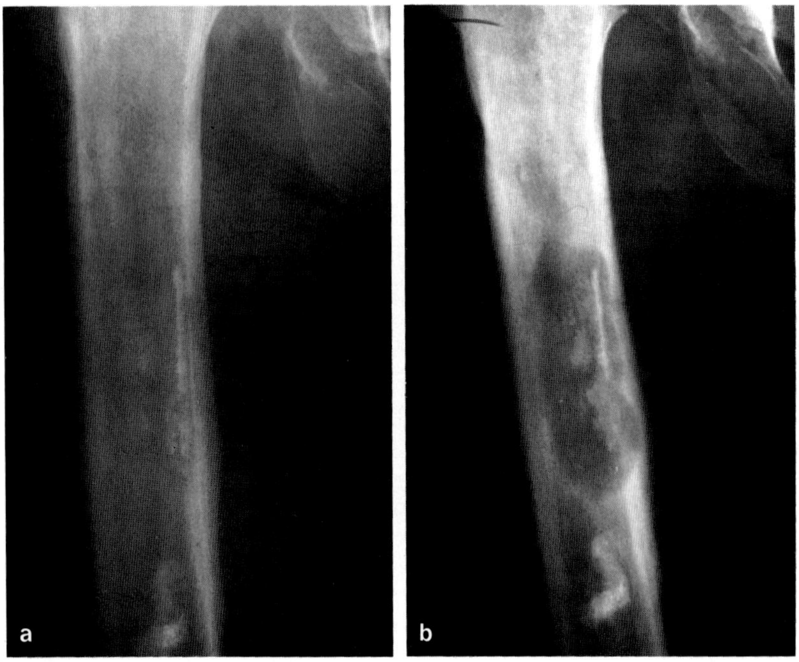

Fig. 8.19 a, b. Residual cement. **a** Following the difficult removal of a prosthesis, a few fragments of cement have been left behind. **b** Almost 2 years later, the patient presented with an acute infection. The roentgenogram shows a central abscess around the residual cement. Further surgery was required

around the greater trochanter that need further surgery, either to drain a central abscess or to excise a segment of necrotic bone.

References

1. Letournel E, Brunet JC (1974) La coaptation trochantéro-iliaque. Actual Chir Orthop 11
2. Marotte JH, Lord G (1972) Coaptation trochantero-iliaque. Réflexions techniques. Nouv Presse Med 1/9: 609–611

8.8 Results of Treatment of Chronic Infection

C. Gaudillat and M. Postel

It is not easy to analyze the results of operations for chronic infection, especially if conclusions being drawn from the study have themselves modified the indications for surgery. The files are very complicated; the cases often involve repeated surgery and do not always end in a situation that is stable enough to enable a perfect assessment to be made. The files have been accumulated over many years, during which the techniques and principles of management have changed considerably. Given that a baseline of controls can be drawn only from a series that (a) is large enough, (b) is homogeneous, and (c) has adequate follow-up, it can be seen that this presents considerable difficulties. However, it is only from this kind of study that a policy can be developed that will give each patient the best chance of a cure and of obtaining the best possible function.

The criteria that we have used in discussing the cure of infection are numerous but clear-cut. They form only a part of the total assessment of the result, the other aspect, of course, being the quality of function of the hip once the infection has been "cured". These criteria are clinical – the disappearance of pain and the resolution of all local inflammation; radiological – the stabilization, or better still, the regression of lesions caused by the infection; and laboratory investigations – a lasting return of the ESR to within the normal range. However, the most important criterion is that the hip should continue to progress satisfactorily over a period of several years.

For a long time we have not considered débridement or other similar procedures to be satisfactory; they are not capable of curing chronic infection. Among the 25 patients who were treated in this way, ten have hips that are tolerable because the acute discharge has diminished, but the infections have not really been cured and the prostheses are still loose. Seven hips have been revised for infected loosening and a new prosthesis has been implanted, and in eight cases the prosthesis has been removed.

Débridement can quieten the acute inflammatory phase and improve a patient's generally poor condition, but it will never be able to cure the infection. Its sole justification today is in old patients who are unfit to undergo more extensive surgery and too badly infected for medical treatment alone to be effective. It may bring them some relief and comfort during their last few months.

It is not fair to compare the results in cases where prostheses have been removed for infection with those in cases where prostheses have been revised, even though this is the real dilemma that faces each patient. A review of the files shows that the situation in which one or the other of these procedures was carried out are markedly different. Thus, one can make only very basic comparisons, as the two populations are dissimilar. Forty-three percent of patients whose prostheses were removed had a fistula, as compared with 18% in the group that were completely revised; 21% of patients in the first group were infected by *Staphylococcus aureus*, compared with only 6% in the second; 42% of hips where the prosthesis was removed contained frank pus, compared with only 18% in the group of revisions. For 88 of 107 (82%) in the first group this was the first repeat operation, while this was so for 92 of 99 (93%) in the second group. It is clear that the surgeon is not so bold when faced with several previous attempts which have ended in failure.

The postoperative management was also different. The infection was serious enough for irrigation to be set up in 83% of those hips where the prosthesis had been removed, compared with 28% where the prosthesis had been changed, and postoperative antibiotic therapy was maintained for more than 6 months in 9% of the first group as compared with 66% in the second.

These facts alone show that there is a large disparity between the two populations. There are other features that are not so amenable to comparison: the poor general condition of the patient, whether due to age or to the infection, and the psychiatric state of patients who, at any price, want the operation that will have the greatest chance of curing the infection, whatever its subsequent effect on function.

Taking all these factors into account, what can we learn from these two major procedures? As might be expected, the straightforward removal of the prosthesis resulted in a high rate of cure of the infection – 85%, two-thirds of the patients having been followed up for at least 4 years after the last operation (Fig. 8.20). However, function was generally poor, and

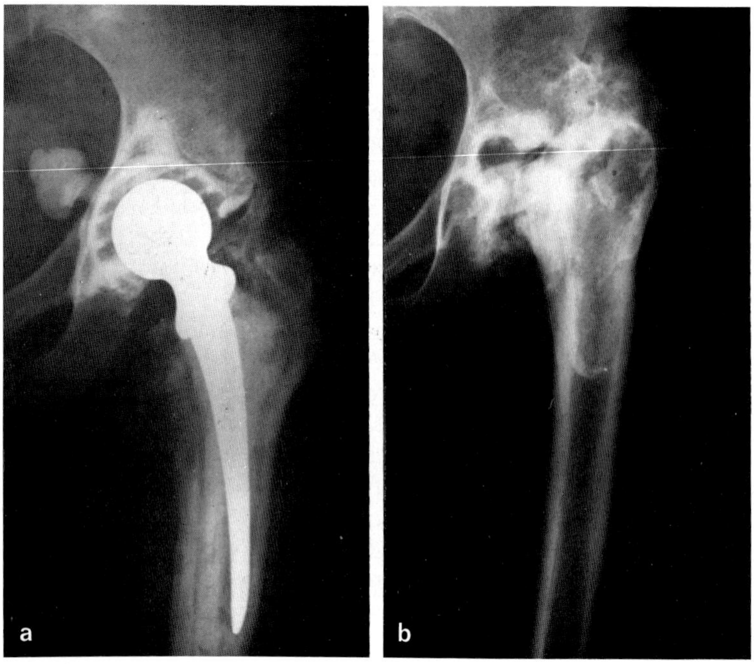

Fig. 8.20 a, b. Removal of the prosthesis. **a** A left Lagrange-Letournel prosthesis that is loose and infected. In view of the extent of the bony damage and the presence of a streptococcal infection, the prosthesis was removed (1972). **b** Radiograph 10 years later: a pseudocoaptation has developed. The functional result is good. There is no pain and the patient can walk for a considerable distance with one cane

three-quarters of these patients had an overall score of 15 or less. This method of assessing the result can be rather misleading in some cases, as complete pain relief and a large range of movement (which is really hyperlaxity) will score 12 points. In fact, several of these patients are virtually bedridden, and the most active can walk a maximum of 2–3 km a day with the aid of a stick. In practice, the majority are grossly disabled.

As might be expected, the results following revision of infected total hip replacements are not as good concerning the cure of the infection.

The series studied involved 99 revisions of both components of the prosthesis. Among these patients, two-thirds of whom had been followed up for 4 years or more, there were 72 straightforward cures; ten were still doubtful, and three had persistent infections for which they had not yet been re-operated upon. Fourteen patients were awaiting further surgery; 11 of these cases involve removal of the prosthesis (by which it can be understood that the patient, the surgeon, or both have given up) and in three cases the prosthesis will be exchanged. One can therefore deduce that, taking into account the varied nature of these cases spread over 10 years, three-quarters of these patients have been cured of their infection by a revision procedure. This is, of course, less than the proportion of those from whom the prosthesis was removed, but it is nevertheless a figure that one would not have dared to hope for 12 or 15 years ago (Fig. 8.21 a–c).

Persistent infections or recurrences present quite early. The majority are seen during the first 2 years following revision, and none were seen after more than 4 years among the cases that we have studied.

No deaths could be directly related to these revision procedures. Of the four patients who died in the years following surgery, only one death can possibly be linked to the infection. It occurred soon after the removal of a prosthesis following the recurrence of infection after a previous revision.

The quality of the functional results is most encouraging, as two-thirds of the hips scored 16, 17, or 18, these being good or excellent results. A score of 16 corresponds here to a hip that is generally without pain, that flexes to nearly 90°, and that is only slightly unstable. Overall, one-third were scored at 6,6,6.

These overall results show that the chances of curing the infection during the period when these patients were being treated were greater when all foreign material had been removed. However, the superiority of the functional results of the revisions is such that we believe that this method should always be used, as long as it is not contraindicated by the general or psychological condition of the patient or by extensive local damage resulting from the infection. We are geratly encouraged by the results of revision as long as the treatment is carried out carefully and the major principles are respected. This involves full débridement at the same time as the components are exchanged and

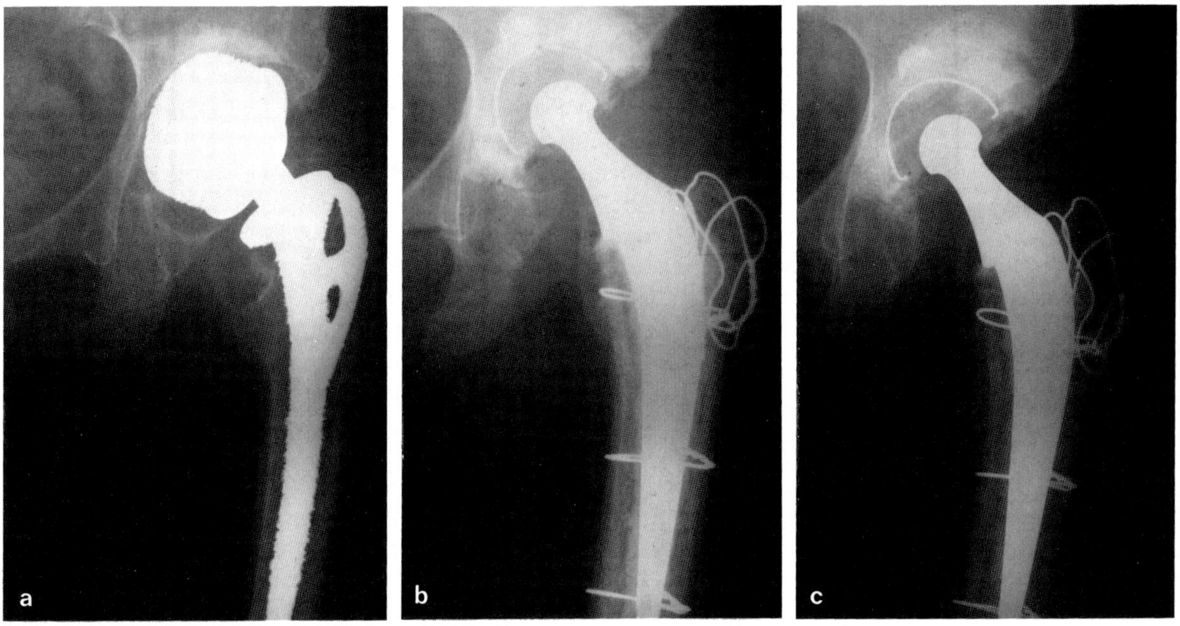

Fig. 8.21 a–c. Exchange of the prosthesis. **a** An infected "porometal" prosthesis. In spite of the envisaged problems and the presence of a streptococcal infection, it was decided to implant a new prosthesis (1979). **b** Postoperative roentgenogram. A long window had to be cut over the lateral surface of the femur, which was held in place by four cerclage wires. **c** Three years later, there are no deleterious radiological changes and the ESR is between 12 and 31. There is good function

the long-term administration of local and systemic antibiotic therapy.

We have not, up to now, treated these patients in two stages, the first being débridement and the second the implantation of a new prosthesis a few months later. We believe that the risk of re-awakening infection would be just as great during the second stage as it is when everything is done at the same time. Also, the additional local damage involved in a second procedure (scarring, muscle damage, osteoporosis) could have only an adverse effect on the new arthroplasty. However, several patients who have been transformed by the cure of their infection following removal of their prosthesis have become dissatisfied with the poor function of their hips. They have returned to ask us to implant a new prosthesis and we have not always refused to grant them their request or regretted having done so.

8.9 Development of Treatment of Chronic Infection in Total Hip Replacement - Present Indications

M. Kerboul

Before defining the present indications for the different operative procedures it is instructive to recall the path that we have taken over the past 18 years.

Until 1969, chronic infection of a total hip replacement was synonymous with failure. This failure did not occur immediately, as function could be maintained, with or without antibiotic treatment, until or sometimes after the components of the prosthesis became loose, and one was in no hurry to remove them. However, the final outcome was inevitable, and when a fistula appeared the surgeon and the patient came to a mutual decision. The prosthesis and cement were removed and the hip was left, either as a Gilderstone procedure or with a trochantero-iliac coaptation. This was not always a disaster as regards function, but it was nevertheless a failure of the arthroplasty.

Revision procedures for loosening had, of course, been performed prior to this. The infection had usually passed unrecognized, as frank pus had not been found. There was the appearance of inflammation around the hip, but this was readily attributed to the presence of loosening. Occasionally, a staphylococcus was isolated, but it was called a "nonpathogenic" contaminant and was not considered to be relevant. When postoperative antibiotic treatment was given, it was only for a few days and, as it did not delay the renewed onset of loosening, which was soon followed by fistula formation, the above view was reinforced.

Until 1969, all operations but one that were carried out in ignorance of the presence of this chronic infection ended in failure. The discovery of a streptococcus isolated from direct culture resulted in a patient being treated with systemic antibiotics during a prolonged stay in the hospital, and this, by change, was effective. As nobody had given instructions for the treatment to be stopped, the antibiotivs were continued during convalescence and then by the general practitioner until the patient discontinued them himself 4 months later. Thus, it was purely by chance that this first patient with septic loosening was cured after the exchange of his prosthesis by a course of antibiotic treatment that at the time would have been thought to be unnecessarily prolonged.

As far as we know, the first revision of an infected prosthesis to be carried out as a planned procedure was in 1970. The organism was a *Pseudomonas aeruginosa* and it had been isolated from a aspirate prior to surgery. A cure seemed to have been effected after 1 year of treatment with gentamicin, although the levels may well have been high, as the patient developed vestibular problems. After 4 years, the hip was perfect both clinically and radiologically. The success of this bold attempt, which was initially kept secret for fear that it would be labeled as heresy, was a strong incentive to repeat the procedure.

Gentamicin was first added to cement in 1971 and, at the meeting of the French Society for Orthopedic Surgery and Traumatology in 1974, we reported 12 successful results among 30 attempts. From this study the advantages of effective, long-term antibiotic therapy were already emerging, together with the determination to persevere with this line of treatment, as it seemed definitely possible to dry a chronically infected prosthesis while preserving excellent function.

The classical approach that sacrified function to eliminate infection nevertheless remained the most prudent solution, especially when the damage caused by the infection, the virulence of the organism, or the poor general condition of the patient made attempts at preservation of the prosthesis too risky or the result too unpredictable. However, in other cases, where the patient was young, fit, and capable of withstanding a long, hemorrhagic procedure, when the extent of the bony damage was limited or could be repaired without difficulty, and when the organism was sensitive to a suitable antibiotic, then it was worthwhile attempting to preserve the prosthesis, and our series gradually grew.

By 1977 we had a series of 52 patients, 43 of whom had retained their prostheses. On closer inspection, however, there were only 27 real successes, and not all looked as if they would be long lasting. With 27 successes among 52 patients we had nevertheless improved on our 1974 success rate of 40% and had crossed the 50% barrier (52%).

The study of 100 revised infected total hip replacements, carried out in February 1980, highlighted certain principles that were essential if the procedure was to be successful. The criteria necessary to cure the infection are (a) the hip must be completely debrided and cleaned and (b) the antibiotic treatment must be effective and prolonged.

Complete débridement and cleaning of the hip means that in each case, *all* infected tissue must be excised. Both components and all of the cement must be removed even if one of the components is well fixed and even if neither of them is loose.

All of the cement must be removed. There is no question of leaving a particularly adherent fragment of cement in the femur, of leaving a plug of cement that is too far down, of allowing a fragment of cement to migrate toward the distal extremity of the femur, or of neglecting a plug of cement that is inside the pelvis.

All infected soft tissue must be excised. This includes not only the tissue involving the fistula but also any soft tissue abscesses within the thigh that have come from an infected perforation through the cortex. This may occasionally extend as far distal as the knee. It may be demonstrated by roentgenography of the fistula or by arthrography. This is the only real indication for arthrography in loosening, and in such cases it is of great help and almost indispensible.

Local antibiotic treatment is essential and can be useful if added to the cement. *Systemic antibiotics* must be effective and should be continued for 6 months.

When all these conditions apply, a successful result is almost guaranteed. Unfortunately, this was the case for only 36 patients in the series, but among them were 34 successes (the two failures being infected with *Staphylococcus aureus*).

We already knew that an unsuccessful revision did not necessarily denote an absolute failure, as in 1980 a second revision was successful in five out of ten patients. Since then the two patients with recurrent *Staph. aureus* infections seem finally to have been cured following a further procedure, one having been followed up for 20 months.

We have also learned that bony reconstruction is as necessary in infected as in aseptic situations, and that one must re-establish the best possible conditions for fixation if the prosthesis is to be durable. It is more important than ever to use a low-friction prosthesis whose components are perfectly adapted to the bone; otherwise the function will remain poor and reloosening will set off the infective process once more (Figs. 8.22 and 8.23).

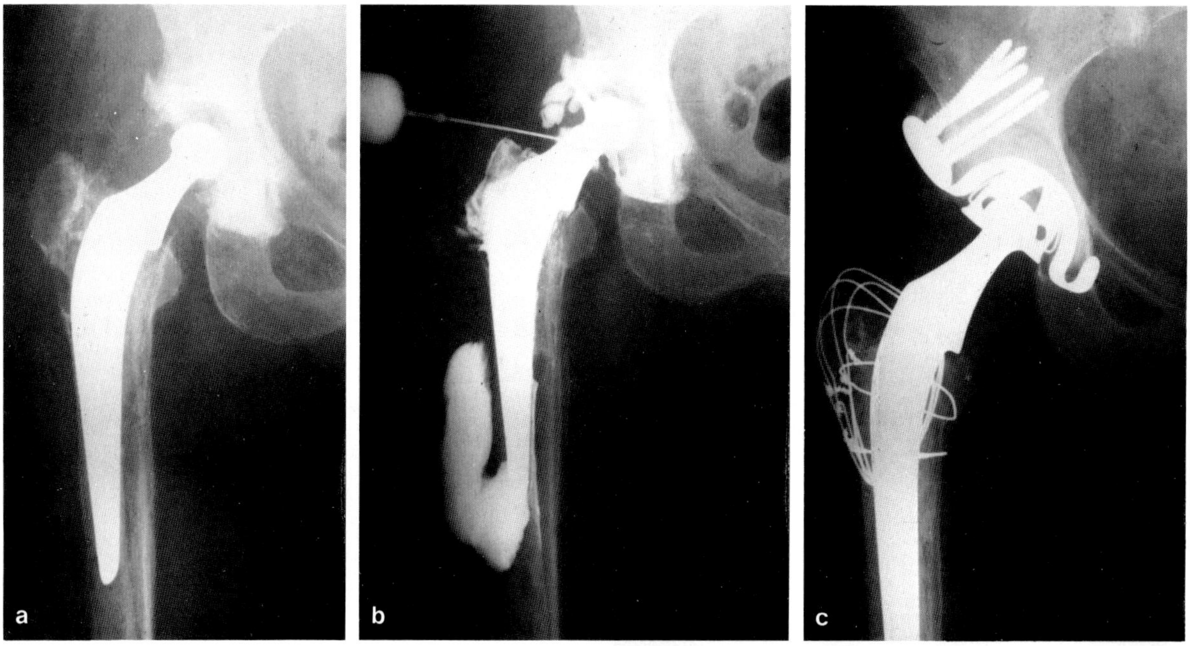

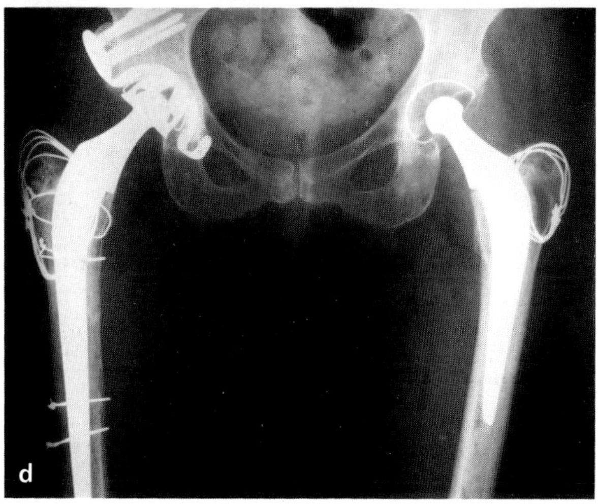

Fig. 8.22 a–d. After 10 years of septic evolution due to *Staph. aureus*, multiple reoperations (one early revision and one revision for chronic sepsis), there is new loosening of both pieces with significant femoral and acetabular osteolysis **(a)**. The arthrography (large abscess extending from distal part of the femur) shows the diffusion of infection to soft tissues **(b)**. Third attempt at conservation with rebuilding of the acetabulum by homograft **(c)**. Two years later, the X-ray provides grounds for hope and infection seems be clinically and biologically healed

Of course, one must not be stubborn and inflexible. Neither should one routinely attempt to preserve the prosthesis in chronic infection, even though we made undoubted progress between 1974 and 1980; the rate of success increased from 40% to 60%, and today it is no doubt 75%.

There are still hopeless cases that will benefit from simply removing the prosthesis and all of the cement from the outset. The patient may have presented too late with irreparable bony damage; there may be extensive infection of the soft tissue; the organism may be virulent and resistant to antibiotics; or the general condition of the patient may be poor. The operation is then a salvage procedure to eradicate the infection. The final function will no doubt be poor in absolute terms, but overall it will be incomparably better than it would have been a few years ago.

After one or two attempts to preserve a prosthesis that has failed, one must be able to accept the failure and stop the advance of an infection, which could flare up and lead to disarticulation at the hip or slowly progress to a fatal outcome.

Are there still indications for carrying out primary troachtero-iliac coaptation at the same time as removing the cement and the prosthesis? No longer, for if the patient is fit enough to withstand such a proce-

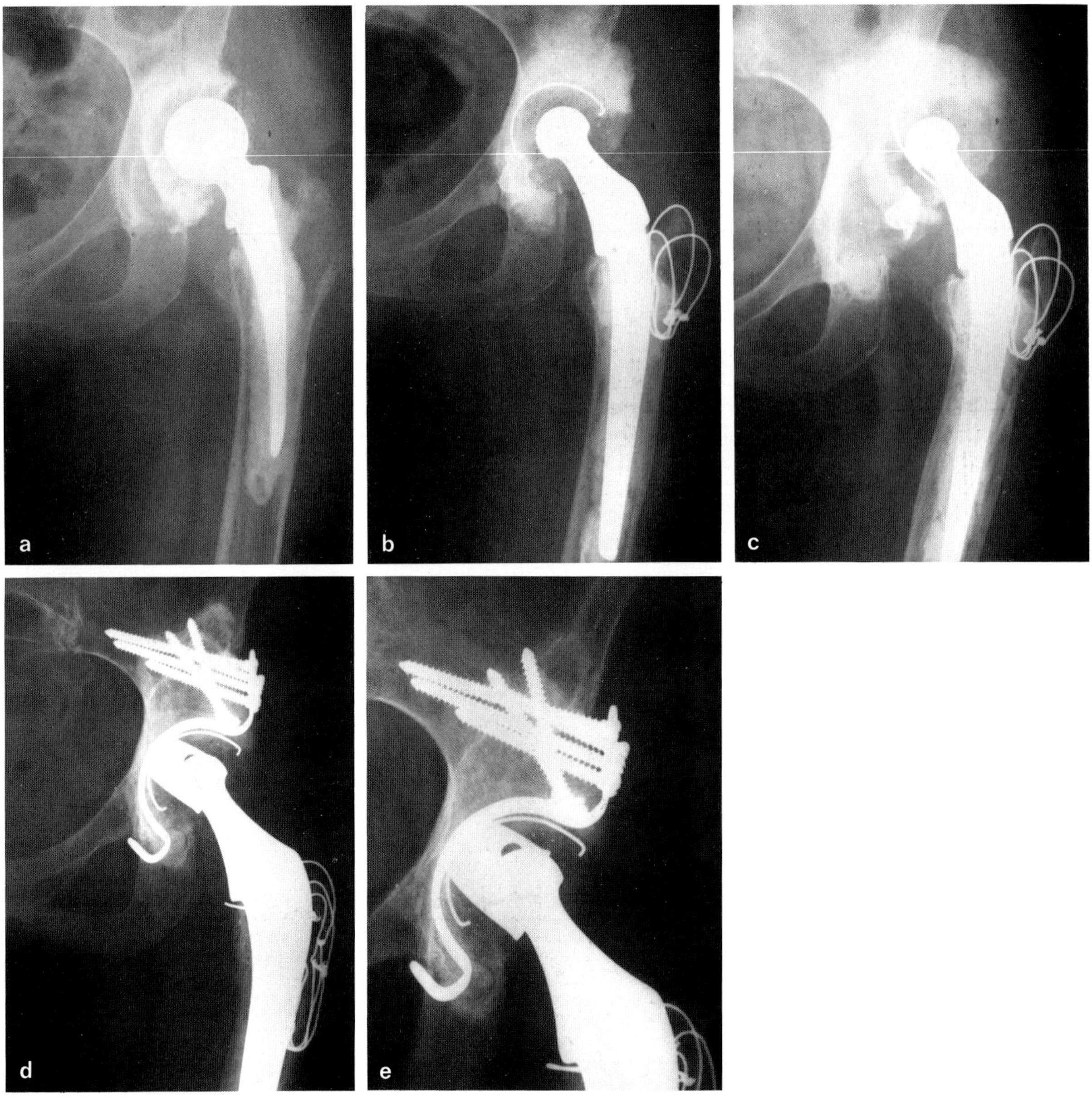

Fig. 8.23. Acute primary sepsis due to *Staph. aureus*. Despite a surgical revision, the sepsis became chronic, and loosening of the acetabulum ocurred. **(a)** A first revision with exchange of the prosthesis failed to heal the sepsis, which led to another loosening of the acetabulum with severe bone destruction **(c).** Another attempt with acetabular reconstruction by homografts and cruciate plate **(d)**: 5 years later, function is good, the ESR is normal, and the X-ray shows excellent consolidation of the grafts **(e)**

dure, and if the quality of the bone is good enough to enable it to be done, then one can just as well make an attempt to preserve the prosthesis.

Are there indications for coaptation as a secondary procedure? This may be so when infection persists in spite of removal of the cement and prosthesis. However, the source of the infection is usually bone, rather than the hypothetical space left in the acetabulum after removal of the cup.

Should coaptation be considered when the hip is dry but very unstable? It may then be perferable to consider reimplanting a new prosthesis, but starting all over again may be one start too many.

"In all things, one must know when to stop."

8.10 Prevention of Infection

J. Evrard

It is, of course, preferable to reduce the incidence of infection following total hip replacement rather than to improve on the methods of treatment, and this is possible, as is shown by the progressive improvement in the rate of infection seen in the published figures. The present figure to be improved upon is 1%, and it is approaching 0.5%.

We shall briefly review the causes of infection in order to give a better understanding of the different means of prevention. Without enumerating all the many types of bacteria, it must be emphasized that the distinction between pathogenic and saprophytic organisms is often blurred. *Staphylococcus epidermidis* and the *Corynebacteria* are both responsible for infection, although until recently they were thought to be innocuous.

Bacteria that contaminate surgical wounds can come from three sources:

1. The surgeon and his assistants, via their hands (through small, occasionally microscopic holes in their gloves) or respiratory tracts (through conventional masks, that can become permeable)
2. The patient himself, from his skin (the difficulty of decontaminating the perineum is well known)
3. The air in the operating room, which is not usually sterile. It carries dust particles of different sizes, and those of 5 μm can carry bacteria and are capable of forming colonies. These can be collected on culture plates and counted. In a conventional operating room there are between 70 and 350 such particles per cubic meter of air, and 1% carry *Staphylococcus aureus* [6].

Postoperative contamination of the operative field may follow a transitory bacteremia from the digestive or urinary tract and less commonly from the lungs. However, it cannot be called a true clinical infection if there are significant predisposing factors, such as a reduction of the patient's natural defenses. Many factors can contribute to a lowering of the patient's resistance: preoperatively – a change in the patient's general health, pre-existing conditions such as diabetes, or the use of steroids or immunosuppressants; during surgery – the anesthetic has been incriminated by several authors in that it retards the patient's natural defenses; after surgery – anything that disturbs local perfusion has an adverse affect.

By what means can we reduce the incidence of operative infection?

1. Preoperative precautions have already been discussed. However, a few points deserve special emphasis: Patients whose general condition is poor should not be operated upon, especially if there is a marked and unexplained rise in the sedimentation rate, in which case a full medical assessment must be made. The treatment of any known infective focus is an essential preliminary to all hip replacement. Patients with dental caries must be referred for the appropriate treatment. Urinary tract infections require assessment by a urologist and possibly a prostatectomy, and biliary tract disease should also be investigated. The patient must be in a physiologically stable condition before surgery, and hyperglycemia, anemia, and hypoproteinemia must be corrected. Obese patients should be encouraged to lose weight.

2. The classical aseptic technique remains the cornerstone of prevention of wound contamination during surgery and of postoperative infection. Routine precautions still provide the most important protection: local preparation of the operative field (iodine remains the best skin antiseptic), scrubbing up (considerable advances have been made in new antiseptic soaps), the surgeon's clothing (there is still room for improvement in the protection of the hands and head), isolation of the operative field (with large adhesive drapes that encircle the the lower limb), and protection of the instruments which should only be exposed just prior to their use).

The importance of adhering to a strict operative routine cannot be overemphasized, and the principles of the classical antiseptic technique must not be broken.

3. Decontamination of the Atmosphere. In a conventional operating room the air usually passes through a "bacteriological" filter and is exchanged 20 times or more per hour. However, this system still allows several hundred colony-forming particles (CFP) per cubic meter to be isolated from the atmosphere during surgery. To improve on this, Charnley developed his "tent", in which air is filtered to 2 μm and exchanged 300 times per hour. The number of CFP then fell to between 1 and 10 per cubic meter and the level of infection dropped markedly (Fig. 8.24). Operating rooms were further improved by the introduction of laminar flow, which had already been used in industry, particularly in the field of electronics. So-called absolute filters were developed, down to 0.3 μm, and these removed virtually all dust from the air, trapping 99.9%. This system had two drawbacks: (a) the noise of the powerful motors that were needed to force the air through the filters, which had a high resistance;

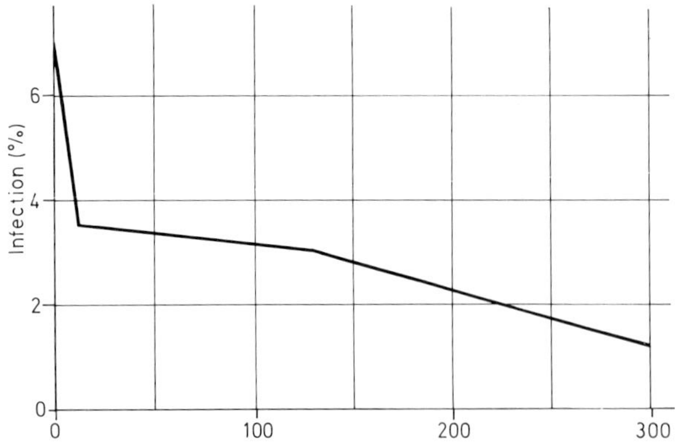

Fig. 8.24. The reduction of the rate of infection in relation to the rate of exchange of air in the operating room. The percentage of infected cases is plotted against the number of exchanges of air per hour. (After Charnley [12])

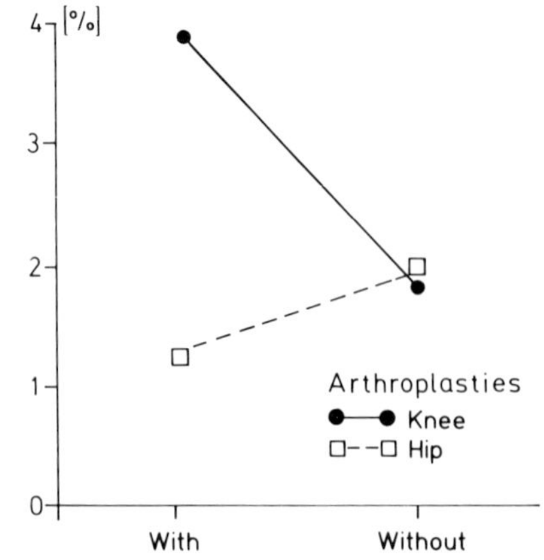

Fig. 8.25. The effect of laminar flow. The percentage of infection after total knee and hip replacement in relation to whether the operating room was equipped with horizontal laminar flow. (Salvato et al. [5])

(b) filters soon became blocked by the accumulation of dust and needed frequent renewal and constant maintenance. Finally, it was far from clear whether such a sophisticated system was really necessary, as the size of the particles producing infection was about 5 μm. This justified the proposals of Joubert et al. [5], who produced filters up to 3 μm that were very effective against those particles that could produce colonies. These "hypersterile" operating rooms, of whatever design, significantly reduced the level of operative infection.

Reviewing a series of 1650 total hip prostheses implanted from 1968 to 1979, Picault [9] showed an infection rate of 0.51% in those patients operated on under laminar flow, compared with 1.47% in those treated in a conventional operating room. Lidwell et al. [7] reviewed 8055 hip and knee prostheses implanted in various hospitals. Using comparable figures, he showed an infection rate of 0.6% when the operation was carried out under ultrasterile conditions compared with 1.5% elsewhere. Salvati et al. [10] recently produced more disturbing figures (Fig. 8.25). The use of horizontal laminar flow had reduced the incidence of infection among total hip replacements. On the other hand, infection had increased among total knee replacements. The authors attribute this to the position of the surgeons in relation to the direction of flow of the filtered air, and suggest that vertical laminar flow is preferable. However, it is difficult to understand why the level of infection should have increased rather than remaining constant in relation to that found in a conventional operating room. One wonders whether this anomaly is the result of a relaxation in the classical aseptic precautions that sometimes unfortunately accompanies improvements in technique.

4. *Prophylactic Antibiotics*. After being out of favor for a long time, antibiotics are once more considered to be an effective way of preventing operative infection. Antibiotics are therefore given before surgery, so that

Table 8.13. Results of randomized therapeutic trials of antibiotic prophylaxis in orthopedic surgery

Reference	Type of operation	Antibiotics	No. of patients given a placebo	Percent of infection	No. of patients given antibiotics	Percent of infection	Statistical significance
Boyd [1]	Fractured femur	Nafcillin	145	4.8	135	0.8	$P=0.041$
Pavel [8]	Orthopedic surgery	Cephaloridine	704	5.0	887	2.8	$P=0.025$
Carlson [3]	THR	Cloxacillin	58	24.1	60	3.3	$P=0.01$
Tengve [11]	Fractured femur	Cephalothin Cephalexin	71	16.9	56	1.8	$P=0.01$
Burnett [2]	Fractured femur	Cephalothin	126	4.7	135	0.7	$P=0.05$
GETPIA [4]	THR	Cefazolin	1067	3.3	1070	0.9	$P=0.001$

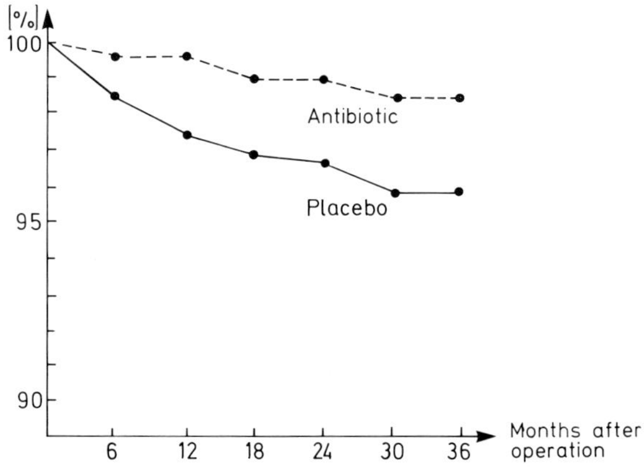

Fig. 8.26. The level of infection in relation to treatment. (After Evrard et al. [13])

the patient has a high serum level of the chosen antibiotic during the procedure (usually a penicillin or a cephalosporin). Since 1973, several clinical series have been studied under controlled conditions. All have shown a reduction in the rate of infection in the antibiotic group compared with the group taking placebos (Table 8.13). We have participated in a large clinical trial with the Association for the Study of the Prevention of Infection in Arthroplasty (GETPIA). Over 2000 patients have taken part in a randomized double-blind trial, taking either a placebo or a cephalosporin (cefazolin), the dose being 1 g i.m. every 8 h over 5 days. Eighty percent of the patients were reviewed 2 years after surgery. There were 3.3% with infections in the placebo group compared with 0.9% in the group that took antibiotics. This difference is higly significant ($P < 0.001$). It is even more significant if we consider only those patients operated upon in a conventional operating room: 5.2% compared with 0.7%.

The fear of seeing a larger number of late infections appear among patients treated with prophylactic antibiotics has proved to be unfounded. This can already be extrapolated from the present curve that goes up to 36 months (Fig. 8.26). This will probably be confirmed after we have assembled the 5-year results of all the revisions carried out among our patients. In our department 415 total hip replacements were performed (using the GETPIA protocol) from October 1975 to February 1978. To date, 11 of these have become infected. All but one belonged to the placebo group, and this gives the following figures: there were 4.8% infections (early and late) among patients operated upon in a conventional operating room with no antibiotic prophylaxis, and 0.5% among patients operated upon in the same conditions but receiving prophylactic antibiotic treatment. Although this shows the efficacy of antibiotics, the best treatment regimen is still debatable. We therefore undertook a second trial to compare two basic treatments: 5 days of cefazolin, using a new low-dose regimen, and cefamandole for 2 days, which has the advantage of being easier for the patient and is also cheaper. It was not possible to make a clinical comparison of the results. As the number of infections occurring under antibiotic treatment was very low, this would have required a large number of patients and a widespread therapeutiv trial that would probably not have produced any significant results. So we looked for another means of comparing the two protocols. The first trial had shown that about 10% of Redon's drains were contaminated when they were removed. This contamination was a useful prognostic indicator, as 4.5% of infections occurred in patients whose drains had a positive culture and only 2% in those with negative cultures ($P < 0.05$). On the other hand, the organisms grown from the drains were much more frequently resistant to cefazolin in those patients who had received prophylactic antibiotics than in the placebo group. The aim of our second study was therefore to determine if treatment with cefamandole for 48 h (a second-generation cephalosporin) would result in a reduction in the number of resistant organisms grown from the drains without increasing the number of positive results. We therefore carried out a new randomized, double-blind trial (after 48 h, the cefamandole group was given a placebo for 3 days), involving 966 patients who had received total hip replecements.

The following results were obtained: Clinically, there was no early infection in either group. There was no significant difference in the number of drains that were contaminated: 35 (7%) in the group that received cefamandole for 2 days, compared with 44 (9%) in the group given cefazolin for 5 days. However, from the qualitative point of view, there was the difference that we had hoped for. There were fewer gram-negative organisms in the cefamandole group (23% as compared with 44%) and fewer organisms that were resistant to the antibiotic that they had received (30% as compared with 61% in the cefazolin group).

In conclusion, it seems that 2 days' treatment with cefamandole is as effective as 5 days of cefazolin and has the advantage of producing fewer resistant organisms.

The fight against infection must continue to be a major concern in prosthetic surgery. At the present time we have a wide range of different methods of treatment enabling us to limit the incidence of infection, which is particularly unacceptable in this branch of surgery where the aim is to improve function.

References

1. Boyd RJ, Burke JF, Colton T (1973) A double blind clinical trial of prophylactic antibiotics in hip fractures. J Bone Joint Surg [Am] 55: 1251-1258
2. Burnett JW, Gustilo RB, Williams DN, Kind AC (1980) Prophylactic antibiotics in hip fractures. J Bone Joint Sùrg [Am] 62: 457-461
3. Carlson AS, Lidgrens L, Lindberg L (1977) Prophylactic antibiotic against early and late deep infections after total hip replacement. Acta Orthop Scand 48: 808-813
4. Evrard J, Mazas F, Flamant R, Acar J et les membres de GETPIA (1981) L'antibiotherapie préventive en chirurgie orthopédique Rev Chir Orthop [Suppl II] 67: 56-59
5. Joubert JD, Coupry A, Bonnet M (1976) Etude d'une nouvelle conception de bloc opératoire du point de vue de l'aérobio-contamination. Ann Orthop Quest 8: 105-116
6. Lidwell OM, Noble WC, Dolphin GW (1959) Use of radiation to estimate numbers of micro-organisms in airborne particles. J Hyg (Lond) 57: 299
7. Lidwell OM, Lowbury EJL, Whyte W, Blowers R, Stanley SJ, Lowe D (1982) Effect of ultraclean air in operating room on deep sepsis in the joint after total hip or knee replacement. Randomized study. Br Med J 285: 10-14
8. Pavel A, Smith RL, Ballard A, Larson IT (1977) Prophylactic antibiotics in elective orthopedic surgery. South Med J [Suppl II] 70: 50-55
9. Picault C (1979) Une expérience du flux luminaire horizontal. Communication au Colloque International sur le Concept des Blocs Opératoires, Lyon
10. Salvati EA, Robinson RP, Zeno SM, Koslin BM, Brause BD, Wilson PD (1982) Infection rates after 3175 total hip and total knee replacements with and without a horizontal unidirectional filtered airflow system. J Bone Joint Surg [Am] 64: 525-535
11. Tengve B, Kjellander J (1978) Antibiotic prophylaxis in operations on trochanteric femoral fractures. J Bone Joint Surg [Am] 60: 97
12. Charnley J (1972) Post-operatove infection after total hip replacement with special reference to air contamination in the operating room. Clin Orthop 87: 167-187

9 The Future of the Polyethylene Cup

M. Postel and J. P. Courpied

Fixation of the Charnley cups has proved reliable in our patients with the longest follow-ups of 12–14 years. It is most unusual to see loosening of late onset. When it has occurred, the fixation of the cup was already unsatisfactory on roentgenograms for a long time. This confirms Charnley's own experience and that of those who have used his prosthesis for many years. Ten years ago, one would hardly have dared to hope for such good results. This leads us to think that this type of fixation will continue much longer, as there is no reason why such a stable, unchanging, mechanical situation should suddenly change after 15 years. At the present time, methylmethacrylate cement (together with a small head) provides the best guarantee, both of a good initial result and of a fixation that will be long lasting. The durability of the fixation of the cup does not seem to be a problem for the immediate future. However, there are other problems that can be grouped under the term "wear" and which form a major area of uncertainty concerning the future of total hip replacement.

What we usually call wear is, in fact, the combination of two phenomena. The first is creep. This simple deformation, which is nonelastic and therefore permanent, is believed by Rose et al. (1980) to be the most important early cause of the head boring into the cup. The second is true abrasive wear that is caused by particles of polyethylene. Over the 10- to 14-year period under review, these two factors have caused the head of the prosthesis to bore inward into the cup, although this is on the order of only 2–3 mm at the most. Deeper penetration of the head or perforation is seen only where there have been gross errors, either in the manufacture of the cup or in the choice of polyethylene. This inward migration of the head seems to have little effect on the degree of friction within the new joint as long as it is not too advanced. However, it can finally reduce the range of movement of the joint and will give rise to serious stresses if the neck impinges against the margin of the cup. This also causes wear of the rim of the cup and increases the amount of polyethylene debris produced. This has led Wroblenski (personal communication) to consider reducing the diameter of the neck of the prosthesis to limit the adverse effects of inward boring of the head. However, true wear has another, more serious effect before impingement occurs: Particles of polyethylene are released, and these cannot be resorbed, but become surrounded by a foreign-body granuloma. It is likely that this has serious biological effects which may perhaps be the source of the major long-term problems with these prostheses.

Apart from the ceramic prostheses, all total hip replacements are at present made of metal and polyethylene. They are all subject to the same problems of wear; the larger the diameter of the head, the greater the extent of wear.

9.1 Measurement of Wear

In accordance with present-day usage, we shall use the term "wear" to mean the combination of both wear and creep, as this is the only parameter amenable to measurement. Many different methods of measurement have been described. Some make use of large numbers of specially centered roentgenograms, while others require complicated calculations. This makes them difficult or impossible to repeat, if one wishes to follow the progression of these features. They are also of little use in a retrospective study. In practice, we measure wear from a routine AP view of the pelvis by drawing the following lines (Fig. 9.1). The midpoint of the line joining the two ends of the metal marker ring is the original center of rotation of the new hip and is also the center of the cup. Although the position of the metallic marker can vary from one hip to another, the midpoint of this line is always very close to the original center of the cup. The center of the head of the prosthesis is calculated by a simple geometric construction. The cords of two arcs of the circumference of the head are drawn. The perpendiculars constructed at the midpoint of these two cords will intersect at the center of the head. Initially, the center of the head coincides with that of the cup. They become relatively displaced as wear progresses, with

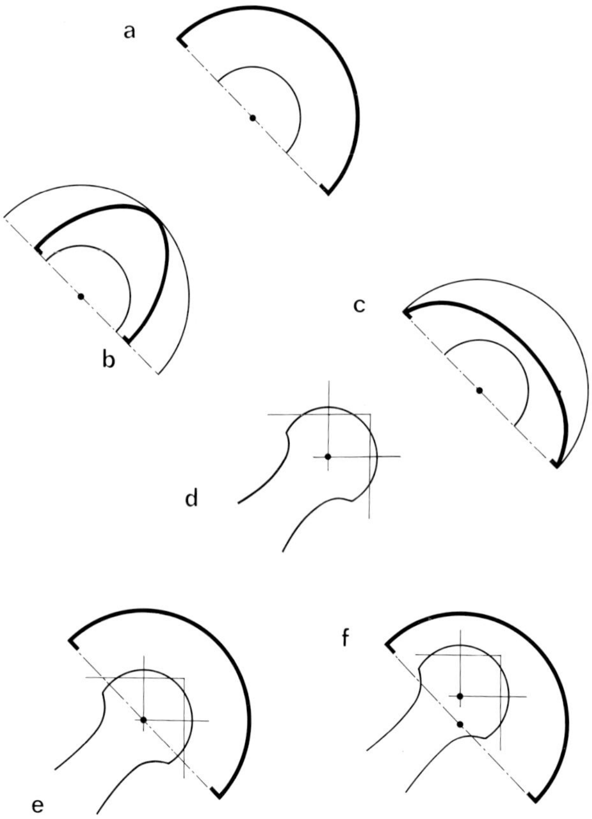

Fig. 9.1. **a–c** In a prosthesis with no wear, the midpoint of the line joining the two ends of the metal marker, whatever its position, is the center of the cup. This is also the center of the head. **d** The center of the head can be found by drawing the chord of two arcs on its circumference and constructing a perpendicular at the midpoint of each chord. These two perpendiculars bisect each other at the center of the head. **e, f** In a cup that is worn, the same method will determine the original center of the cup and the center of the femoral head that has been displaced as a result of wear

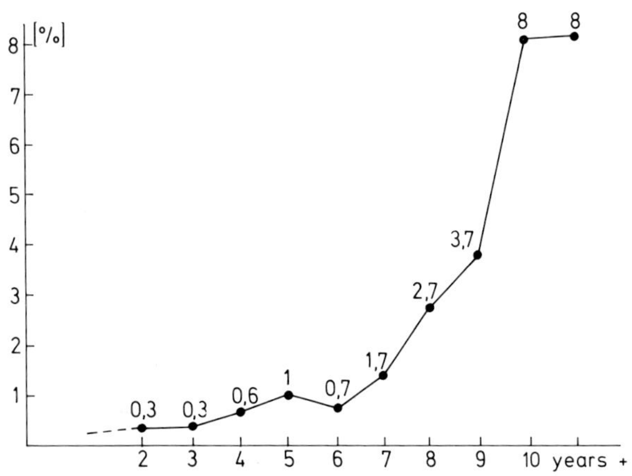

Fig. 9.2. The development of wear

the inward migration of the head. It is not difficult or time consuming to mark out these lines. They can be repeated on every control roentgenogram taken of the same hip, year after year. They are little affected by small variations in the angle of incidence. Of course, this gives only an anterior view of the migration of the head, which in fact moves upward, medially, and anteriorly, and so is slightly less than the true figure. However, this technique seems to give a good assessment of what is happening and how wear is progressing.

9.2 Incidence of Wear

Among the 640 prostheses that have been followed up radiologically for 6–13 years, there was measurable wear in 67 patients (10.5%). Of the 184 prostheses with a 10-year follow-up, wear was measurable in 39 patients (22%). Of the 118 prostheses followed up for more than 10 years, wear was seen in 35 cases (29%). Not surprisingly, the number of prostheses showing wear increases with time (Fig. 9.2).

When Does Wear Become Apparent?

The curve begins to rise sharply after 8–9 years, and there is nothing to indicate that this will not continue. It is to be expected that all cups will become worn after a sufficient period of time (Fig. 9.3).

However, it is interesting to note that while wear occurs more frequently after the 8th year, it may occasionally be seen prior to this. Two unusual cases presented after the 2nd year.

There are only nine cases of wear exceeding 2 mm in this series. As expected, they all began early, before 6 years, which was much earlier than the average. There are at least two possible explanations for these early cases of wear. One may be the surgeon. The polished head of the prosthesis, that has been machined to within 1 μm, is very delicate. It may be damaged simply by a scratch from a metal instrument during surgery, and this may have a serious effect on the polyethylene. This is only a hypothesis. To try and confirm this, we looked to see if an increase in wear had occurred in those cases where the operation file commented on a difficult reduction, as this may have caused damage to the head. The figures are not significant and the hypothesis remains unproven. The other explanation could be the lack of homogeneity that is now known to exist in the layers of polyethylene from which the cups are made. There are zones of low molecular weight within these layers that are less hard

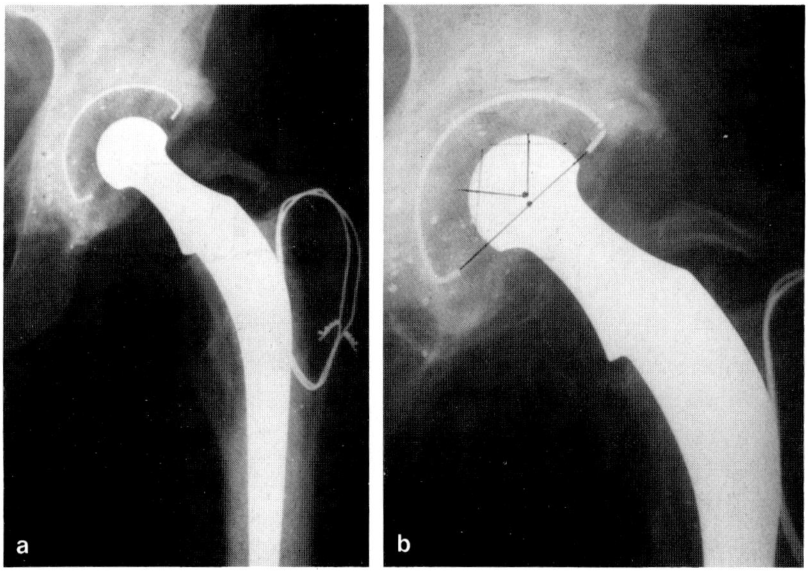

Fig. 9.3. **a** One year after surgery the cup is perfect; **b** 12 years later there are 2 mm of wear

and so are more susceptible to wear. The number of cups that have had to be removed because of wear is still much too low to implicate the quality of their constituents as a problem.

What Other Factors Have an Effect on Wear?

The *age* of the patient is of course of no significance in itself. However, it is possible that the greater activity of young patients may be a factor in producing wear. The average age of patients in the series is 64.5 years, and that of those whose hips developed wear was 59.7 years at the time of operation. These figures are in agreement with what one would expect if activity were to have an effect, but they are not significant, especially the latter, which relates to a very short series. Charnley found that the *weight* of the patient had an effect. This was not recorded often enough among our patients for it to be assessed. The *position of the cup* could also be a factor. Too vertical a cup would correspond to a dysplastic acetabulum that is known to predispose to arthrosis. There was no significant difference in our series.

9.3 Association of Wear with Abnormalities of Fixation

One can postulate two types of reaction between wear and the fixation of the prosthesis: (a) An abnormality at the bone-cement interface could release particles of bone or cement, which could become abrasive to the cup and lead to wear. (b) The particles that are released during the "normal" wear process and become incorporated into a granuloma could attack the bone-cement interface.

Among the 185 prostheses followed up for over 1 year, 130 showed not the slightest sign of a lucent area around the cup at 3 years, and at 10 years only 23 showed evidence of wear (17.7%). On the other hand, 55 patients had partial or extensive lucency at 3 years, and at 10 years 16 showed wear (29%), especially when the lucent zone was extensive. Conversely, some cups that were worn at 10 years had no lucent areas at 7 years, and none developed subsequently. Other cups that were worn at 10 years had a lucent zone at 7 years which remained constant, with no change in its width or extent. One could therefore say that wear does not seem to have any effect on the appearance of lucent zones around the cup, nor does it cause those already present to become more extensive. There does not seem to be any correlation between wear and femoral fixation in our series. Among a total of 18 femoral loosenings, 15 were not accompanied by any signs of wear. Three loose prostheses were associated with wear, and among the 39 worn prostheses that were followed up for 10 years or more there were only two loose femoral components.

Overall, the quality of the fixation seems to have a slight influence on the early appearance of wear. Conversely, from the figures available to us, wear could not be incriminated in the development of loosening.

However, two things are lacking in this study: a longer follow-up, using a larger number of patients to give true statistical value to the figures, and a more exten-

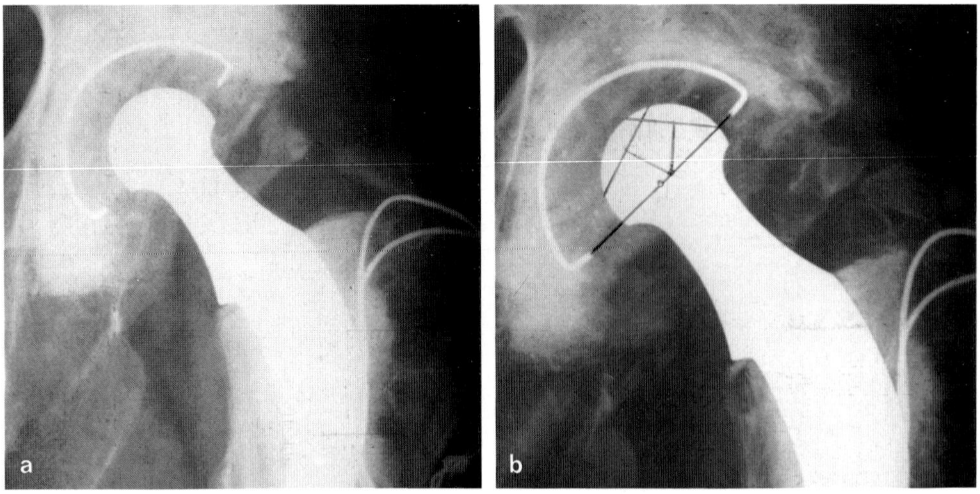

Fig. 9.4. **a** One year after surgery the cup is not worn and the femur is normal; **b** 10 years later, there is wear of 2 mm and a cyst showing resorption of the calcar, with no effect on function

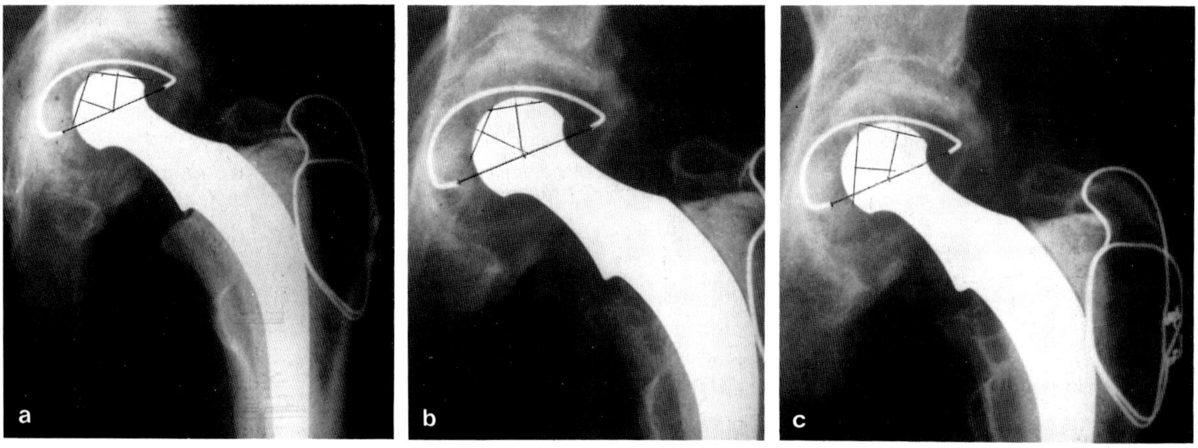

Fig. 9.5. **a** One year after surgery. In spite of the abnormal position of the marker on the cup, the two centers remain superimposed. **b** Seven years later there is no wear, but some resorption of the calcar is seen. **c** Ten years after surgery: marked wear and extensive resorption

sive anatomical study of the membrane found at revisions, in order to determine the part played by polyethylene in the formation of granulomas around prostheses.

This last point is probably of great long-term significance, but it is one that can only be assessed in the years to come. Whatever its theoretical importance, we shall be able to gather this information only very slowly.

9.4 Response of the Femur

In a few sporadic cases we noticed resorption cavities around the calcar, which Charnley described as "cavitation". We prefer to call them "granulomas". These lesions are not the same as lucent zones or signs of loosening (Figs. 9.4 and 9.5). They are situated at the part of the joint where one imagines that debris produced by wear would accumulate. At 10 years, these areas of resorption are present in 20% of cases among the series overall and in 59% of worn prostheses, which seems to incriminate wear debris. However, they are also present without any measurable signs of wear. They also seem to occur more frequently when the neck is cut high, at more than 1 cm above the lesser trochanter. It seems logical that there may be a peroperative vascular factor that increases the resorption of necks that are too long. It is possible that it is caused by a combination of both these factors. If this series is divided into four groups according to whether the residual femoral neck is short or long and to whether the cup is worn or not, then granulomas of the calcar are seen 2–3 times more frequently in the group with a long neck and a worn cup than in the other three. These lesions take different forms. Many are 2–3 mm in diameter and seem to have been present for a long while with no mechanical sequelae. In a few rare cases where they are more extensive, they have already given rise to complications.

Reference

Rose RM, Nusbaum HJ, Schneider H, Ries M, Paul I, Grugnola A, Simon SR, Radin EL (1980) On the true wear rate of ultra high-molecular-weight polyethylene in the total hip prosthesis. J Bone Joint Surg [Am] 62: 537–549

10 Response of Local Tissue to Total Hip Replacement

M. Forest*

In order to classify the types of reaction of bone and the periarticular tissues to total hip replacement, an analysis must be made of the cellular and tissue lesions that occur. These are very complex and depend on the type of arthroplasty, on how long it has been implanted, and on the mechanical forces acting on the joint.

The pathologist must have adequate information concerning the clinical and radiological features of the hip. He must also be familiar with the histological appearance of connective tissue that has been subjected to a variety of mechanical stimuli and with the cellular response to debris produced by wear. The lesions found around the Moore and Judet prostheses give a simpler picture, but it is invaluable for an adequate understanding of the lesions that are seen around cemented total hip replacements.

Although the lesions seen in tissues that are subjected to mechanical stress progress only slowly, the cellular response to wear debris changes over a period of several years, especially in its pattern and intensity [1].

Some morphological investigations involve special techniques that pose considerable problems. They require the precise identification and preservation of the junctions of bone or connective tissue with cement or the prosthesis, whether for macroscopic studies or for histology.

The orthopedic surgeon must appreciate that the study of specimens taken during surgery captures only a moment during the progression of changes that occur in the tissues. It is often impossible to describe a pathophysiological pattern of loosening without repeated specimens and multiple sections. The surgeon must realize that the same basic lesions are often found, whether the prosthesis is securely fixed or not, and that the information provided by the specimens is of relevance only when taken in its clinical and radiological context.

* In collaboration with A. Carlioz, P. LeFloch, M. Daudet Monsac (CNRS). Département d'Anatomie et de Cytologie Pathologiques, U.E.R. Cochin-Port Royal, Paris

This variation in morphology that is seen with different implants is now being increasingly supplemented by the use of microprobe analysis and by studies of the ultrastructure of the interposed membranes [13, 21, 31, 37, 43].

We shall base this review on histopathological studies of routine specimens taken during revisions of total hip replacements at Cochin. This has been supplemented by the study of joints that have been removed post mortem, and by the analysis of specimens of bone and cement following the implantation of special prostheses in the treatment of tumors. All suitable bone specimens have also been studied with high-definition roentgenograms.

The pathologist is frequently asked three questions:

1. Why are the tissues surrounding the joint so hyperplastic?
2. Is wear debris present, and of what does it consist?
3. By what mechanism is bone resorbed, whether in contact with the cement or with the prosthesis?

We shall therefore study the newly formed structures around the joint, their morphological appearance, the difficulty in the identification of wear products, and, finally, the different features of the bone-cement interface.

10.1 Newly Developed Structures Around the Joint

These are the most common source of biopsies taken during hip revision. Their structure is important, as it most frequently reflects the composition of the tissue membrane that will finally form around the cup or the femoral component. Localized osteolytic lesions such as cysts or areas of resorption around the tip of the stem have the same histological appearance.

They consist of two distinct elements: one is the tissue changes caused by surgery or by the underlying pathology and the other is the appearance of a florid histiocytic foreign-body reaction, or granuloma.

10.1.1 Periarticular Changes Caused by Surgery or by the Underlying Joint Pathology

These are characterized by dense sclerotic layers with relatively reduced capillary vascularity. This sclerosis is sometimes refractile and often hyalinized. There are often cavities containing residual synovial structures or broken-up areas of new synovium. This newly differentiated synovial tissue is often extensive and appears early on. All the transitional stages between young fibroblasts and multinucleated synoviocytes are seen. It is not uncommon to see a marked cellular hyperplasia similar to that of rheumatoid synovitis (Fig. 10.1).

There are often areas of metaplastic bone or cartilage associated with the layers of collagen around the capsule. Smaller islands of metaplastic chondroid tissue may be seen on the fringes of residual atrophic synovial tissue whose outline may have disappeared.

On the surface are sclerotic nodules; these are the remains of old fibrinous exudates that have become organized.

Incrustation by bone and cartilage is minimal and has often been partly resorbed. Hemosiderin deposits are similarly limited. One may occasionally see islands of mucous degeneration within the connective tissue, or fatty deposits that probably result from fibrinolysis or tissue destruction.

10.1.2 Histiocytic Cellular Response

The histiocytic response normally determines the special morphological appearance of the tissue around the prosthesis (Fig. 10.2). The development of this histiocytic reaction is qualitatively identical, whatever the type of debris that has been phagocytosed (polyethylene, methylmethacrylate, metal).

The morphology of the granuloma is dependent solely on the size of the particles. Particles of 2–5 nm are intracytoplasmic, being taken up by mononuclear histiocytes. Larger particles elicit a marked giant cell response.

The histiocytes are arranged in thick layers that are

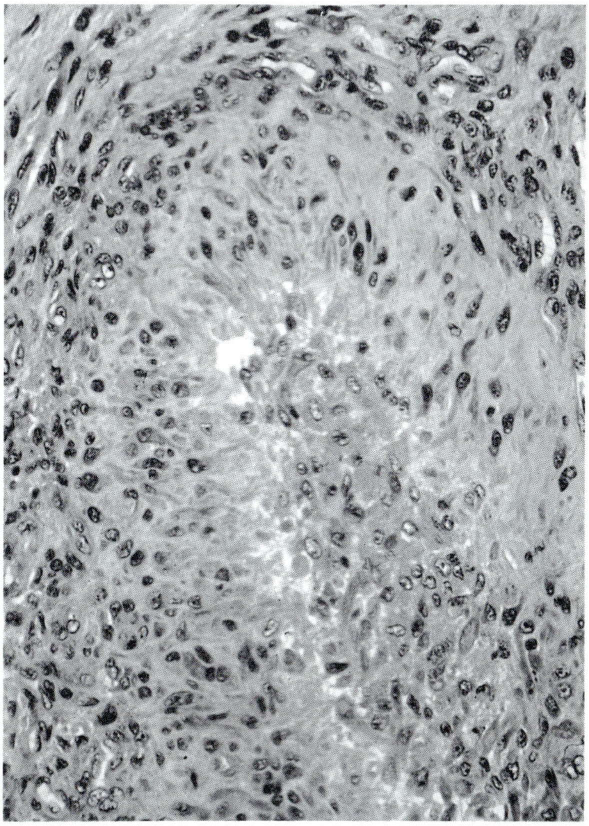

Fig. 10.1. Newly formed synovium contained in a recess in the new capsule. H & E, ×66

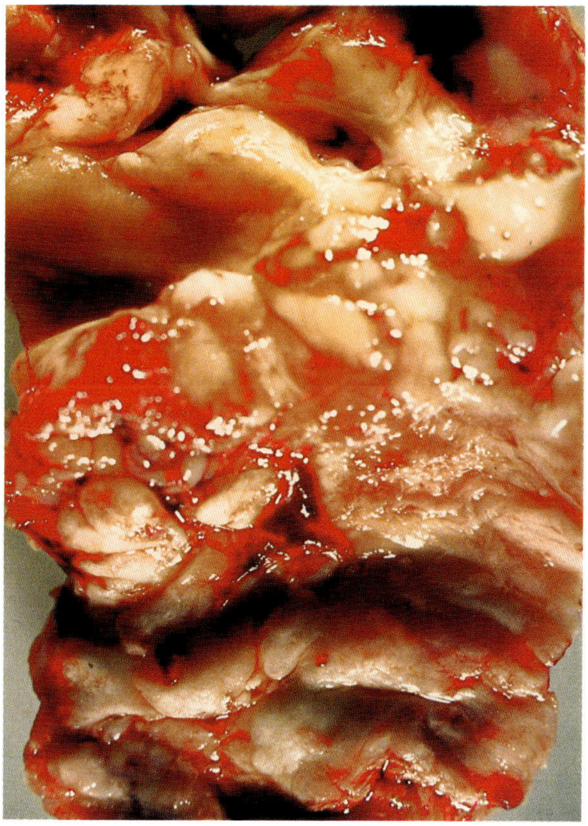

Fig. 10.2. The new capsule. Hyperplastic appearance; yellow coloration due to lysis of the histiocytic granuloma; superficial fibrinous exudate

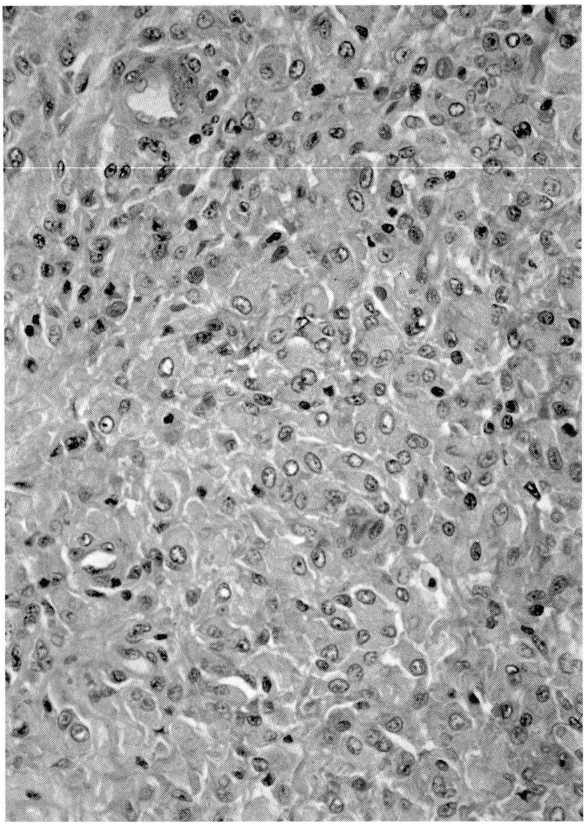

Fig. 10.3. Histiocytic granuloma (polyethylene). Densely cellular with active mitoses. The superficial areas are less vascular. H & E, × 66

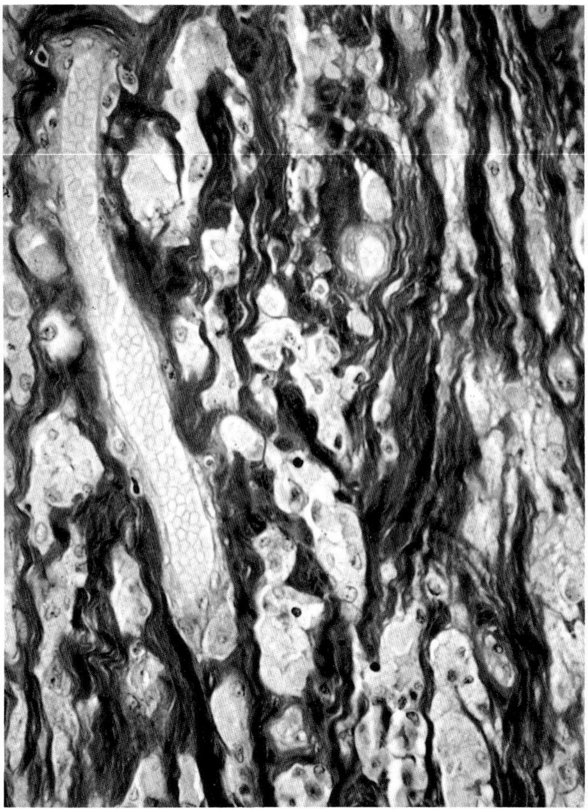

Fig. 10.4. Progressive organization of the granuloma. Trichrome, × 66

poorly vascularized and protrude into the joint cavity (Fig. 10.3). Within sclerotic areas, the histocytes follow the paths of the capillaries or arterioles.

In the majority of cases, the histiocytic granuloma becomes remodeled, and it is this that produces such a distinctive macroscopic appearance.

Cytolysis occurs in the large sheets of histiocytes that are often packed full of small particles. This results in broken-up layers of cells that are either superficial or embedded within sclerotic tissue. Cytolysis of giant cells is less common. These areas of necrosis frequently produce (a) release of lipids and cholesterol crystals that result in the secondary production of fat granulomas [22], and (b) secondary fibrosis. The collagen fibers frequently become hyalinized, forming outgrowths of coalescent nodules (Fig. 10.4).

These histological lesions are responsible for the overall macroscopic appearance of the periprosthetic tissue. There is a shell of hyperplastic fibrous tissue, with yellow areas that are rich in lipids and broken-up areas of necrosis that may lie superficially or deep.

The granuloma is often diffuse, extending into the periarticular fat and the surrounding muscle fibers. When extensive, it gives rise to pseudotumors or newly formed bursae (metal-on-metal prostheses).

10.2 Wear Products and Their Identification

We shall consider methylmethacrylate, polyethylene, and metallic debris, which frequently occur together. The reliability with which they can be identified depends on the number of specimens taken, their correct orientation, the use of polarized light, and an understanding of the commonly occurring artifacts.

10.2.1 Methylmethacrylate

These cement particles may occur in isolation or they may coalesce. They are dissolved by the fat solvents used in routine histology, and then appear as pearls or vacuoles whose average size is 10–30 nm. This is very variable, and some of 2–5 nm are found within giant

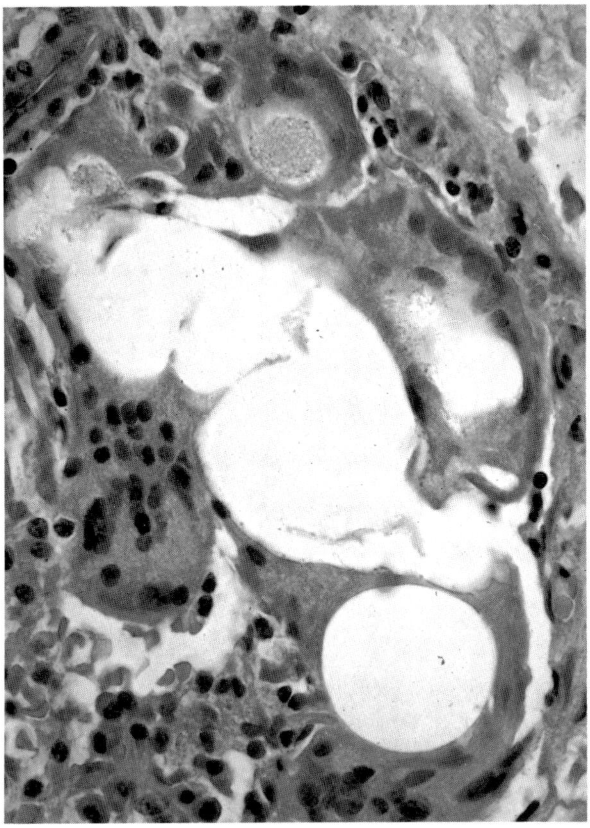

Fig. 10.5. Coalescent pearls of methylmethacrylate. Histiocytic reaction. Residual focus of granular material (barium sulfate). H & E, × 132

cells. Others are embedded within the sclerotic tissue or form particles that are several millimeters in diameter, especially when the cement has extruded outside the capsule. Granules of barium sulfate 1–2 nm in diameter may be seen in the larger vacuoles filling the whole cavity, or just on the periphery, and this can be an aid to diagnosis.

Examination by polarized light is of course negative in this instance, but it may be useful in showing the outline of the collagen fibers around the particles.

Cement typically produces a giant cell response, and extensions of giant cell cytoplasm envelop the cement particles (Fig. 10.5).

Phase-contrast microscopy is helpful in determining the relationship of the particles to the cytoplasm and the distribution of barium sulfate. The identification of pearls of cement by frozen section using fat stains is a lengthy and unreliable procedure (12–24 h), as some particles of polyethylene will also take up the stains [32, 47].

Cement can also be identified by tissue-imprint cytology if the particles are intracellular. The larger specimens adhere to the blade and are difficult to cut.

We have also reproduced the disappearance of false birefringence by heating debris from the cement sheath. This technique is useful when there is incomplete dissolution by xylene [15].

Does "wear" of the cement occur? Some theories favor the formation and migration of particles during surgery. The sheaths or casts of cement that we have examined show no superficial defects on macroscopic high-power examination. This is confirmed by studying blocks of cement taken at autopsy that do not show obvious wear. The histological identification of large particles that are deeply embedded in successive layers of collagen is an additional argument supporting this theory.

The most frequent *errors in diagnosis* are as follows:

- One may overlook particles of cement that are free or are embedded within layers of fibrous or necrotic tissue and that have not been sectioned.
- Particles of cement may be confused with fat vacuoles; the differential diagnosis is not easy.
- False polarization (always incomplete) of cement particles, produced by recrystallization in a supersaturated xylene solution, may lead to confusion with polyethylene [12].

10.2.2 Polyethylene

On routine staining, polyethylene has a cloudy or translucent appearance. There is characteristically very bright birefringence in polarized light.

The size of particles is very variable. Particles of 2–5 nm produce a response of mononuclear histiocytes, while larger fragments (several hundreds of nm) just become enclosed within the surrounding tissue (Fig. 10.6). They have a sharp outline, and the larger particles may have been damaged during sectioning. The small polyethylene particles produce a marked histiocytic response.

Errors of diagnosis are not frequent, but it should be pointed out that (a) particles of polyethylene may be broken up or disappear during preparation and leave vacuoles that may then be confused with cement, and (b) debris that is produced by wires lying just outside the section may lead to confusion [29].

10.2.3 Metallic Debris

Macroscopically, the new joint capsule or interposed membrane usually appears bluish-black (Fig. 10.7).

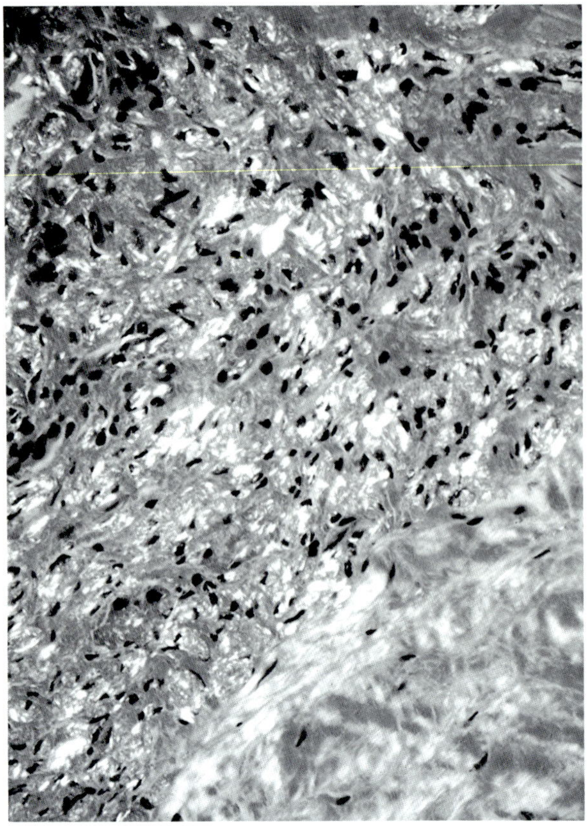

Fig. 10.6. Marked mononuclear macrophage response to polyethylene particles. H & E, polarized light, × 66

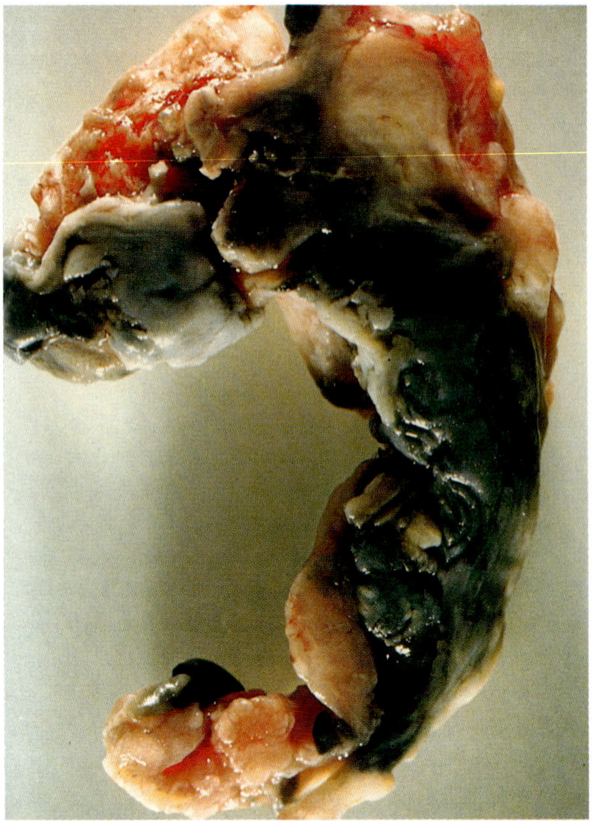

Fig. 10.7. New capsule affected by metallosis (metal-on-metal prosthesis)

The extent of the metallosis depends on the type of the prosthesis and on how long it has been implanted.
On histological examination, the small particles (1–2 nm) of ground-up debris may be intra- or extracellular. They often produce a marked mononuclear histiocytic response (Fig. 10.8).
Perls' reaction is variably positive. Bright polarization is often seen, but this is less marked than with polyethylene (Fig. 10.9).
Some particles cannot be seen by polarization; more rarely, others have a rectangular shape of 5–10 nm and show polarization only around their borders [36].
Two points deserve emphasis in relation to metallosis:

1. There is often extensive necrosis of the histiocytic granuloma, with subsequent secondary release of metallic particles. The whole granuloma may undergo necrosis.
2. There may also be a lymphocytic response that is limited to the granuloma. This reaction is most marked at the periphery where the granuloma is extending. Occasionally, there are islands of lymphoid tissue with clear centers (a type-IV allergic response due to cellular hypersensitivity?). This seems to be just a later stage of the overall response, as in the first series of 30 revisions of metal-on-metal prostheses, no such lesions were seen [23].

Particle size and the appearance of particles on polarization may result in confusion with fragments of polyethylene, especially when the particles are small. The macroscopic appearance will then enable the diagnosis to be made.
Pigmentation caused by formalin and the presence of nonrefractile hemosiderin deposits do not usually cause diagnostic problems.

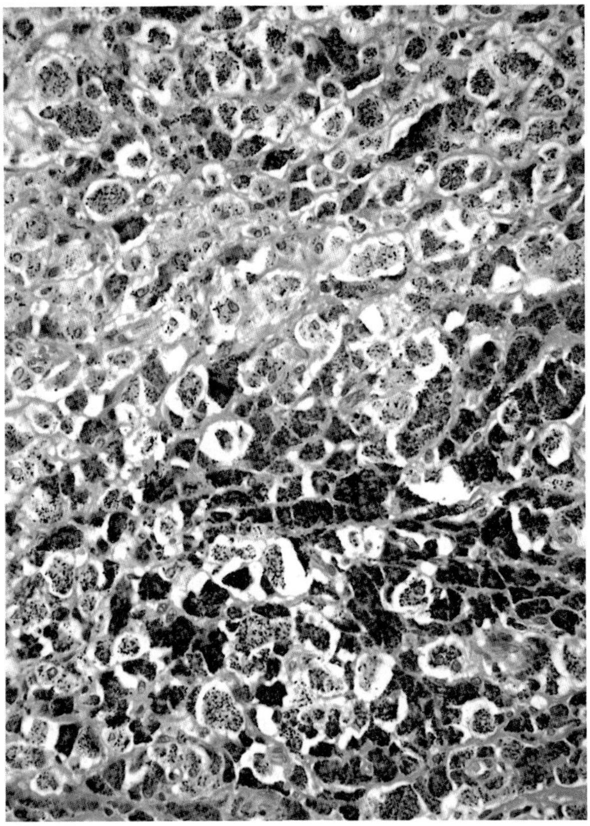

Fig. 10.8. Marked mononuclear histiocyte response to metal. H & E, × 66

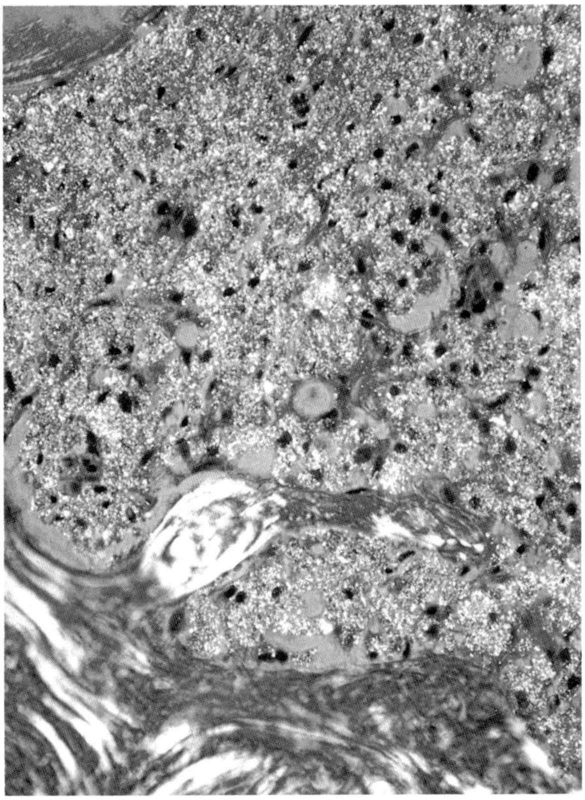

Fig. 10.9. Metallosis within lacunae of medullary bone. H & E, polarized light, × 66

10.2.4 The Quantification of Wear Products

Is there any value in quantifying this debris occurring within the tissues [28, 29, 33]? We have found that there are too many variable factors. Can we be sure that the biopsy taken during the revision gives a quantitative representation of all the structures around the joint and of the interposed membrane? How should the specimen be orientated for histology when the tissue is often fragmented and the debris is embedded within necrotic or fibrous tissue? We have therefore limited ourselves to a qualitative approach.

10.3 The Bone-cement Interface and Aseptic Loosening

We shall look in turn at the structural changes that occur in a clinically satisfactory fixation, at the lesions that are seen in loosening, and at the histological theories proposed to explain the different physiopathological mechanisms of bone resorption.

10.3.1 Histological Features of Prostheses with Good Fixation

The assessment of fixation combines both the clinical result and an understanding of the nature of the tissues around the prosthesis. The latter can be determined only by the use of postmortem material (Figs. 10.10, 10.11). We have studied the progression of changes in the tissues around the cup and femoral component from 2 months up to 4 years, and found the following: After 2 years, there is only direct bone-cement contact around one-quarter of the available surface of the cup. A thin layer of fibrous tissue separates the remainder of the cup from the underlying medullary bone. Within this sclerotic tissue are partially resorbed sequestra that result from the original surgery. Bone remodeling has resulted in large surface irregularities where the cement has left hollowed-out imprints.

This resorption of bone produced by surgery is superficial and alternates with areas of new osteons within the sclerotic bone. There are always some areas of fi-

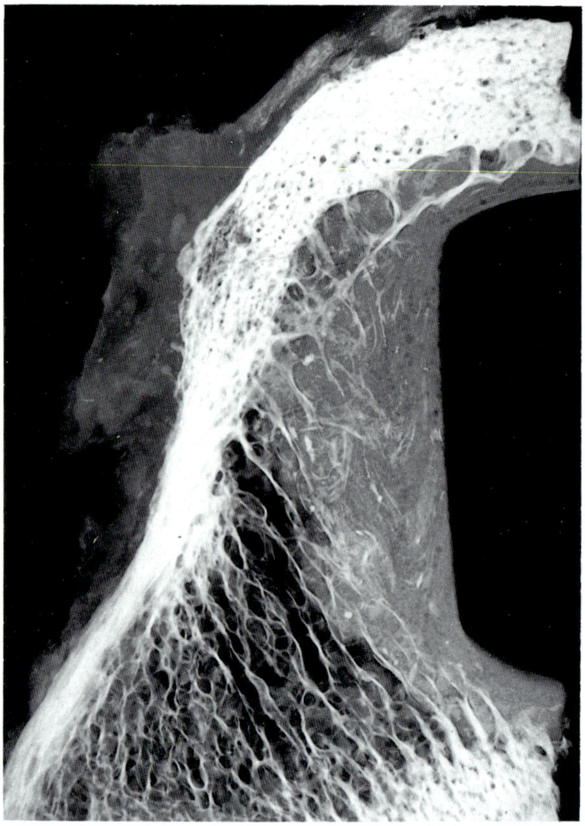

Fig. 10.10. Bone-cement interface. Relationship of cement to the cancellous bone of the femoral metaphysis. A cemented Charnley prosthesis, 4 months postoperatively

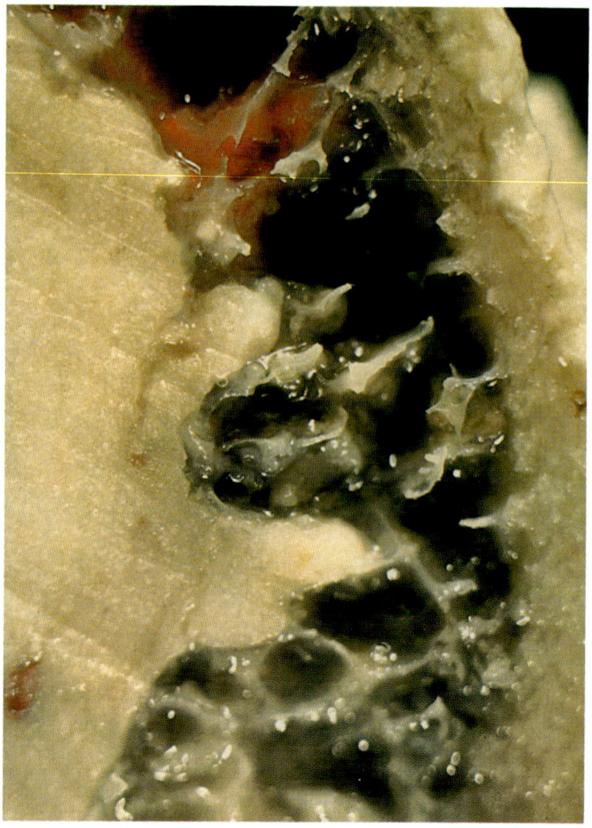

Fig. 10.11. Bone-cement interface. Relationship of cement to the cancellous bone of the acetabulum. A cemented Charnley prosthesis, 4 months postoperatively

brocartilage, but these are irregular and not extensive.

A histiocytic response to the cement is always seen in the medullary tissue of the acetabulum, and isolated macrophages occur within sclerotic areas. Extensive lysis was seen on only one occasion.

The histiocytic response is most marked in areas of least stress [7, 9]. In our material it is closely related to breaks in the medullary bone of the acetabulum.

Cancellous bone around the keying points of the acetabulum is in direct contact with the cement, but two-thirds of this surface consists of a thin layer of fibrous tissue. The histiocytic reponse is variable and is related not to the size of the lucent zone, but to the nature of the surrounding medullary bone and especially to its vascularity.

Areas of necrosis produced at the time of surgery by the exothermic polymerization reaction were very small, not greater than 5-600 nm.

On the femoral side, in both the metaphysis and diaphysis there were some areas of remodeling that were in direct contact with the cement and that alternated with a fibrous or fibrocartilaginous membrane. This membrane was present over nearly half of the available bone-cement interface in those cases with clinically satisfactory fixation. It was not continuous, but was often broken up by zones of cancellous bone that still contained osteocytes. The areas of fibrocartilage were not extensive. Focal areas of histiocytes were seen within the cancellous bone and had not undergone lysis. They were poorly vascularized. Areas of sclerosis were present, especially around the stem of the prosthesis. Newly formed haversian systems appear next to histiocytic infiltrates. Sclerotic bone also surrounds regions of dead bone some distance from the cement.

The morphological changes seen in our material are similar to those described in the literature [8, 25, 43] and can be divided into three successive phases:

1. A period of *necrosis* during the first few weeks. This involves the bone as well as the medullary tissue. It is always associated with a fibrinous exudate that may be quite marked.

2. A phase of *bone remodeling* occurring after 2 months. There was active osteoclastic resorption, together with areas of necrosis and osteoblastic activity.
3. A phase of *bony adaptation* at the end of 2 years. Although some areas were still devoid of osteocytes and the cancellous bone was porotic, the layers of bone around the femur were parallel to the cement sheath.

10.3.2 Anatomical Appearance of Loose Prostheses

The gap that develops between the bone and the cement has the radiological appearance of a clear band outlining the margin of the cement. This lucent zone becomes wider as a result of osteolysis, separating the cement from the bone over the whole surface with which it is in contact [19].

Morphologically, it most frequently consists of a layer of interposed tissue, made up of a fibrous membrane or shell that is macroscopically similar to the newly formed capsule.

The tissue interposed between the cement and the acetabulum has the same histological appearance as the new capsule. It consists of layers of collagen, with a variable histiocytic reaction, together with regions of necrosis and islands of metaplastic bone or cartilage.

The tissue interposed between the cement and the cancellous or cortical bone of the femur is usually not as thick, with layers of fibrocartilage and islands of chondroid tissue. Histiocytic responses are present, though more in the surrounding medullary tissue than in the fibrous shell itself.

In aseptic loosening a third membrane is occasionally seen between the cement sheath and the femoral prosthesis [18]. This is sometimes present only as a thin, unbroken layer of poorly vascularized, dense collagen (Fig. 10.12). It is thicker at the metaphysis and is continuous with the layer surrounding the neck of the prosthesis, extending into the new capsule. It is characterized by its fibrin content and may be the site of metallosis.

Histologically, the interposition tissue is of two main types that frequently occur together:

1. The granulomatous type. Layers of histiocytes, particularly around the joint itself, result in sclerotic hyperplastic tissue, usually following the organization of areas of cytolysis. This sclerosis increases by the incorporation of fibrous tissue and exudative lesions from the surrounding medullary tissue.

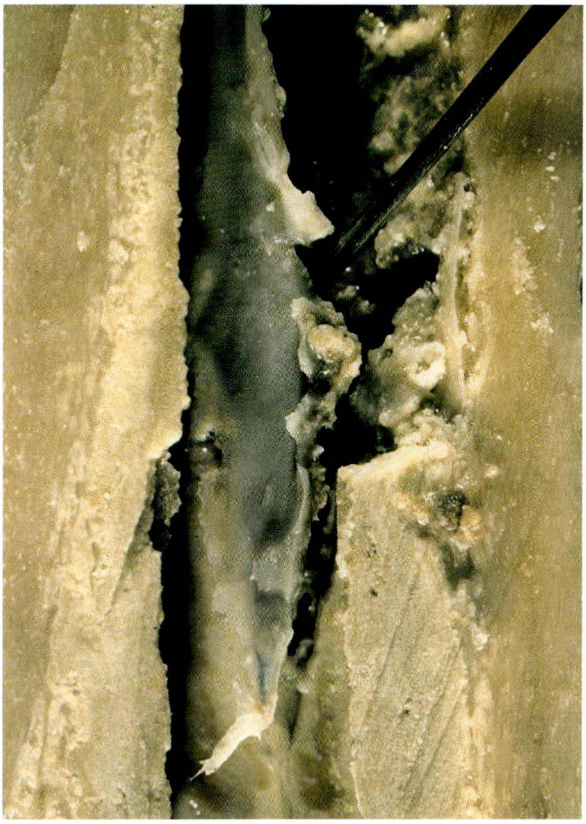

Fig. 10.12. Membrane interposed between prosthesis and cement (loose prosthesis, 4 months postoperatively)

2. The "mechanical" form, in which the fibrous shell contains few cells. When present, the histiocytic response is less marked, and there are scattered macrophages. Islands of metaplastic chondroid tissue are seen. There are also broken-up areas of new synovial tissue that are directed toward the cement surface and not toward the bony structures. These are inconstant, and are often seen only as outlines, not having the characteristic hyperplastic appearance of joint synovium.

A study of the bone of the acetabulum and femur must include the relation of bone to the interposition tissue and to the granuloma, together with the remodeling of bone and the sites from which bone is resorbed.

The connective tissue that forms the interposition membrane is of varying composition, according to the nature of the underlying bone. When connected to cancellous bone it is continuous with the fibrous tissue of the medulla. When adjacent to osteosclerotic or cortical bone it often has planes of cleavage and islands of mucoid degeneration that seem to be mechanical in origin.

Whether the granuloma is found with collagen tissue or not, it is often in direct contact with bone which may or may not contain osteocytes. It may also surround areas of osteogenesis, and osteoblastic zones are mixed with histiocytes. In the cortex, histiocytes are often found in haversian canals without having destroyed their blood supply or affected the deposition of osteoid. Other areas where resorption is occurring are often packed with sheets of histiocytes.

Bone that is being remodeled differs little from that around a well-fixed prosthesis. We have never seen ischemic lesions or microfractures within the cancellous bone.

The most important feature is the increase in the number of bone resorption sites, whether related to the interposed membrane or to the cement. Some are inactive and are probably related to the effects of surgery, while others are associated with large numbers of osteoclasts. Predominant osteoclastic activity is usually associated with a reduced osteoblastic reaction. Such osteoclastic resorption seems related to the state of local vascularity. This is especially evident at areas of resorption in the acetabulum.

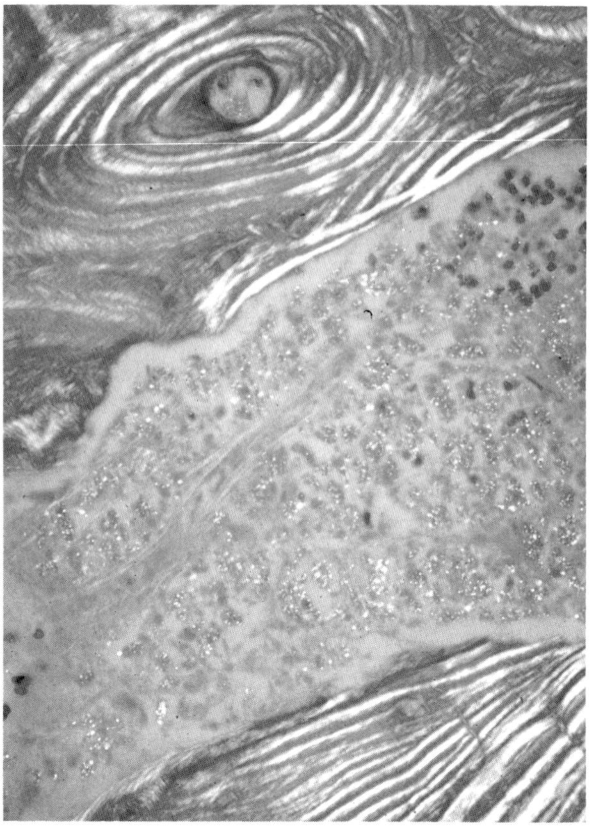

Fig. 10.13. Permeation of a metal granuloma within the cortex, with areas of resorption. H & E, polarized light, × 66

10.3.3 Histology and the Different Physiopathological Theories for Bone Resorption

Following the identification of these tissue changes (osteonecrosis, histiocytic granulomas, new synovium, osteoclastic activity), various theories of resorption have been put forward and have more recently been supported by enzyme studies [20, 22, 24].

These hypotheses must be tested with the histological findings. Three factors must be considered:

1. The identification of the causative factor (histiocytic granuloma, new synovial tissue, or osteoclastic activity) together with its importance relative to other structures
2. The site of the causative factor, not only in relation to bony structures but also in relation to the cement sheath, the positioning of the prosthesis, and the joint cavity
3. The identification of the signs of bone resorption, such as areas of active or inactive resorption and the disappearance of osteocytes. These lesions must be differentiated from the consequences of surgery itself.

We shall consider the different possible mechanisms of bone resorption in the light of the morphological findings from our own study.

Physical factors are of primary importance and should not be neglected. These are (a) movement or mechanical forces acting on bony structures and stimulating osteoclastic activity [29]; (b) the physical effect of the newly formed interposed tissue, whatever its histological structure.

This hypothesis is concerned primarily with interposition tissue that is of a mechanical origin, whether it consists solely of collagen or has been formed by the organization of a histiocytic granuloma.

This tissue produces a disturbance of the bony microenvironment and especially causes resorption. These morphological theories confirm the presence of bony remodeling rather than a process of isolated and passive osteolysis.

The effects of *necrosis or changes of local vascularity* are also implicated [17]. Osteonecrosis occurs at the time of surgery, but it is limited and does not increase with time. We have never seen massive bone necrosis. As for the destruction of the local blood supply by the granuloma, especially in a florid histiocytic response to metal or polyethylene, this is refuted by the pres-

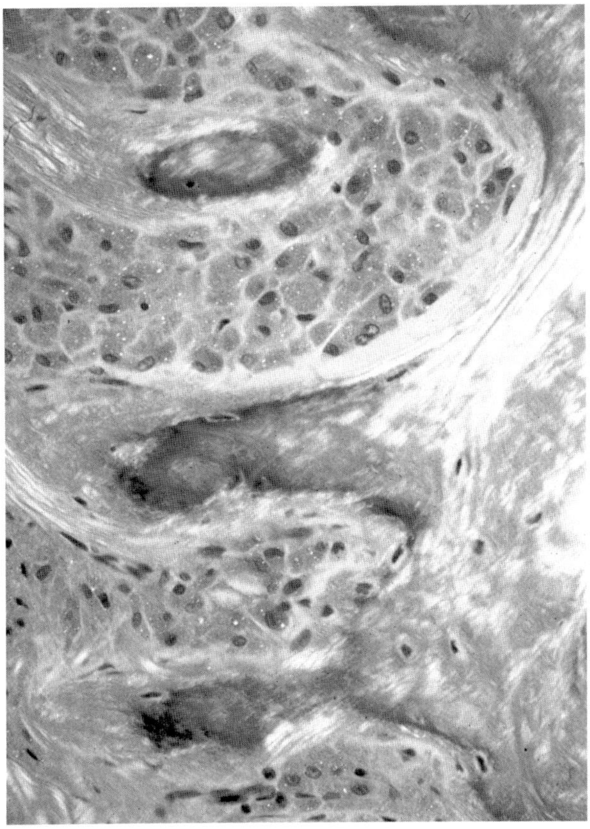

Fig. 10.14. Osseous metaplasia within the new capsule. Histiocytic granuloma (metal) in direct contact with osteoid. H & E, polarized light, × 66

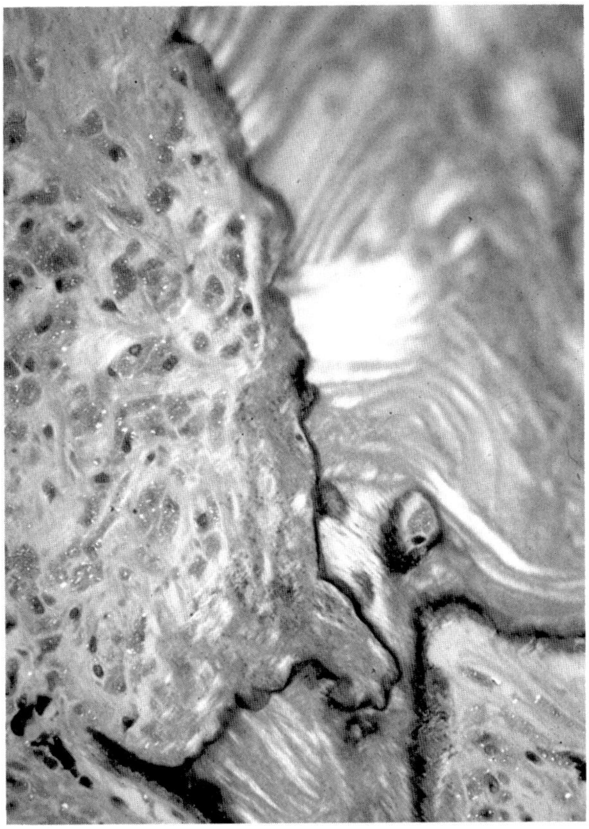

Fig. 10.15. Histiocytic granuloma (metal) around new sites of bone resorption with empty lacunae. H & E, × 66

ence of bony structures that are completely surrounded but whose osteocytes remain intact. With regard to the metal-on-metal prostheses in particular, we saw no vascular lesion in our series.

The *direct action* of the histiocytic granuloma on bony resorption is more frequently proposed [43]. Morphological studies demonstrate layers of histiocytes within areas where large amounts of bone are being resorbed (Fig. 10.13).

Techniques of cytoenzymology have shown that the granulomas are rich in acid phosphatase [22, 24]. In the metal-on-metal prostheses, where lysis of the granuloma is especially active, lysosomal proteolytic enzymes are released which produce osteolysis [23].

Certain morphological features are contradictory, however: the lack of correspondence between the granuloma and the area of resorption or absence of osteocytes, and the predominance of acid phosphatase in giant cells and not in the more numerous mononuclear histiocytes.

It should be emphasized that topographic correlation is often difficult in isolated biopsy specimens. Here we come up against the problem of orientation. In order to determine the role of the granuloma in resorption we have undertaken a morphological study of metaplastic ossification in capsules that have been removed during total hip revision. These lesions give us a true experimental model in vivo. The newly formed bony structures show active osteogenesis, often with marked osteoid at the periphery. They are in direct contact with, and are often surrounded by a histiocytic granuloma.

Osteoblastic activity and marked osteoid formation is seen in association with a histiocytic response to metal or polyethylene, whether this is on the periphery of the bony lamellae (Figs. 10.14, 10.15) or within the haversian systems of the newly formed sclerotic bone.

Sites of active resorption are created only by osteoclastic activity (Fig. 10.16). As the osteoclast has a short life, these sites of resorption are secondarily filled with neighboring histiocytic granulomas. Whatever may have stimulated the osteolysis, the predominant factor is the role of the osteoclasts.

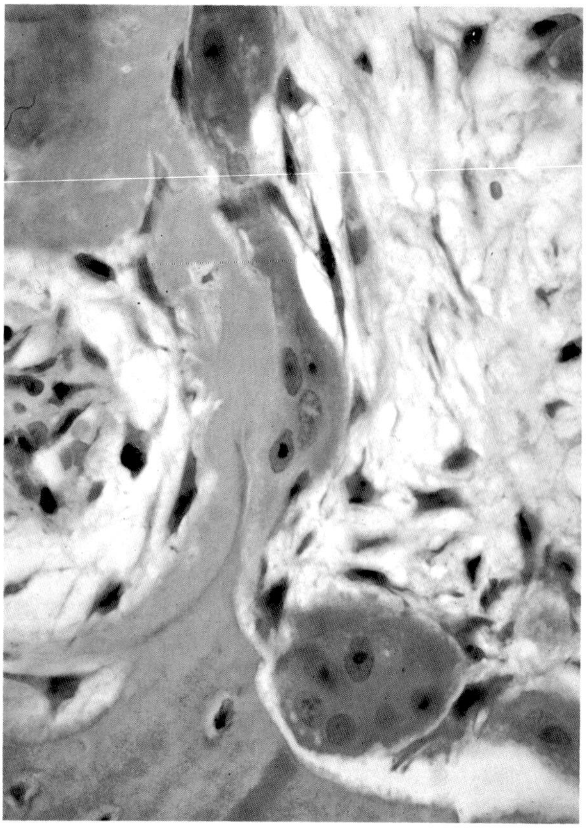

Fig. 10.16. Active osteoclasts. Osseous metaplasia in the new capsule, within a surrounding granuloma. H & E, × 132

Mention should be made of the *newly formed synovial tissue*. Extensive areas of it may be found around the joint cavity, and it is also found in association with the tissue membrane around the femur. Recent studies have shown that it contains the same enzymes as true synovium and can produce prostaglandin E_2 and collagenase [20].

Is this structure involved in bone resorption? Some morphological theories are equally contradictory. Around the joint cavity its macrophage activity is virtually nil.

Newly formed synovial tissue is not always found with the femoral membrane and may be present in small, patchy fragments. On the other hand, it is always orientated toward the cement. It is also most frequently seen in interposition tissue that is dense, hyalinized, and of an apparently mechanical origin.

In fact, our findings favor the *indirect role* of the granuloma in bone resorption, the active element being the osteoclast. Above all, the granuloma induces osteoclastic activity by the secretions from activated lymphocytes or by prostaglandins, it promotes the differentiation of osteoclasts from the store of mononuclear phagocytes, and it helps in the phagocytosis of the debris produced by the osteoclastic resorption of bone [30].

References

1. Abelanet R, Forest M, Durigon M, Postel M, Kerboul M, Meynet JC (1975) Les réactions tissulaires locales aux arthroplasties de hanche. Arch Anat Cytol Pathol 23: 47–56
2. Abele M, Steinhauser J (1972) Histomorphologische Untersuchungen zur Spätlockerung des Pfannenteils bei Totalprothesen der Hüfte. Z Orthop 110: 412–417
3. Benecke G, Kuprasch R (1973) Die Reaktion der Gelenkkapsel nach Totalarthroplastik des Hüftgelenkes. Arch Orthop Unfallchir 75: 289–301
4. Bullough PG (1973) Tissue reaction to wear debris generated from total hip replacement. In: Evarts CM (ed) Hip society: The Hip, vol. 1. Mosby, St. Louis, pp 80–91
5. Charnley J (1964) The bonding of prostheses to bone by cement. J Bone Joint Surg [Br] 46: 518–529
6. Charnley J (1970) Tissue reactions to implanted plastics. In: Acrylic cement in orthopaedic surgery. Livingstone. Edinburgh, pp 1–9
7. Charnley J (1970) Long-term histology of acrylic cement in bone. In: Acrylic cement in orthopaedic surgery. Livingstone. Edinburgh, pp 47–66
8. Charnley J (1970) The reaction of bone to self-curing acrylic cement. J Bone Joint Surg [Br] 52: 340–353
9. Charnley J (1979) Cement-bone interface in low-friction arthroplasty of the hip. Springer, Berlin Heidelberg New York, pp 25–40
10. Charnley J, Crawford WJ (1968) Histology of bone in contact with self-curing acrylic cement. J Bone Joint Surg [Br] 50: 228
11. Charnley J, Follaci FM, Hammond BT (1968) Long-term reaction of bone to self-curing acrylic cement. J Bone Joint Surg [Br] 50: 822–829
12. Charosky CB, Walker PS (1973) The microstructure of polymethylmethacrylate cement. Clin Orthop 91: 221–224
13. Charosky CB, Bullough PG, Wilson PD (1973) Total hip replacement failures. J Bone Joint Surg [Am] 55: 49–58
14. Cotta H, Schulitz KP (1970) Komplikationen der Hüftalloarthroplastik durch periartikulare Gewebsreaktionen. Arch Orthop Unfallchir 69: 39–59
15. Crugnola A, Schiller AL, Radin E (1977) Polymeric debris in synovium after total joint replacement: Histological identification. J Bone Joint Surg [Am] 59: 860–861
16. Draenert K (1978) Histomorphology of bone-cement contact. Chirurg 49: 276–285
17. Evans ME, Freeman MAR, Miller AJ, Vernon Roberts R (1974) Metal sensitivity as a cause of bone necrosis and loosening of the prosthesis in total joint replacement. J Bone Joint Surg [Br] 56: 626–642
18. Fornassier VL, Cameron HU (1976) The femoral stem/cement interface in total hip replacement. Clin Orthop 116: 248–252
19. Freeman MAR, Bradley GW, Revell PA (1982) Observations upon the interface between bone and polymethylmethacrylate cement. J Bone Joint Surg [Br] 64: 489–493
20. Goldring SR, Schiller AL, Roelke M, Rourke CM, O'Neill DA, Harris WH (1983) The synovial-like membrane at the bone-cement interface in loose total hip replacements and its

proposed role in bone lysis. J Bone Joint Surg [Am] 65: 575–583
21. Heilman K (1974) Morphological changes in tissues surrounding alloarthroplastic hip prostheses. Light and electron microscopic studies. Verh Dtsch Ges Pathol 58: 403–407
22. Heilman K, Diezel PB, Rossner JA, Brinckmann KA (1975) Morphological studies in tissues surrounding alloarthroplastic joints. Virchows Arch [Pathol Anat] 366: 93–106
23. Langlais F, Postel M, Berry JP, Le Charpentier Y, Weill BJ (1980) L'intolérance aux débris d'usure des prothèses. Int Orthop 4: 145–153
24. Linder L, Lindberg L, Carlsson A (1983) Aseptic loosening of hip prostheses. A histologic and enzyme histochemical study. Clin Orthop 175: 93–104
25. Lintner F (1982) Histological examinations of remodeling proceedings on the cement-bone surface of endoprostheses after implantation from 3–10 years. Pathol Res Pract 173: 376–389
26. Massloff W, Neuhaus-Vogel A (1974) Die Gelenkkapsel nach Alloplastik. Arch Orthop Unfallchir 78: 175–195
27. Meachim G (1976) Histological interpretation of tissue changes adjacent to orthopaedic implants. In: Biocompatibility of implant materials. Sector, London, pp 120–127
28. Mirra J, Amstutz HC, Matos M, Gold R (1976) The pathology of the joint tissues and its clinical relevance in prosthesis failure. Clin Orthop 117: 221–240
29. Mirra J, Marder RA, Amstutz HC (1982) The pathology of failed total joint arthroplasty. Clin Orthop 170: 175–183
30. Mundy GR (1983) Monocyte-macrophage system and bone resorption. Lab Invest 49: 119–121
31. Ohnsorge J (1970) Änderungen der Spongiosafeinstruktur unter dem Einfluß des autopolymerisierenden Knochenzementes. Z Orthop 107: 405–411
32. Pedley RB, Meachim G, Gray T (1979) Identification of acrylic cement particles in tissues. Ann Biomed Eng 7: 319–328
33. Pizzoferrato A, Sozarino L, Lambertini V (1980/81) Histopathological grading suggestion for the evaluation of the intolerance in hip joint endo- and arthroprostheses. Chir Organi Mov 76: 147–171
34. Ranieri L (1979) Reaction of periarticular tissues to products of abrasion of high-density polyethylene. Chir Organi Mov 65: 1–11
35. Revell PA (1982) Tissue reactions to joint prostheses and the products of wear and corrosion. In: Berry CL (ed) Bone and joint disease. Springer, Berlin Heidelberg New York (Current topics in pathology, vol 71, pp 73–101)
36. Revell PA, Weightman B, Freeman MAR, Vernon-Roberts B (1978) The production and biology of polyethylene debris. Arch Orthop Trauma Surg 91: 167–181
37. Spinelli R (1976) A study of the interface between bone and acrylic cement by scanning electron microscopy. Ital J Orthop Traumatol 2: 103–115
38. Vernon-Roberts B, Freeman MAR (1976) Morphological and analytical studies on the tissues adjacent to joint prostheses. In: Schaldach M, Hohmann D (eds) Advances in artificial hip and knee joint technology. Springer, Berlin Heidelberg New York, pp 178–186
39. Vernon-Roberts B, Freeman MAR (1977) The tissue response to total joint replacement prostheses. In: Swanson SAV, Freeman MAR (eds) The scientific basis of joint replacement. Pitman, London, pp 86–129
40. Willert HG (1973) Tissue reactions around joint implants and bone cement. In: Chapchal G (ed) Arthroplasty of the hip. Thieme, Stuttgart, pp 11–21
41. Willert HG, Frech HA (1976) Tissue damage caused by bone cement. In: Gschwend N, Debrunner HU (eds) Total hip prosthesis. Huber, Bern, pp 240–242
42. Willert HG, Puls P (1972) Die Reaktion des Knochens auf Knochenzement bei der Allo-arthroplastik der Hüfte. Arch Orthop Unfallchir 72: 33–71
43. Willert HG, Schreiber A (1969) Unterschiedliche Reaktionen von Knochen und Weichteillager auf autopolymerisierende Kunststoffimplantate. Z Orthop 106: 231–252
44. Willert HG, Semlitsch M (1976) Tissue reactions to plastic and metallic wear products of joint endoprostheses. In: Gschwend N, Debrunner HU (eds) Total hip prosthesis. Huber, Bern, pp 205–239
45. Willert HG, Semlitsch M (1976) Problems associated with cement anchorage of artificial joints. In: Schaldach M, Hohmann D (eds) Advances in artificial hip and knee joint technology. Springer, Berlin Heidelberg New York, pp 325–346
46. Willert HG, Semlitsch M (1977) Reactions of the articular capsule to wear products of artificial joint prostheses. J Biomed Mater Res 11: 157–164

11 Conclusions

M. Kerboul

We hope that the reader will have found something of interest within our account of total hip replacement. We have tried to describe the road that we have taken over the past 18 years. This has followed a relatively straight course and we have tried to make it as safe as possible.

At each stage we tried to recognize everything that was worthy of saving or being improved upon and to quickly discard everything that was dangerous or not helpful. Our aim has always been to make this a better and more reliable operation. Our degree of success is already considerable, as the patient can be guaranteed perfect function in 96% of cases. Of course, there is always the fear of seeing the painstaking work of joint reconstruction being devastated by infection. Fortunately, this is being seen less frequently, thanks to prophylactic systemic antibiotics and to better asepsis and antisepsis during surgery. However, infection is ever present and ready to strike with increased virulence should we cease to fear it. The fact that we have a better understanding of how to repair the damage produced by infection is no argument for lowering our guard.

Aseptic loosening can produce massive bone damage affecting both the femur and the acetabulum. We have now learned how to repair this damage accurately, as well as how to replace the loss of bone with homograft in order to restore the anatomical environment needed for the reimplantation of a new prosthesis. Moreover, we now seem to be able to prevent aseptic loosening, as shown by the rarity with which it occurs today.

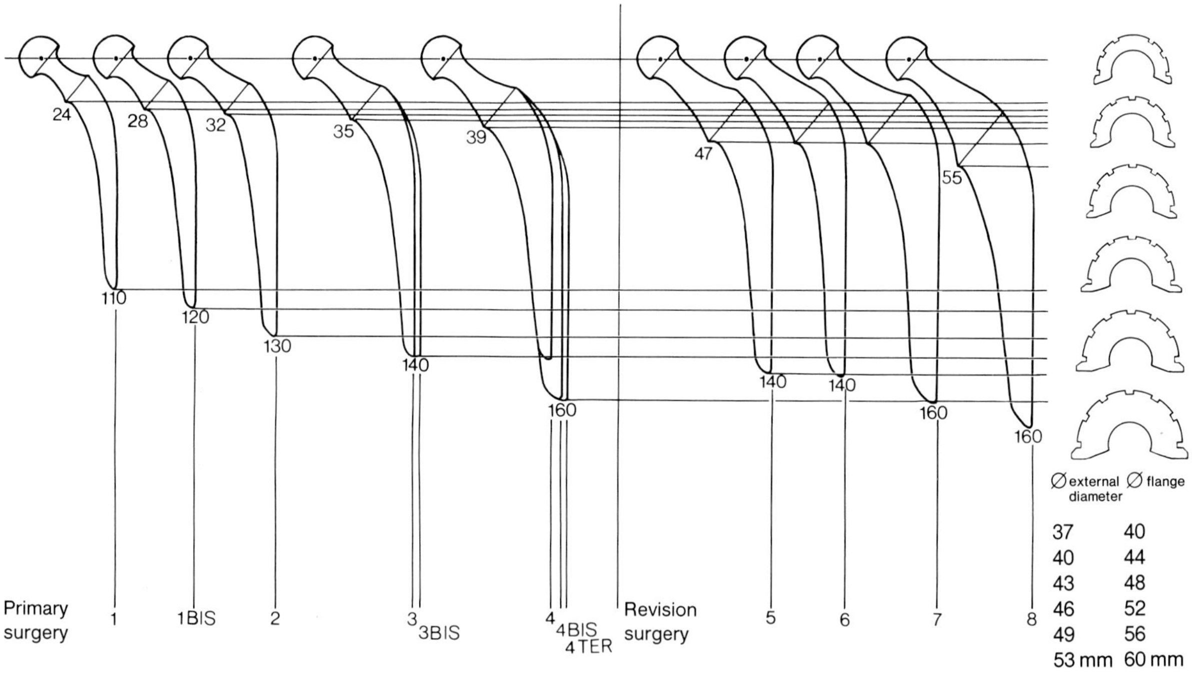

Fig. 11.1. The components that make up the new series of prostheses. *Left:* 12 femoral components of stainless steel. *Right:* six cups of increasing size (HDP)

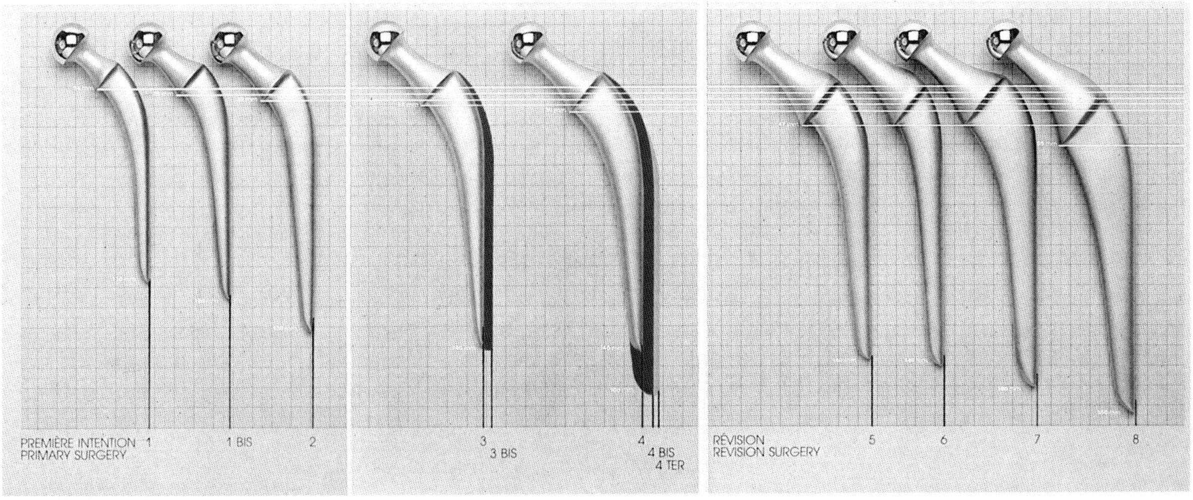

Fig. 11.2. The femoral components

Charnley's idea of reducing the size of the femoral head to 22 mm was a stroke of genius that cannot be overemphasized. There is no doubt that this has been responsible for the high quality and durability of acetabular fixation. Thanks to the modifications made in the femoral components 10 years ago, aseptic femoral loosening has also virtually disappeared. The cement to which we attributed so much blame no longer has any faults, now that we do not expect it to hide or correct the defects of the prosthesis. It ages even better than one could have dared to hope.

However, not everything is perfect, and we believe that there is still room for improvement. With this in mind, we have produced a new series of prostheses (Figs. 11.1–11.3).

On the femoral side, a few intermediate sizes were lacking. Perhaps they are not indispensible, but they provide a welcome addition that completes the series. They make the operation easier by reducing errors that may arise in cutting the femoral neck and by enabling immediate correction to be made for varying neck lengths. By introducing a femoral stem that is oval in cross-section, we have given the prosthesis a tighter fit within the diaphysis. This eliminates high spots and so prevents zones of stress concentration. Although there is no real risk of fatigue fracture of the stem, this better distribution of the stresses acting on the prosthesis will perhaps be transmitted to the bone more satisfactorily. We may then see fewer secondary bony changes of late onset, where the cortices become thickened or are partially converted into cancellous bone. This is often asymptomatic, although it may sometimes be the source of intermittent pain.

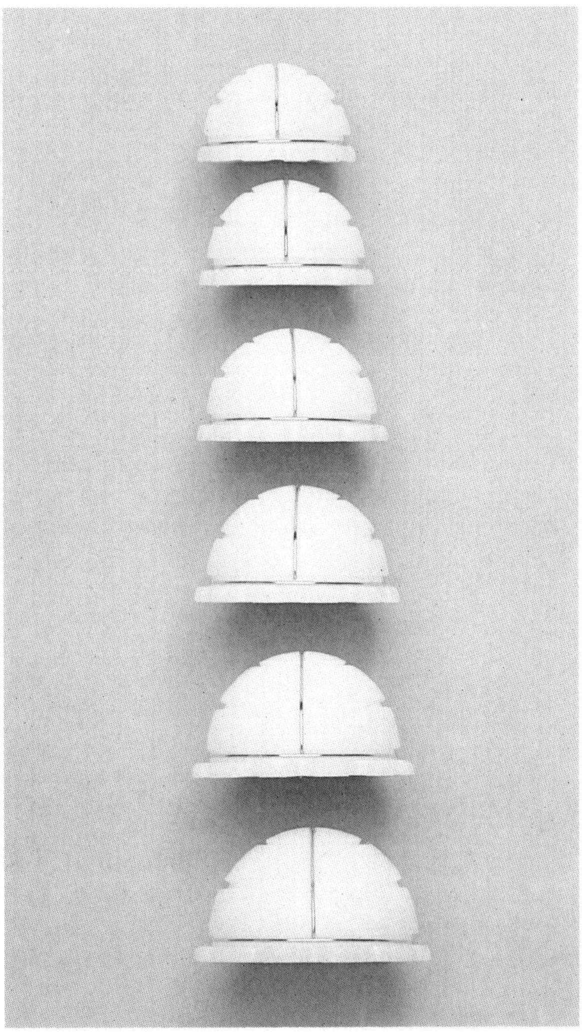

Fig. 11.3. The cups

Finally, there is no doubt that the cups presently in use become worn. This wear is slow and variable, as demonstrated by the fact that 80% show no macroscopic changes on roentgenograms after 10 years. However, the physical and biological consequences of this wear may eventually be disastrous, leading to progressive osteolysis around the cup and femoral neck and resulting in failure. For this reason we are now studying a new type of polyethylene, whose composition should double the life expectancy of the present components. These new cups will soon be available, and it is on them that we base our hope of seeing the life span of total hip replacement being extended to 20 or 30 years.

12 Subject Index

J. Charnley

Low Friction Arthroplasty of the Hip

Theory and Practice

1979. 440 figures, 205 in color, 22 tables. X, 376 pages.
ISBN 3-540-08893-8

E. W. Somerville

Displacement of the Hip in Childhood

Aetiology, Management and Sequelae
1982. 262 figures. XIII, 200 pages.

The Cementless Fixation of Hip Endoprostheses

Editor: E. Morscher

1984. 230 figures. XV, 284 pages.
ISBN 3-540-12254-0

R. Liechti

Hip Arthrodesis and Associated Problems

Foreword by M. E. Müller, B. G. Weber

Translated from the German edition by P. A. Casey

1978. 266 figures, 35 tables. XII, 269 pages.
ISBN 3-540-08614-5

F. Pauwels

Biomechanics of the Normal and Diseased Hip

Theoretical Foundation, Technique and Results of Treatment

An Atlas

Translated from the German by R. J. Furlong, P. Maquet

1976. 305 figures, in 853 separate illustrations. VIII, 276 pages.
ISBN 3-540-07428-7